A professional's view of this groundbreaking book:

Attachment Disability is a fresh and usable book for helping professionals. I wish I had this book thirty years ago; I would have made it required reading for every therapist on my staff.

The author makes excellent use of case studies to substantiate his exciting new theories of attachment disability and is a must-read for anybody working with survivors of trauma. Teachers will quickly recognize those students who hate learning—and why. Therapists will better understand why "incomplete mourning" makes humans "incomplete" in coping with life. It provides excellent explanations for why therapy combined with psychotropics works, and why it doesn't. After reading this book, the reader, lay or professional, will always think twice whenever they hear or read the word "depression." It also teaches why antidepressants have become "antistressants." It should be mandated in all training of mental health professionals.

Dr. Curran's book is so well written that I looked forward to turning the pages to see what he had learned from his many years as a psychiatrist, and to note how easy it was for the reader to learn from him.

—Richard Obershaw, AMW, MSW, LICSW
 Author of the best-selling *Cry Until You Laugh: Comforting Guidance for Coping with Grief*
 Founder and director, Grief Center and Burnsville Counseling, Burnsville, Minnesota

Attachment Disability

Attachment Disability

Volume I:
The Hidden Cause of Adolescent Dysfunction and Lifelong Underperformance

Including a plea for psychiatric diagnostic reform

John Curran, MD, ABPN

Bidwell Learning Institute

Copyright © 2017 by John Curran, MD, ABPN.

All rights reserved. No part of this publication may be reproduced, stored in a retrieval system, or transmitted in any form or by any means, electronic, mechanical, photocopying, recording, or otherwise, without the prior written permission of the copyright holder, except brief quotations used in a review.

The information in this book is presented for educational purposes. It is not intended to substitute for treatment by a psychotherapist or psychiatrist.

Design by Meadowlark Publishing Services.

Cover photo ©IStock.com/stray_cat.

Published by Bidwell Learning Institute
8014 Olson Memorial Highway
Box 452
Golden Valley, MN 55427

Manufactured in the United States of America.
ISBN 978-0-9996028-0-5

Published 2018

To Kitty, the ship of my life

... All anxiety involves the prospect of separation.
   —Dr. Lawrence C. Kolb

Contents

Preface xi
Introduction: Attachment Disability Defined xvii

Part 1: Understanding Attachment Disability
1   Origins of the Idea of Attachment 3

Part 2: Varieties of Attachment Disability
2   Attachment Avoidance: Three Cases 15
3   Attachment Entanglement: Four Cases 57
4   Attachment Acting-out: Three Cases 77

Part 3: Origins of the Theory of Attachment Disability
5   Early Origins 103
6   Later Origins 135
7   More Recent Origins 153

Part 4: Attachment Disability, Anxiety, and Depression
8   Attachment Disability and Anxiety 187
9   Attachment Disability and Depression 215

Part 5: Managing Attachment Disability
10 Management: Strategy and Tactics 247
11 The First Management Principle: Clarification 289
12 The Second Management Principle: Acceptance . . . 329

13	The Third Management Principle: Focus on What Can Be Changed 337
14	Current Psychiatric Assessment: A Plea for Reform. .377

Notes 423
Bibliography 435
Index 447
Author's Note: Introducing Volume 2. 477
About the Author 489

Case Studies by Type of Trauma

Note: Some cases indicate exposure to more than one type of trauma. Parentheses indicate the first page of the case study.

Death of family member, peer, pet:
    Holden Caulfield (35), Helen (45), Amy (57),
    Charles (195), Julie (209), William Styron (228),
    Hans Castorp (308), Peggy (311), Rita (394)

Abandonment:
    Dyllen (15), Georgina (67), the Punker (72), Amanda (85),
    Maya (95), Rebecca (189), Rose (236), Samantha (296),
    Darrell (345), Carla (347), Lara (356)

Neglect:
    Peggy (311)

Abuse, either witnessed or sustained:
    Physical: Charlotte (64), Samantha (296), Carla (347)
    Emotional: Rebecca (189), Rose (236)
    Sexual: Jackie (79), Renée (173), Peggy (311)

Betrayal:
    Renée (173), Maddie (281), Peggy (311), Lindsey (320)

Unknown:
    Charles (195), Owen (254), Ryan (261), Mr. POP (269),
    Rita (394)

Preface

No book is written free of the spirits hovering over it during its creation; mine is no exception. One of these is Brother Julius Winkler, FSC; another is Dr. Greg Heimarck, ABPN. A third is a hallucination. From Brother Julius came inspiration; from Greg, leadership; from the hallucination, decisiveness.

Let's start with the hallucination.

I'm a student at Saint Mary's College in Winona, Minnesota (now Saint Mary's University of Minnesota), and I'm participating in a monthly seminar intended to promote interest in vocations. The idea is, I suppose, to direct attendees' attention to things spiritual and intellectual for a change, perhaps even to a career with the Brothers or the priesthood. I'm certain I have no attraction to either. So why am I attending the seminar? I'm uncertain about my career, I would like to become a psychiatrist, but that would require attending medical school, which would require science courses, which I found so boring that I dropped out of pre-engineering the year before.

Suddenly a voice, unquestionably in my head, emphatically in my mind: *Do it! Be a doctor!* I don't cry out or fall writhing to the floor. Nothing of the sort, but rather a mental nod: *Oh, sure, of course, why not? What's the problem?* So the following semester I sign up for science classes.

Princeton University psychologist Julian Jaynes conjectures that "preceding consciousness there was a different mentality based on verbal hallucinations."[1] In other words, "command hallucinations" enabled preconscious humans to carry out executive action when confronted by a novel situation. Nowadays, Dr. Jaynes notes, hallucinatory experiences, sometimes soothing, sometimes authoritative, still commonly occur, especially in times of stress. When casting about for a career, perhaps I was not in a state of stress, but I certainly was of uncertain mind.

As for the inspiration:

At the end of my first year at St. Mary's I had dropped pre-engineering. A familiar dilemma emerged: now what? The following year I bided my time by signing up for lower division prerequisite courses, one of which was Introduction to Psychology, taught by Brother Julius Winkler, FSC.

He was a slender, slightly stooped figure with angular features and an alert, intense gaze that gave him the air of always being fully present. In the classroom he labored mightily to make "Intro Psych" interesting, but it was mighty dull stuff. Recognizing our apathy, he kept encouraging us not to give up: "It will get more interesting when we get to abnormal psychology in the next course." And it did, in part because our textbook flowed like an adventure novel as we were introduced to Freud, Jung, Adler, and other bold explorers of the modern psyche, and because Brother Julius seemed to live the quest with them. Reading the work of these pioneers, I was transfixed. Thus, the inspiration: *wouldn't it be exciting to see if I could create a meta-theory of abnormal behavior? A unified field theory of human dysfunction? What a challenge! What a life goal!*

Finally, the leadership.

Brother Julius suggested I apply for a Rhodes Scholarship, and said he would provide a recommendation. Waiting for my interview at the University of Minnesota with a dozen or so other applicants, I introduced myself to the fellow in the next seat. He was Greg Heimarck, a senior at St. Olaf College in Northfield, also interested in medicine, also interested in psychiatry, also interested in philosophy. We chatted for ten minutes, my name was called, we exchanged the usual gestures of worthy competitors, and I advanced to meet my destiny. Well, I emerged bloody and bowed.

I returned to my seat next to Greg. As we talked, he was excited to discover I was taking a course in Existential Philosophy; our "conversation" consisted of Greg talking and me nodding my head. That was the essential Greg: gregarious, curious, forthright, open, enthusiastic, energetic, informed, cultured. I suppose he sounds too good to be true, but that is how I found him then and ever after.

I wasn't called back for a second interview (no surprise there), but Greg was (also no surprise). I waited to see how his second interview worked out. He didn't make the cut either. I never learned what he felt about the rebuff, but I felt relieved about mine. I had no interest in studying abroad since I had already mapped my future: finish up at Saint Mary's, then medical school and psychiatry at the University of Minnesota.

Greg and I kept in touch. After graduation he and his soulmate, Claire, exchanged vows and moved to New York where he had been accepted at Columbia University's College of Physicians and Surgeons (P&S). I returned to St. Mary's and was accepted at the University of Minnesota Medical School.

About six weeks into the school year I received a note from Greg about P&S. He loved it and told me I should apply. Why not? I figured. So I did ... and heard nothing for months. In mid-January I received a telegram: "Pleased to offer you position class of '61. [Signed] AE Severinghaus, Dean, College of Physicians and Surgeons." I wrote back, saying that I wouldn't accept unless I received a scholarship. Another telegram arrived: "Not sure I completely understand your letter, but pleased to offer you a $500 scholarship. [Signed] AE Severinghaus, Dean."

What a delight it was to write Greg and Claire with the news.

During the first months at P&S I was pretty homesick. Greg and Claire had an apartment just a few blocks from school and I got in the habit of dropping by unannounced at lunchtime. Always gracious, they would invite me in and share their meal, Claire the quiet one, Greg coaching me what to expect in class, loaning me his old textbooks, things of that sort. I think they had a better fix on my loneliness than I.

Greg was a bundle of interests and initiative. He introduced me to a host of ideas and books beyond the traditional psychiatric curriculum: for example, Erik Erikson's notion of "identity crisis" as depicted in his book *Young Man Luther* (1958), and Magda Arnold's *Emotion and Personality* (1960), her attempt to recast emotion as an organizing rather than disorganizing cognitive experience. And to give you an idea of the breadth of his curiosity, he also loaned me his first edition hardcover copy of Tolkien's *The Lord of the Rings*. Another example of his leadership was finding me work, first with him at a hospital laboratory, then later at a mental health clinic.

After my residency training I moved back to Minnesota while Greg remained in New York to undergo further training at the Columbia University Center for Psychoanalytic Training and Research, where he later served as adjunct professor. For years he also taught psychiatry and religion, a lifetime interest, at Union Theological Seminary, an affiliate of Columbia.

Greg died in 2010. And this book is part of his legacy, for without his enthusiasm and leadership, I would never have ventured forth from Minnesota to P&S, then to New York Psychiatric Institute, where I had the good fortune to be subject to the exacting demands of its director, Dr. Laurence Kolb. During a chance encounter, which I describe in chapter 8, Dr. Kolb happened to comment that "all anxiety involves the prospect of separation." It took me years to accept the truth of this proposition. And even more years, as I also describe in chapter 8, to realize that he had given me the unifying concept for which I had been searching and that now provides the foundation of this book:

> *Separation either enables — the anxiety it activates motivates learning — or disables. A frequent cause of disabling anxiety is trauma from death or loss or abandonment or neglect or abuse, resulting in wounded trust, dissociation and difficulty learning from experience, what I term the "trauma trilogy." Consequently trauma victims demonstrate difficulty maintaining or establishing relationships. That is, they exhibit an emotional disability, which in this book I call "Attachment Disability."*

And this is where my book begins.

From Brother Julius to Greg to P&S to PI to Dr. Kolb to what turns out to be a unified field theory, not of human dysfunction but of human functioning. What an unlikely consequence of a hallucination!

Introduction:
Attachment Disability Defined

*Psychotherapy is education, replacing maladaptive
learning with adaptive learning,*

The goal of this volume is to provide an introduction to Attachment Disability and its causes. Injured trust, dissociation (reduced awareness of reality), and maladaptive learning—what I call the "trauma triad"—are the basis of a unique form of emotional disability: Attachment Disability. It specifically identifies the inability to form and maintain stable relationships because of trauma associated with abuse, neglect, abandonment, betrayal, or loss.[i]

By definition, trauma is "unbearable and intolerable."[1] Victims survive only because their bodies respond automatically, encapsulating and walling off otherwise overwhelming sensory stimulation. But their confidence in themselves and others does not survive undamaged. Trust is injured. Affected children and adults seek to relate to others, to be sure, but their relationships are tentative, insecure, unstable, and

---

i. The notion of "Trauma Triad" is not equivalent to the diagnosis of Posttraumatic Stress Disorder as set forth in the *Diagnostic and Statistical Manual of Mental Disorders, Fifth Edition (DSM-5)*, American Psychiatric Publishing, Arlington, VA, 2013, 271, although it may feature some elements of the latter. It is a broader, dynamic and more useful concept.

ridden with sadness, guilt, and anxiety as well as unpredictable angry outbursts. Unfortunately, the protective quality of these defensive behaviors is not recognized as such but is frequently misdiagnosed, pathologized, and mismanaged. This further obscures the underlying trauma while aggravating distrust and promoting maladaptive learning.

Contrary to conventional opinion, recent research suggests that the consequences of child maltreatment are broadly equivalent.[2] Thus many youngsters bring to school a deficiency of trust because of their early traumas, regardless of type. Others find that the school experience itself exposes them to a different sort of maltreatment: bullying. In either case, a child's ability to assess life's issues is contaminated by a tendency to blame—either themselves or others. To be sure, this is a natural tendency of early childhood as youngsters seek to comprehend the adversities that are inevitably part of growing up. But if the adversity is trauma related, their blaming becomes entrenched and difficult to modify through subsequent happier experiences. They do learn but such learning is maladaptive rather than adaptive.

Underperformance is an early sign of the trust deficit, and dropping out is a later sign. For some troubled youngsters, however, the disability or vulnerability persists into young adult and adult life because, not surprisingly, such early life trauma leaves its mark. In a thoughtful editorial, public health scientist Dr. Benjamin Lahey reviews the robust if unhappy evidence that troubled youngsters are at high risk of becoming troubled adults.[3] While Dr. Lahey has in mind two specific childhood disorders, Oppositional Defiant Disorder and Conduct Disorder, in my experience these labels typically signal misdiagnosed Attachment Disability. Other research indicates that by their late twenties, both childhood bullies and their prey are at high risk of developing psychiatric disorders.[4]

Dr. Lahey discusses the virtues of various prevention options, including "reducing factors that cause psychopathology across the life span." As I see it, one such preventive measure would be to reconsider our traditional psychiatric categories, which at present frequently ignore or misinterpret the trauma triad. I will discuss this option at length below.

Another preventive measure would be to abolish mandated school attendance, which, as I will discuss in the second volume of this series, risks aggravating the suspicion and distrust that are the inevitable fallout of early life trauma. Damaged youngsters may learn to hate learning. Thus they enter adulthood with two disabilities: one emotional, the other educational.

Attachment Disability Ignored

The concept of attachment and its vicissitudes was developed by two British psychoanalysts and child psychiatrists, John Bowlby and Donald Winnicott, based on their observations of children and adolescents raised in foster homes, in orphanages, or by biological relatives during the turmoil of World War II. Their notions regarding attachment impairment and its later consequences were a prominent feature of my psychiatric training in the 1960s.

But mysteriously, their ideas lost traction. Consequently a generation or more of psychiatrists, child care specialists, and teachers sustained an education gap when it came to the understanding and management of Attachment Disability. That is, while the underperformance and dropping out remained all too visible, its major cause—attachment-impaired trust—escaped detection. Although invisible and hidden, it nonetheless continued its pernicious work into later life.

So the question is, what happened? Why were Bowlby's and Winnicott's valuable contributions to child care and development neglected?

In part this is because sufferers are trapped in a Catch-22 situation: to acknowledge such concern to another requires the very presence of the trust and security that are absent. While their emotional disability eventually becomes obvious, the underlying causes—distrust of closeness and fears of abandonment—remain concealed.

But Attachment Disability goes undetected for another reason: professional disinterest.

1. First of all, until very recently Attachment Disability has been overlooked by child care services, at least in the United States. Perhaps this may be related to the overseas origins of the idea of attachment impairment. Moreover, the original reports of the consequences of child-parent separation were published more than sixty years ago. Indeed, it would appear that only in the last quarter century has a wider interest in attachment theory and practice flourished, primarily among child development theorists, researchers, and therapists. An example of this is an excellent handbook, *The Attachment Therapy Companion*, published in 2009.[5]

It is most relevant that of the approximately 231 references cited in the handbook, my tally finds only six from the 1970s and earlier, sixteen dated in the 1980s, fifty-seven in the 1990s, and the rest in the 2000s, apart from nine references to publications between 1944 and 1981 by the originator of the attachment concept, John Bowlby. Moreover, the handbook is vague about the applicability of attachment therapy to adolescents and adults. There is one 1988 reference to attachment issues of late adolescence, plus 1987 and 1995 references to follow-up studies of childhood Posttraumatic Stress Disorder. There is a description of a semistructured assessment interview, the Adult Attachment Interview (p. 107), for age sixteen and older individuals, but its clinical use seems limited to assessing mothering styles. Interestingly, there are no references whatsoever to Donald Winnicott.

I will leave it to observers of the US child care culture to account for this historical amnesia.

2. More importantly, attachment concepts are ignored and neglected by our psychiatric establishment. For example, the persisting emotional and cognitive consequences of relationship trauma are minimized in standard psychiatric textbooks and nomenclature. Indeed, the 2013 edition of the American Psychiatric Association's *Diagnostic and Statistical Manual of Mental Disorders, Fifth Edition (DSM-5)*, while retaining a Reactive Attachment Disorder category, limits it to withdrawn and inhibited behavior only, while recommending "the diagnosis should be made with caution in children older than 5 years." The former Reactive Attachment Disorder, Uninhibited is renamed Disinhibited Social Engagement Disorder, which to my mind serves only to obscure its traumatic origins. However, the manual does recognize that the condition can persist into middle childhood and adolescence, yet "has not been described in adults."[6]

Fortunately, in recent months this narrow vision of Attachment Disability may have been modified because of research studying possible long-term consequences of childhood and adolescent trauma. Prospective studies of adolescent brain function reveal that youngsters with a history of life stress display possibly permanent limbic lobe abnormalities plus increased threat sensitivity, creating a vulnerability to later Depression. Moreover, whether clinically Depressed or emotionally vulnerable or not, they remain at risk of lifelong underperformance, so to speak, never realizing their full potential.[ii]

---

ii. Swartz JR et al. "Developmental Changes in Amygdala Reactivity During Adolescence: Effects of Family History of Depression and Stressful Life Events." *American Journal of Psychiatry*. 2015; 172 (3):276–83. An accompanying editorial by Hamilton JP (214) notes, "This study is emblematic of a maturing neuroscience of depression and reflects the growing realization that the pathophysiology of major depression manifests itself more over the course of decades than months." See also Van Dam NT et al. "Childhood maltreatment altered neurobiology, and substance use relapse severity via trauma-specific reductions in limbic gray matter

Introduction

But a timely and focused prospective study of this sort is only a beginning. By itself it cannot hope to negate and reverse the larger issue: an overreaction by later twentieth-century American psychiatry to the earlier influence of Freudian "depth" theorizing about the origins of mental and emotional problems. In its enthusiasm to develop and promote a more "objective" nomenclature, our psychiatrist establishment abandoned all dynamic—that is, cause-effect—assessment of symptom development. Psychiatric residencies marginalized the relevance and importance of psychodynamic formulation and assessment; consequently, interest in counseling techniques withered. And with it attachment theory and practice.

I will discuss this at length in chapter 14.[iii]

3. And to be frank, I myself, after employing Winnicott's notions in designing a very effective adolescent and young adult inpatient program, proceeded thereafter to forget his insights for almost four decades. I have searched my office records and

---

volume." *JAMA Psychiatry*. 2014; 71(8):917–25.

The *amygdala* is a portion of the brain which, in conjunction with another closely associated brain structure, the *hippocampus*, scans environmental input for signs of a deviation from the routine. (Park S and Ichinose M, "Amygdala on the Lookout." *American Journal of Psychiatry*. 2015 (8);704–5.) Cf. chapter 7 for a discussion of how early life stress can also predispose to chronic pain, and chapter 9 for a discussion of why I prefer the notion of "stression" rather than Depression when describing the consequences of life's stresses.

iii. This verdict derives from my perspective of fifty years as a consulting psychiatrist providing services in a wide range of venues: state and private mental hospitals, county and private mental health centers, nursing homes, and residential treatment centers for adolescent sexual offenders and adult alcoholics, plus a few years of clinical research after completing my psychiatric residency, as well as forty-four years of private practice. Readers who wish to obtain a more historical perspective of the genesis of this book might want to begin with chapter 14 before turning to the clinical perspective of the earlier chapters.

found that the earliest mention of attachment issues in them dates from 2006. However, Dr. Bessel van der Kolk, in a comprehensive review of his thirty years' experience investigating and treating the enduring psychosomatic consequences of trauma, *The Body Keeps the Score*, notes that a 1974 standard psychiatric textbook put the frequency of incest at about one in a million, also that it might protect against subsequent mental illness.[7] Obviously I was not alone in my obtuseness. I discuss my amnesia below in chapter 9.

The goals of this book, therefore, are twofold:

1. To provide a reintroduction to the understanding and management of Attachment Disability, emphasizing its major psychological features: damaged trust, dissociation, and maladaptive learning.

2. To advocate for psychiatric reform. In my experience, many psychiatrists do not understand—and thus misinterpret—the clinical manifestations of trauma triad. They diagnose disease rather than recognize disability, with the result that the disability is pathologized rather than normalized. I will provide examples of this below. Therefore in chapter 14 I plead for revision of psychiatric assessment practices that too frequently promote dysfunction by misinterpreting and mismanaging Attachment Disability.[iv]

---

iv. In volume 2 of this series I also advocate for education reform, needed because of the emergence in post–World War II America of what might be a novel human species: the Teenager. Today's adolescents may very well be something new under the sun. The authority that regulates their behavior originates in cue sensitivity to media driven peer group values and tastes rather that rituals or rules that governed social development throughout human history. Motivation is now dominated by anxiety rather than guilt or shame. Unless in the midst of this social upheaval adults provide *strong and insightful parental and educational leadership*, attachment-troubled youngsters may stall out and drop out because of

Introduction

In short, it is time to move beyond the boundaries of conventional psychiatric practices. It is time to go outside of the box. We have to make some changes.

It is unrealistic to expect even interested psychiatrists to devote their energies to becoming skilled in the therapy of attachment-disordered children, adolescents, and young adults. Nonetheless their focus must become attuned to *not making things worse*.

But all of us—parents, sponsors, health-care professionals—have a stake in the management of these unhappy children and young adults, even if we have the good fortune to enjoy a life untroubled by the burden of dealing with them in our home, classroom, or office. Their dropping out, with its risk of a lifetime of underperformance, while tragic in itself, blights both them and our society because of the social and economic costs of their unfulfilled potential. Humanitarian considerations aside, we cannot afford to waste our most precious commodity. Therefore I urge everyone to develop some awareness of attachment issues and join with me in my plea for psychiatric reform.

---

learning avoidance, underperform throughout life, and be at risk of chemical dependency. Hence in volume 2 I will recommend the abandonment of mandatory school attendance. This antiquated nineteenth-century century educational policy makes it too easy for parents and sponsors to cop out from the responsibilities of leadership. Forced school participation accelerates attachment issues in floundering youngsters because *they tend to avoid the classroom*. But today's adolescent needs no incentive to learn. They are always learning, flooded as they are by peer group sentiments. The issue therefore is never *are they learning?* Rather it is just what are they learning?

Introduction

Overview

First Goal: Recognizing, Understanding, and Managing What Drives Attachment Disability: Damaged Trust

This book is my attempt, derived from my five decades of evaluating and treating youngsters and adults, to make explicit what is hidden in the unhappy lives of attachment-disabled youngsters and adults in order to facilitate early recognition and management of their distrust and separation issues. It is intended for the professionals—teachers, counselors, therapists, nurse practitioners, family physicians—whom parents will call on for help, and for those parents and sponsors who wish to develop a deeper understanding of attachment issues.

I have divided the book as follows: history the concept of attachment (chapter 1), examples of Attachment Disability (chapters 2, 3, and 4), validity of the concept of Attachment Disability (chapters 5, 6, and 7), understanding Attachment Disability (chapters 8 and 9), management of Attachment Disability (chapters 10 through 13), and a plea for psychiatric diagnostic reform chapter 14).

But first some guidelines.

1. After reviewing an early version of this book, my dear older brother recommended I include a glossary because it is impossible to avoid technical terms when discussing Attachment Disability in general or with respect to the individual cases I present herein. However, after a lot of deliberation, I have decided not to include one. In great part this is because most of the language of psychiatry is ambiguous, which is why I consider this book as "outside the box." Inside the box of psychiatry we find a confusing landscape indeed.

For example, consider the term "depression," the various meanings of which I discuss at length in chapter 9 but will preview here for illustrative purposes. To begin with, there is the popular, generic use that refers to a kind of uncomfortable feeling or behavior. In this book I signify this use by quotes: "depression." Then there is the conventional use as defined in standard psychiatric textbooks, which I signify by upper case: Depression. Finally, in the context of this book, is the technical meaning I employ to designate *persistent self-criticism*, a psychological phenomenon, denoted by italics: *depression*. Thus:

- Popular use—some kind of uncomfortable feeling or behavior, signified by quotes: "depression."
- Technical use—as defined in standard psychiatric textbooks, signified by uppercase: Depression.
- My use—persistent self-criticism, a psychological phenomenon, signified by italics: *depression*.

To complicate things further, there are at least four Depressive subtypes, plus a host of sub-subtypes. Further yet, certain medications termed Antidepressant, which might lead you to assume they are so designated exclusively for treatment of Depression, can also be used to treat a number of other conditions: Anxiety Disorders, Sleep Disorders, Chronic Pain, and so on. The same is true of the Antipsychotics, presumably defined by their use in the treatment of psychosis, but that in fact are also employed similarly. It would require an appendix the size of a book chapter to fully explore the multiple significations of such terms.

In my presentation and discussion of the case studies in this book, I will make use of this generic/conventional/technical convention. If clarification of a term is otherwise needed, I suggest Wikipedia and the references therein, or one of the standard psychiatric reference works.

2. By "parents" I have in mind not only the biological mothers and fathers of attachment-disabled children and adolescents, but

Introduction

the astounding host of figures who also provide the equivalent of parental support: grandparents, foster parents, older siblings, teachers, aunts and uncles, stepparents, peer parents, and others. So when I refer to "parents," this encompasses a broad array of surrogates so crucial to the nurturing of troubled youngsters. On occasion I will also use the term "sponsors" to reemphasize that more than just biological parents play a part in the management of these unhappy kids.

3. My preference for the terms *understanding* and *management*.

Whether medical or psychological, disability is usually discussed from the viewpoint of *diagnosis* and *treatment*. A comprehensive mastery of both domains requires extensive study and training specific to the disability of concern. Attachment Disability is no exception. However, the average professional and interested sponsor will rarely have the time and energy to cultivate such expertise. In view of this, my plan is to depart from the usual model by presenting adolescent and adult Attachment Disability from a different angle: *understanding* and *management*.

These are concepts I have extracted from my experience as one of six brand new first-year psychiatric residents assigned to work on the inpatient wards at Columbia-Presbyterian Hospital Center. We were charged with providing consultation to the hospital staff regarding management of patient problem behaviors. Typical problems included noncompliance with hospital rules, refusal of consent for procedures, threats to sign out Against Medical Advice (AMA), hostility, withdrawal, psychosis, dementia, feigning illness, severe depression, and so on. As consultants we were to review medical charts and records, interview both staff (nurses, residents, medical students) and patients, perhaps even relatives if available, and then present our findings to our supervisor, Dr. Donald Kornfeld, and the other residents for discussion.

Now, as you subsequently peruse this book, you will note a

distinct similarity between adolescent behaviors in the office and patients in the hospital. And you will discern another similarity: in both situations the thrust of the consultation is not primarily directed to the problematic adolescents and young adults but to their support system—the hospital team for inpatients, family and therapists in office settings. In hospitals this type of service is designated *consultation-liaison* (C-L). I have adopted this term here, recognizing that for our purposes the liaison is with families, sponsors, relatives, and concerned professionals.

Dr. Kornfeld proved to be an energetic, supportive mentor with a unique approach and remarkable leadership qualities, just what we psychiatric greenhorns needed (at least I did).

As former students and interns, we were comfortable with hospital customs and patient care. And we had thoroughly assimilated the traditions of medical education: hit the books. We imagined we were to promptly become knowledgeable about things psychiatric: diagnosis, medications, treatment options, that sort of stuff. But Dr. Kornfeld, while not explicitly disavowing such expectations, followed a different path. I am sure he assumed we needed no encouragement to study; otherwise, how else could we have survived the rigors of medical school and internship? Furthermore, we were a pretty mature bunch: most married, several parents. Instead his interest was in us learning to investigate the problem behavior not in isolation but in context, in relation to the environment where it had emerged. He encouraged us, most of whom had enjoyed excellent health, to look at things from the patient's point of view: isolated, surrounded by other sufferers, dependent on strangers who used a bewildering lingo, expected to obey directions without resistance, and so on. His talent was to extract relevant facts from the stream of our presentation and build an uncanny reconstruction of a patient's protective posture as he or she attempted to cope with, in essence, the foreign country that is a hospital ward. That is, we were to view the "problem" as a misfired adaptive response. Once it was so formulated, he would then explore with us what recommendations we might make to the patient's treatment team. In short, his emphasis, as I recall it, was on what I term *understanding* and *management*, less on diagnosis and treatment.[v]

I now employ these terms to dramatize two simple but vital principles without which effective Attachment Disability remediation is unlikely.[vi]

Understanding

Instead of diagnosis, I choose this term for two reasons. First, to promote constant awareness that we are dealing with an individual whose *ability to trust is wounded* because of trauma due to separation or abandonment or loss or abuse, alone or in combination. And second, to emphasize that trauma is the *disease*—an altered brain/body configuration as suggested by the above reports and by Dr. van der Kolk's investigations;

---

v. I am recreating this wonderful adventure some fifty years later. I hope I am doing justice to his leadership and instruction. Those who wish to have him speak for himself might consult Albert H. and Kornfeld D. "The Threat to Sign Out Against Medical Advice." *Annals of Internal Medicine*. 79: 888–91, 1973. The authors summarize their experiences with twenty-eight patients manifesting such threats, presenting vignettes of four to illustrate the variety of dynamisms that precipitate such desperation: overwhelming fears, anger, or psychotic processes. One of the case reports describes a dying patient desperate to sign out because of her abandonment concerns about her aging foster mother. Who would care for her later? Such concerns are one type of trauma consequence and will be discussed at length throughout this book. The authors conclude that "dispassionate investigation" and "management" set the stage for enhanced cooperation as well as later return of many who had left AMA.

vi. In my view these principles apply to *all* disability regardless of the specifics of *any* individual situation: for example, the disability of chronic pain. Cf. chapter 7 for a more extended discussion of this topic.

impaired trust is the *disability*. Distrust is not always obvious. Therefore subsequently I will present in great detail a number of case studies to illustrate the many faces of wounded trust.

Management

I use this term to highlight the second principle: *avoid making things worse.* Attachment Disability implies vulnerability. Fear of subsequent relationships is a *normal* response to any of the above unhappy life events. Consequently, subsequent offers of support may elicit wariness and concerns about being hurt again and, in extreme situations, generate distrust bordering on paranoia. *But it is important not to mistake disability for disease.* Rather, the goal here is to normalize apparent pathological behavior, which I discuss at greater length in chapter 10.

For now I note that the concept of normalizing vs. pathologizing distrust is developed in a recent document from the British Psychological Society, "Understanding Psychosis and Schizophrenia."[vii] Its authors note that paranoid distrust and

---

vii. As reported by Luhrmann TM. "Redefining Mental Illness." *New York Times Sunday Review.* January 18, 2015, SR5. The report also contains a timely critique of our current psychiatric diagnostic nomenclature, well deserved in my opinion. This occasioned an impassioned rejoinder from psychiatrist Ronald W. Pies, editor in chief emeritus of *Psychiatric Times,* in which his comments, "The War on Psychiatric Diagnosis," appeared (April 2015, 38). Ordinarily thoughtful and insightful, on this occasion Dr. Pies was a bit shrill, as the above title suggests, implying the BPS report was an attack of sorts, possibly even "anti-psychiatry." I guess my reaction is, why so touchy? Our current nomenclature is an Establishment creature, therefore automatically a target. Whether it stands or falls depends on the strength and structure of its internal validity, not the potshots of outsiders. And even highly qualified insiders, for example, Dr. Thomas Insel, former director of the National Institutes of Mental Health, consider it a matter of informed opinion rather than science. See chapter 14.

hallucinations, while not uncommon, may represent a reaction to deprivation, trauma, and abuse. While such experiences may be distressing, mental health professionals should not categorize them as illness but as a variety of human experience that needs to be processed rather than treated as abnormal.[viii] This does not rule out the role of medication, which some may choose to minimize their disability.

In other words, to slightly reformulate and extend the Society's rather extreme position, it is time for a different approach, time for outside-of-the-box thinking when it comes to "treatment" of the distrust that is the inevitable consequence of relationship injury. In medicine we carefully distinguish between disease and disability: for example, between an injury and its associated pain. We are taught to view the latter as a sign of tissue damage imposed by the former. Pain signals tissue damage, and when patients complain of pain, we search for disease. However, sometime psychiatrists muddle the distinction; they come to view emotional pain and suffering, i.e., the disability itself, as the basic problem, and stop their search for the underlying trauma. It seems to me this is the Society's basic message: distrust signals emotional damage.

In the comprehensive case studies of chapters 11 through 13, I present examples of what I consider the three principles of Attachment Disability management: *clarification, acceptance,* and *focus*. Experienced therapists and counselors will immediately recognize these as the foundation of all effective psychotherapeutic strategies. However, as I note above, the majority of attachment-disabled children and adults will not have the benefit of such expertise. In my experience their care, by design or default, will fall to professionals, sponsors, and family members unfamiliar with such concepts. These will need

---

viii. See the case presentation of Mr. POP, chapter 10, a Paranoid Schizophrenic by the usual criteria. At discharge he complained of being "out mentalized" after we employed a management dialogue to neutralize his anger and uncooperativeness, which we understood as disability, not disease.

management guidelines. It is my hope they will find helpful the rudimentary instruction in this book.

Second Goal: Remediation

The experience of trauma does not inevitably precipitate Attachment Disability. Indeed, one enduring theme of world literature and drama is the hero or heroine who rises to an exceptional level despite abuse, separation, or loss, perhaps even motivated by it.[ix] Others are not so fortunate, perhaps because of neurological residuals of the type noted above in the Swartz and Van Dam publications. They enter school and, later, young adult life with enduring functional disabilities.

If we assume Attachment Disability is a persisting residual, then the three principles of public health—*identification, treatment,* and *prevention*—would apply. Taking into account the precepts I have proposed above, the first two principles would translate to *understanding* and *management*. On the other hand, *prevention* is an impossible ideal.

And for this reason: even if children are raised in an environment without abuse or trauma—a "good enough"[x] environment, in other words—they cannot escape loss. For example, as I will describe in great detail in chapter 2, Holden Caulfield experienced during adolescence the death of his younger brother; Dyllen also lost his brother during adolescence; and Helen's mother died when she was six.

---

ix. See Charles, whose case I present in chapter 8. Or the American artist Terry Redlin, who was voted America's most popular artist for a number of years because of his remarkable wildlife and outdoor paintings. At age fifteen he lost his leg when he was run down by a motorcyclist, forcing him to surrender his ambition to be a forest ranger. He used a disability scholarship to attend an arts college, where he learned painting, which launched his career.

x. The term was originated by psychoanalyst Donald Winnicott, whom I will discuss in chapter 1.

Children and adolescents cannot avoid the risk of these and other losses as peers die or move away, or beloved grandparents age and die, or pets die or go missing, or as they change schools when moving from junior to senior high, or transition to college, and so on. Moreover, when the environment is not "good enough," when there is also abuse or trauma, either witnessed or sustained—sometimes both—again, *prevention* is impossible. True, *intervention* may occur when things become too extreme to be ignored by family or society, but too late to avert damage. In short, with prevention beyond reach in either a good or not-so-good environment, our task becomes more complex. It becomes one of *remediation*.

The term *remediation* comes from the domain of education, not medicine or psychiatry. I was introduced to it by Dr. Frederick Sheridan, principal of an Alternative Learning Center (ALC) for dropouts; I will write about his work in more detail in volume 2 of this series. He explained it has two meanings: improving skills and reversing damage.

Remediating Psychiatry

Attachment Disability is seldom recognized as such. It is misdiagnosed variously, for example, as Oppositional Defiant Disorder (Holden Caulfield, chapter 2), Borderline Personality Disorder (Jackie, chapter 4), Persistent Depressive Disorder (Rebecca, chapter 8), and Recurrent Major Depressive Disorder (Julie, chapter 8). And frequently undetected is its contribution to other diagnostic categories such as Panic Disorder (Dyllen, chapter 2, also Charlotte, chapter 3, and Charles, chapter 8), Bipolar II Disorder (William Styron, chapter 9), and Rapid Cycling Bipolar I Disorder (Rose, chapter 8).

In my view such assessment errors are a delayed consequence of an overhaul of psychiatric nosology in the 1970s that was too extreme. Perhaps a correction of psychiatry's prior emphasis on a psychodynamic "explanation" of symptom manifestation was called for. However, in the midst of the new enthusiasm for an "objective,"[xi] tangible diagnostic nomenclature, psychiatric leadership minimized the role of life events—especially life traumas. Subsequent residency programs graduated a generation of psychiatrists proficient in the mechanics of labeling and prescribing but deficient in the arts of what I term *understanding* and *management.*

No better illustration of the fallout from such lopsided training can be found than in a clinical vignette that appeared in the March 2015 issue of *Psychiatric Times* by its editor in chief Dr. Allan Tasman, professor and chairman, University of Louisville Department of Psychiatry and Behavioral Sciences.

Titled "Remember That Drive-by Shooting?" Dr. Tasman's article describes what he discovered during a fifteen-minute precepting interview with a single mother of two, diagnosed with Paranoid Psychotic Disorder and under the supervision of a nurse practitioner and one of "our best residents." Her extreme fears of a break-in had not been allayed by hours of nightly safety rituals, nor had they responded to increasing doses of an Antipsychotic medication.

Following the lead of his empathic response to her, with a few questions Dr. Tasman established that a notorious drive-by shooting of a nine-year-old had occurred on the patient's front porch, where the victim had been playing with the patient's own nine-year-old. She had never mentioned the tragedy before because she did not think it was relevant—also because no one had inquired. With her basic issue identified, she was off medications and symptom free in six weeks. He concludes, "I've often wondered how many other patients I've seen (that all of us have seen) are unlisted and undiscovered victims of violence?"[xii]

---

xi. It turned out that certain of the so-called "objective" criteria were actually reported rather than observed, therefore "subjective": for example, duration of symptoms.

xii. Dr. Tasman has expressed such concerns before:

Introduction

I strongly recommend every reader of this book access Dr. Tasman's report, which, vignette as it may be, is too extensive to reproduce here. It deserves careful scrutiny at length not only for the richness of his insights but because it epitomizes my concerns that straitjacketed thinking impairs the potential of psychiatry to contribute to Attachment Disability remediation.

And I have another concern as well. In recent years there has been movement to promote the integration of psychiatry with primary and family practice: *integrated psychiatry*. The idea is to provide in-clinic consultation to other professionals—liaison consultation, in other words. I believe this is a very promising step. But to make this transition work, it is critical to allow for the differences in caseload between the two venues.

The typical family practice or primary care clinic is physically isolated, deliberately so in most cases, to provide service outreach and ease of contact. Major psychosis and major Mood Disorder are rarely seen and even less likely managed in-clinic. They are referred out—properly in my opinion—for inpatient or outpatient specialty care. I was fortunate to witness complete integrated care during my ten years of part-time consulting at Mayo Clinic Health Systems, Austin, Minnesota, Hospital Division. Our mental health department was sited within the hospital where all services enjoyed direct and timely access to each other. Even at the Austin Hospital, which served as a regional catchment area, it was unusual for a major psychiatric issue to present or emerge in the outpatient clinics. In such an instance the patient would be sent or escorted to the ER,

---

Tasman A. "Lost in the DSM-IV checklist: empathy, meaning and the doctor-patient relationship." *Academic Psychiatry*. 2002;26:38–44. In addition to the demands of diagnostic diligence, trainees are also distracted by the energies required to create a concurrent electronic medical record. Rasminsky S et al. "Are We Turning Our Backs on Our Patients? Training Psychiatrists in the Era of the Electronic Health Record." Editorial, *American Journal of Psychiatry* 2015 August 1;172(8):708–9.

inpatient psychiatry, or our reservation desk for an appointment. Of course, such options are otherwise not immediately available to family practice, primary care, and nurse practitioners, nor are they needed.

What is needed, on the other hand, for effective integrated care is psychiatrists trained to provide a meaningful C-L evaluation ("curbstone consult" per Dr. Tasman). That is, psychiatrists who are not constricted by and chained to our shopworn psychiatric *DSM* lingo. In my experience, non-psychiatric medical, nursing, and other professional providers are well informed with respect to the peregrinations of our nomenclature. But they want and need something more for their patients than just another label and medication option.

In particular they need to be informed about and comfortable with attachment concepts and their clinical manifestations and social origins, especially the injured distrust that is always the lingering fallout of loss, abandonment, and abuse. For example, I wonder if trust issues contributed to the silence of the mother featured in Dr. Tasman's vignette. Not only did she discount her trauma; at some level she may have suspected others would as well: how could they possibly understand?

Second, and perhaps more importantly, psychiatrists who choose to work in medical clinics must understand the psychological consequences of the loss of physical independence, due not only to physical and psychological trauma but to advancing degenerative illness. As I discuss at length further on below, some individuals solve childhood/adolescent neglect or abuse by "escaping" into the independence and support offered by hard work and income/career opportunities in the civilian workforce or service in the armed forces, sometimes combined with early parenthood. Their self-esteem is nourished by their objectively productive work, the brother/sisterhood of coworkers, the comradeship of fellow soldiers, marital/parental status, and financial achievement. But the progression of degenerative

Introduction

disease degrades physical independence and threatens to close the "escape" door.

If such "escapees" have, in the interim, enlarged their adaptive repertoire—have developed other escape hatches, so to speak—they are likely to avoid feeling trapped and helpless once again. Their increasing physical limitations are therefore less likely to trigger the psychological and emotional storm that blighted their early years. One such adaptive skill, surprisingly, is a history of having survived prior spells of injury or sickness and disability. They learned that not all authority is abusive and that submitting to its therapeutic powers is worth the indignities and frustrations that inevitably accompany supervised healing.

On the other hand, if they have not developed adaptive flexibility—say, because they have always been blessed with excellent health—even insignificant findings such as mild hypertension or elevated blood sugar with their ominous symbolic content may precipitate paralyzing "anxiety" and "depression." Typically poor responders to successive trials of Antidepressants, they wind up referred to a psychiatrist, misdiagnosed as "treatment nonresponders." In fact they are actually "medication nonresponders" in need of a skill set that goes beyond providing a label and a pill.

The situation is much more ominous if the "escapees" are younger and victims not of degenerative illness but of acute civilian or military injury or trauma. The door to independence is slammed shut before they have a chance to fully exercise, explore, and capitalize on life's promise and options. Their despair and hopelessness are silent and profound. This might contribute to the shocking suicide rate among veteran returnees from deployment in Iraq and Afghanistan.[xiii]

---

xiii. Some research suggests childhood abuse may also be a factor since there is evidence that abuse survivors are more likely than others to sign up for military service. Tracie O. Afifi et al. "Association of Child Abuse Exposure With Suicidal Ideation, Suicide Plans, and Suicide Attempts in Military Personnel and the General Population in Canada." *JAMA Psychiatry.* 2016; 73(3);229–38.

Introduction

The psychiatric establishment (aka APA) has much work to do if it is to fulfill the promise of integrated care. I discuss this in chapter 14.

Part 1

Understanding Attachment Disability

… to be human is to cultivate attachments

1

Origins of the Idea of Attachment

In the middle decades of the twentieth century certain psychoanalysts revised and extended Freudian concepts of psychological development. These individuals, the "neo-Freudians," had trained with Freud and his disciples but later modified classical psychoanalytic concepts. Rather than focusing solely on intrapsychic structures—ego, superego, id—as the source of conflict, their interest was more extrapsychic. In their view, conflict was related to the strength and consistency of parental or surrogate nurturing (or lack of thereof) during infancy and childhood. That is, quality of childhood nurturing foreshadowed quality of life relationships. Psychological development was less the consequence of an unfolding father-mother-child triad; much more relevant was whether there were parental relationships to begin with.

Of the many revisionists, here I will briefly review two figures whose elucidation of the vicissitudes of child development is absolutely crucial to the understanding of Attachment Disability and, by extension, the management of adolescent dysfunction and underperformance.

John Bowlby (1907–90): Attachment Defined

Attachment is a term originated by the British psychoanalyst and pediatrician John Bowlby, derived from his pioneering studies of childhood development.

During World War II he investigated what happened to children who had been separated from their familiar caregivers during the war. He studied orphans, youngsters who had been evacuated to the countryside to live with relatives, children raised in communal nurseries, and even those separated from their families during brief hospitalizations. He concluded that any early life separation could have a profound and lasting effect on all subsequent relationships. The child's ability to develop trusting and stable relationships—*attachments* was the term he used—was impaired. Anxieties and concerns about loss and abandonment prevailed, sometimes openly, sometimes hidden.[1] Once in school, as security concerns sapped their energies, they tended to fall behind. The security of relationships consumed their attention. How teachers and peers looked and what they did, not what they said, were paramount.

On this side of the Atlantic, attachment-disordered kids came to be understood as the product of extreme deprivation—orphans adopted from abroad, for example—or extreme turmoil: youngsters raised in crack houses or subject to frequent placements. Attachment problems were therefore seen as an issue of early childhood. In youngsters of that age, Attachment Disorders are relatively easy to recognize, especially if the youngsters come from backgrounds of flamboyant neglect, deprivation, turmoil, or abuse.

Eventually Bowlby's notions were incorporated into our psychiatric diagnostic terminology as *Reactive Attachment Disorders*. Two polar types are identified: *inhibited* and *uninhibited*. The child either connects with no one or everyone. The latter condition is especially dangerous because it renders the child

Origins of the Idea of Attachment

very vulnerable to persuasion: for example, likely to wander off with a passing stranger.[i]

However, in recent years it has become apparent that not all attachment problems appear in early childhood, nor are they all accompanied by a history of dramatic neglect or abuse. Some develop in later childhood or early adolescence when a figure who has earned trust is lost because of such causes as illness, death, separation, or divorce.

Moreover, such later attachment disruption does not inevitably result in Attachment Disability. This is because children, although vulnerable, are tough and adaptable. Their needs drive them to seek and restore the lost relationship. If things work out, they find a replacement who earns their trust—an aunt or uncle or older sibling or step-parent or sobered-up parent or special friend. They learn that the world is not totally chaotic. If that figure remains present and stable, they may learn to extend their trust to others whom that figure seems to trust. Thus they begin to find security in other relationships. They become able to manage transitions and the anxieties that transitions inevitably engender. In short they learn to manage *separation anxiety*. The loss and sense of abandonment are more or less repaired. It is not that they "get over" what has been lost—one never really "gets over" a lost love; rather, they learn to accept the pain without blame. Acceptance releases energy and motivation previously consumed by blame. Wounds heal, although a scar remains, and youngsters move forward to explore new attachments. The impossible now seems possible.[2]

But sometimes the turmoil of separation and abandonment sustained during later childhood and adolescence is not repaired. Disturbance and turmoil evolves into disability.

There are three possible outcomes, or corners of the dis-

---

i. In the latest edition of the American Psychiatric Association's *Diagnostic and Statistical Manual (DSM-5)*, the uninhibited type is renamed Disinhibited Social Engagement Disorder, 268.

ability triangle: Attachment *Avoidance,* Attachment *Entanglement,* and Attachment *Acting-out.* The first two may be understood as delayed manifestations of the inhibited and uninhibited early childhood behaviors Bowlby first described. The third apex of the triangle, however, was first recognized by his contemporary, Donald Winnicott, whom I will discuss in the next section.

Attachment Avoidance

In this situation wounded youngsters fail to heal, and their life grinds to a halt. Their school performance suffers and their grades decline. They close up and withdraw from or spurn friendship. Their attitude becomes sour and negative; they radiate a sense of hopelessness and despair. In short, their ability to replace the lost relationship has atrophied. They now avoid reaching out and withdraw from the opportunity to do so: they now *fear* attachment. J. D. Salinger's portrayal of the aimless Holden Caulfield, who has yet come to grips with the death of his beloved younger brother three years before, is a textbook description of *Attachment Avoidance*.[3] In most cases the disability, while enduring, is not deadly but occasionally can evolve into severe Depression and suicide risk.

Attachment Entanglement

This corresponds to the uninhibited type of Attachment Disorder seen in early childhood. Here adolescents deal with their miseries by becoming emotionally overattached, so to speak, to others—especially peers and family—feeling increasingly responsible for their welfare.[ii] Their appreciation of their own needs and feelings becomes engulfed and smothered—*entangled*—by their perceived sensitivity to the needs and feelings

---

ii. Therapists often describe this attachment style as *enmeshment*.

of the other. They report worrying about "everything." Cutting is always a sign of entanglement, ping-pong suicidal behavior between peers an extreme sign. In my experience adolescent girls are more likely than boys to develop this attachment style. If they manage to navigate their adolescent and early adult life without a life disaster, they typically are attracted to careers in nurturing professions — medicine, veterinary medicine, teaching, counseling, and so forth—and occasionally in criminal justice—police, probation officer, for example.

Donald Winnicott (1896–1971)

Bowlby did not consider acting-out behavior—*externalizing behavior* is the more contemporary term—to be an attachment issue. This notion comes from the work of his contemporary, Donald Winnicott.

Like Bowlby, Winnicott was a psychiatrist and psychoanalyst. He, too, studied and commented on the vicissitudes of children evacuated to the countryside during the Blitz.[4] He originated the notion of the "good-enough" mother. As he saw it, the developing child did not require heroic attentiveness or perceptiveness from its mother to develop normally. Constant tangible skin-to-skin contact and fondling of the child were not necessary prerequisites for social development. Some constancy was "good enough." In fact the behavioral principle of *intermittent reinforcement* soundly supports his position.[iii] An infant frustrated by the lack of an immediate response to its unmet needs does not give up but proclaims its problem with increasing vigor. Hopefully a caretaker, not necessarily its

---

iii. I will discuss the concept of reinforcement (reward) at length in volume 2 of this series. For now, consider the difference in behavior evoked by operating a slot machine versus a candy bar dispenser. If the latter fails to produce what we select we may try once again before giving up, obviously not true when playing the slots.

mother, will respond, creating the potential for trust building and perseverance: socialization, in other words.[iv]

Of particular interest to this book, however, is that Winnicott viewed the emergence of "antisocial" behaviors characteristic of the later stages of child and adolescent development as the youngster's "claim" on its environment.[5] As he saw it, such behavior represented an attempt to correct for deficient mothering; that is, mothering that had not been "good enough." The disruptiveness was a disguised plea for help, a demand for need fulfillment from the larger world, an attempt to repair mothering failure.

In my view his perceptive insights have stood the test of time and are constrained only by his limited notion of "mothering." His observations were derived within a society where most children were born and raised by two adults united in wedlock. In our postmodern society, an increasing percentage of children are born out of wedlock and raised by an array of figures. "Mothering" now incorporates nurturing from unwed and often single parents, their partners, teachers, grandparents, older siblings, relatives, stepparents, neighbors, sitters, day care staff, and more. Relationships with nurturers are therefore more equivocal, shifting, and evanescent. On the one hand this bestows resilience and protection because of the increased security to be found in a potentially wider support network. On the other hand it bestows vulnerability if a vital support is lost and the network, such as it is, is too fragile and disjointed

---

iv. Fifty years later epidemiologic and genetic research strengthens Winnicott's hypothesis. Scholar Charles Murray, citing two such exhaustive studies, reluctantly concludes, "... it increasingly appears that once we have provided children with a merely OK [read "good-enough"] environment, our contribution as parents and as a society is pretty much over." Murray C. "Parenting's minimal impact on IQ: Home environment and socioeconomic status are even more irrelevant to kids' intelligence." Minneapolis Star Tribune. November 28, 2014:A17. In other words, things go better if we avoid making things worse, which is the premise of this book.

to respond to the unmet needs of a youngster who perceives the lost relationship as abandonment.

But too frequently the subsequent search for need relief is unfocused, misfires, and takes the form of angry, even defiant demands. What we professionals might define as "oppositional," Winnicott would recognize as a cry for help from the environment. In short, the failed healing takes the form of the acting-out kid.[v] In this respect it is very unfortunate that the traditional concept of acting-out behavior has been replaced by "externalizing behavior" because this deflects attention from considering what unmet needs drive this kind of behavior.

As professionals we must be careful, therefore, when dealing with students, not to misinterpret such a disguised plea for relief. It is important to recognize the underlying attachment issue and direct our awareness toward the youngster's unmet need for (and fear of) "mothering" in the larger sense of the word: that is, as a need for a perceptive attentiveness. Above all, the idea is not to make things worse by our own loss of control in response to the defiant provocativeness that is the signature camouflage of these troubled youngsters.

Attachment Acting-Out

Here a fear of recurrent loss becomes cloaked with anger. The behavior of such youngsters is (not necessarily consciously) designed to keep parents and teachers at a distance, to alienate them, to avoid closeness—in other words, to establish

---

v. Usually diagnosed as *Oppositional Defiant Disorder*. In order to qualify for insurance reimbursement, or to provide a requested official certificate of disability, it may be necessary to provide an official term for the behavior disturbance. However, it is vital that we professionals not be seduced by the use of the label. We must always remain alert that behind the façade of defiance in a frightened youngster, wounded by lost or neglectful relationships, who distrusts and tests offers of support.

an interpersonal boundary. The idea is to establish a wall of behavior behind which the adolescent feels safe. If you are not close to anyone, you are at less risk of experiencing the pain of abandonment, which, as these youngsters now believe, is inevitable. These days such youngsters are more likely the product of a broken home or a serial placement experience than an orphanage or crack house.

Thus they relate at a distance, so to speak, by using behavior to keep others irritated and frustrated. "They enjoy provoking me, bugging me!" sponsors say. (Younger miscreants not infrequently display a guilty smile, and sometimes will fess up when I inquire.) Such disrespectful and defiant behavior serves a second function as well. It is an indirect way of asking for love, which frustrated sponsors express when, flooded with guilt about their own angry response to the provocations, they afterward apologize and try to make up. This kind of failed healing, while more dramatic, noticeable, and provocative, has a *much better prognosis* than the other varieties of Attachment Disability. It is less likely to result in self-mutilating and self-destructive behavior and less likely to culminate in suicide, although such kids may engage in risky behavior with a lethal potential.

Many kids with this background, if they survive into young adulthood without an irremediable disaster—a felony record, say, or a disabling injury—evolve into law-and-order pillars of the community: police officers, attorneys, probation officers, and so on. Some years ago I happened to attend Sunday high mass in my childhood parish on a morning featuring the investiture of three men as Subdeacons, one of the lesser orders of the Catholic Church. At the conclusion of the sermon, which included some instruction on the historic role of the Subdeacon in the Church, with a dramatic flourish the good father called upon the three to step forward and be received into the order. The three, appropriately garbed, reverently approached the altar. I was startled. Two of the three were among the biggest goof-offs of my grade school years.

It is unfortunate that such behavior is now termed "externalizing," as opposed to other adolescent behaviors viewed as "internalizing." The idea of "acting-out" behavior contains an implicit question: what is the underlying dynamism driving the behavior? What is the motivation? But discarding the term in favor of "externalizing" not only risks inhibiting further inquiry, but also risks converting disability to disease: that is, making things worse.[vi]

In Summary

From an evolutionary perspective, attachment promotes survival, but from a social perspective it creates vulnerability. Survival/vulnerability is the yin/yang of attachment. After fifty years I can't say that I fully understand the knots and tangles of adolescent and adult Attachment Disability issues. However, one thing is clear: you can't begin to pick them apart without a constant awareness of this inevitable human predicament.

To be human is to cultivate attachments. Moreover, even when fully developed, attachments require constant nourishment. We think only children require daily reminders that they are loved, but the truth is that all of us need to hear words of love, perhaps even more than youngsters, because as adults we have learned that attachments are not forever. We know that to be attached is to be at risk of loss, to be susceptible to pain. We have learned that not all endings are happy.

But we have also learned that without attachments we could not survive. Like Bowlby's orphans, we would wither away. So to survive, most of us solicit and engage in attachments, risks notwithstanding.

---

vi. The hazards of labeling disability as disease is an issue I will address at length in chapter 14.

Part 2

Varieties of Attachment Disability

... acting-out youngsters are deeply attached but ambivalently so.

As I mentioned earlier, there are three kinds of Attachment Disability: *Attachment Avoidance, Attachment Entanglement,* and *Attachment Acting-out.*

To illustrate each variety, I will present case histories of troubled adolescents and young adults. In each case I will highlight the significance of certain behaviors as symptoms or signs of a hidden attachment issue. Regardless of the specifics, however, all cases feature a common emotional disability: injured trust. Moreover, the distrust extends both outward and inward: outward toward relationships, inward toward feeling states. Both situations acquire an aura of danger that is not always consciously appreciated. But threat awareness is present in all cases, having been programmed into the nervous system by trauma experience(s).[1]

One caution. I have chosen these cases because they are in large part a prototype of the variety of disability I am describing. In fact, however, most attachment-disordered youngsters demonstrate a mixture of all three types. For example, Holden Caulfield, the protagonist of Salinger's *The Catcher in the Rye,* is nearly a "pure culture" of Attachment Avoidance, yet he acts out by going on the run. It is important, therefore, when dropped-out or underachieving kids sit before you, to sift through their behaviors and identify the attachment variety that appears to be most disabling.

2

Attachment Avoidance: Three Cases

[CASE STUDY]
"Dyllen": Solving Panic with Avoidance and Addiction

Dyllen's story is a composite of attachment-driven underperforming and dropout behavior I have encountered in young male adults who seek help years after leaving high school. His experiences illustrate how attachment and abandonment issues can also generate addiction risk, and how teacher recognition of risk might avoid its magnification. Dropout and addiction prevention begin the first day of school, a topic I will briefly discuss here within the limits of a single case study, but which will be the subject of volume 2 of the series, *Attachment Disability: The Hidden Cause of Dropping Out and Addiction*.

Note: I will begin by recounting Dyllen's story as I would learn it during an initial interview and then follow up with a more detailed look and analysis.

Dyllen is a twenty-two-year-old single male who requests a psychiatric evaluation. He is attentive, cooperative, compliant, not unattractive, casually dressed in clean but worn clothing. He is restless, a bit on edge, waits for inquiries. In reply to questions he is descriptive, providing answers rather than unresponsive explanations, although as a historian he is bland and vague. There are undertones of shame but little blaming of self or others.

The problem is anxiety. A while back—maybe six months ago, maybe a year or so—he began to cut down on pot and alcohol after years of using. In fact, he has not used at all for four or five months. But he's noticed he's become anxious, increasingly so. In addition, he's had an occasional panic attack and is more reluctant now to leave his apartment. He prefers to shop at night, with a companion if possible. He dreads having to stand in line. And when he's out he worries constantly about what others might be thinking of him. Also, lately thoughts of dying have been popping into his head. Not that he would ever commit suicide, but why is he thinking of it? He's always been a poor sleeper but recently it's been worse. He has strange dreams where someone is in trouble—he's not sure who—but he's helpless to do anything about it. He's most comfortable when working, He's a mechanic with a dirt track team; they leave him pretty much alone because he's good at setting up engines.

Otherwise his health is okay. He takes no prescription medications and does not have a physician, even though he just qualified for health care. He has never seen a psychiatrist before.

I ask if he has ever had panic attacks before. Yes. The first one was at age nine when his teacher asked him to recite. He made a big fuss and she turned to someone else. After that, whenever it was his turn to go to the blackboard or recite, he would act up so he wouldn't have to be in front of everybody. After a while his teachers stopped asking and left him alone.

He can't remember if he had any more panic attacks after that, but the recent ones brought it all back.

He doesn't know if there is a family history of panic. His father was an alcoholic; in fact, that's why his mother left his father. She pretty much raised him. Also in the house was a brother eight years older, a half sib, a bit of a gearhead. They got along okay, but he moved out as soon as he could to join the army. That was a shock.

I ask if he ever witnessed or sustained any abuse: physical, sexual, or emotional. He has to think about the question. Nothing sexual, but his parents fought a good deal, shouting, yelling, things of that sort. She might have called the cops once or twice, it's pretty hard to remember, he doesn't think about that stuff much.

His mother had to work. Maybe his father would send money now and then. He visited his father a few times but that petered out after a while. He's not heard from him in years but as far as he knows he is still alive. Neither his brother nor his mother talks about him.

He got along with the two of them okay. But they were both busy, his mother working, his brother with his friends. So he was pretty much on his own. He had a few buddies, that's where the pot and alcohol started, maybe sixth or seventh grade or thereabouts, he's not sure. He didn't shoplift like they did or take money from his mother's purse, too scary. His brother would slip him a few bucks now and then. Also, he used to hang out with a neighbor who worked on cars. He would help him out, run errands, it was kind of fun.

He is vague about school—not much of a problem. He was never held back, never was in Special Ed. He drifted along, tried out for basketball, made the B squad, but he dropped out. He never studied much. His grades were poor because he never did or turned in homework assignments. He usually did well on exams because he listened and had a good memory, but the missing assignments dragged him down. Once or twice teachers told him he had potential, especially in drafting class, and should study harder. Otherwise they left him alone. Maybe he talked to a school counselor once or twice, but he didn't like her, although she did not confront him about his poor record. And she never asked him why he bothered to come to school in the first place. She invited him to keep seeing her, but there was not much to talk about. So he stopped going. They would pass in the hallway but he would avoid looking at her.

By now he was using pot pretty much every day. He began to cut school and was sent to court. He was assigned a truancy officer, told to get some counseling. His mother raised the roof, so to keep her happy and the officer off his back he stopped skipping. But things didn't change. He just sat in class waiting until he was sixteen when he could drop out and go to work because his neighbor lined up a job for him. Nobody made much of a fuss when he stopped going. In fact he was really surprised when his mother said it was okay.

The job was with an auto parts store stocking and delivering parts, a job he really liked. During lunch hour he would browse manufacturers' websites reading recall bulletins. It was amazing what you could find out. He became the go-to guy for the clerks up front when they had a customer question they couldn't answer. He was proud to wear a baseball cap with the company logo. But he got into an argument with the store manager about working up front more, something about his attitude, and quit.

He hung out with a few buddies, going to movies, playing video games. He found a fast food job, but dealing with customers was pretty uncomfortable. He got by on odd jobs, helping his neighbor and friends work on cars—by now he was pretty good at brake jobs and oil changes, and was learning how to swap out engines and transmissions. After a while he started working on stock cars.

Eventually his mother requested he start paying rent so he moved in with some buddies.

About a year ago he met a girl, they began to date. She is a certified nursing assistant, goes to a tech school, wants to become a nurse. He moved in with her about six months ago, about the time he started to cut back on pot. He's crankier, his sleep is restless, they argue more. But she's happy he's using less. When his anxieties built up, she bugged him to get help, said she would come along. In fact she's waiting outside. She's met his mother, they seem to get along.

He worries about his mother. She still smokes at least a pack. She works hard, looks tired and worn out, has a cough. Her back aches. Once in a while his half-brother calls. He's out of the army now, going to school in IT. His brother says Dyllen needs to get his GED and go back to school. He's not sure about this. It would mean dealing with people, sitting in class, which he now realizes makes him feel trapped. Besides, even though he can read okay, he doesn't like to study, and he's not good at writing.

We very briefly discuss the origins of his anxiety, how he has been "treating" it with pot all these years. I talk about treatment, explain that Antidepressants might be helpful for his panic and avoidance. He's heard about them from his lady friend, but he is dubious. In high school he heard how they can make you suicidal. How about Ativan? he asks. Instead I suggest clonidine, as an alternative with no addictive potential, helpful with social anxiety and insomnia. We review potential risks and benefits. He accepts a script, commits to return in three weeks. We'll see.

The Significance of Dyllen's Behavior

I have constructed Dyllen's history to illustrate certain experiences commonly reported by male underperformers and dropouts that contribute to the development of Attachment Disability.

Since his initial history and mental status exam are not

suggestive of a developmental disorder, we will assume that his early development was more or less normal.

True, his father was an alcoholic and no doubt brought into the home all the turmoil of an alcoholic parent: uncertainty, bitterness, arguments, perhaps even physical assaults. Dyllen was not spared. Even if none of the abuse was directed toward him, he did witness it. He tried to ignore it but it left its mark: his vagueness as a historian. Sometimes the hallmark of trauma is vivid; for example, recurrent nightmares or flashbacks. But not infrequently trauma residuals are notable only by what is absent. Often such survivors are bland and expressionless, providing a history that is colorless and sparse. Not infrequently, when questioned about their development, they will respond with off-hand remarks such as "… things are sort of a blank … I don't remember much … some kind of a gap there." This is dissociation at work, a sign of unfamiliarity with the inner world of feeling and emotions, a consequence of trauma.

But there were some positive developments. First of all, his father did leave the household, at what age we do not know. It must have been a relief; it provided Dyllen an opportunity to reestablish a firm connection with his mother. Second, there was his older half sib who remained in the home. I suspect the brother took on a parenting role. Perhaps that is how Dyllen became interested in working on cars, watching his brother tinker with engines. Out of this attachment grew other affiliations, with the neighbor who worked on cars, possibly with cousins or aunts and uncles.

In school things probably went well at first. He must have partially managed the third grade transition to more independent study since he tells me he can read, although when it comes to writing he is not comfortable.

Then his brother joins the service.

Symptoms Cannot Be Explained but They Can Be Understood

Now consider Dyllen in class, trying to cope with his brother's departure, ruminating, perhaps feeling it all must be his fault. *If I had done something different, anything, maybe he would not have left.* In the midst of his preoccupation, his teacher asks him to step to the blackboard. His heart starts to pound, he begins to feel sweaty and hot, he shakes, and he can't think straight even though he knows the answer to the problem she just wrote on the blackboard because he studied it last night, just like his brother told him to before he left. Thoughts spin in his head. *What if I make a mistake, everyone will laugh. What if I get it right, everyone will think I'm a show-off.* He feels sick, starts to cry, collapses into his seat with his head buried in his hands. Everyone laughs. She turns to someone else. He feels very foolish. After that he worries every day on the way to school, wondering, *Will she ask me again?* When she does, he pretends not to hear, or clowns or goofs off, or gets stubborn, or pretends he doesn't know the answer. Eventually she leaves him alone, but he still worries.

"What if" thoughts do not necessarily lead to disability. Some individuals are able to rationally evaluate such a threat and its likely consequences, and respond realistically. For example, Dyllen might have thought something like, *So what, who really cares? I've seen other guys choke and the world didn't come to an end. I can live with being embarrassed.* But others react like Dyllen and begin to ruminate and avoid. They listen to their "Igor," the personification of their irrational voice who always predicts catastrophe.[2]

What caused his fear to conjure up his Igor rather than a rational "friend" can never be explained. Science deals with the general, not the specific, and therefore cannot *explain* the specific. But we can understand what happened.

Thus, at that very critical moment in his life, as he struggled with intense abandonment issues, Dyllen sustained a severe bout of *performance anxiety*—in other words he choked up—when, possibly for the first time in his life, he was confronted by a request to make a change from passive observer to active participant. Or perhaps he was familiar with the routine and yet unaccountably froze up; we don't know why. In any event, his attention was distracted from his prepared answer by the way his body felt, then by worries about how his peers would perceive him. No matter how he performed, one way or another he would lose respect. In his mind he faced additional separation.

On the other hand, his collapse not only "rescued" him, but it also showed him how to avoid similar demands by making a "fuss." And clowning or playing dumb or getting stubborn earned respect from his peers. A double payoff.

It would have been better if Dyllen had reacted to his panic and its underlying sense of separation and loss with more of an angry, blustering, and rebellious attitude. As you may recall from the discussion of Winnicott above, acting-out behavior can be understood as a youngster making a "claim" on its environment to rectify an unmet need. In the midst of his abandonment the child or adolescent, unable to identify and verbalize his discomfort, externalizes it, projects it undifferentiated onto his world. He wants to be rescued, soothed, understood. Had Dyllen's miseries turned in this direction, he might have been identified as in need of a remedial or restorative approach.[3] Anger is more likely to attract a response than is withdrawal.

Too frequently, unfortunately, the environmental response is one of anger, frustration, and rejection. Teachers, sponsors, and the authorities generally do not recognize the fear behind the anger, do not understand that anger and fear are inseparably linked: that is, where anger is manifest, you look for the hidden fear and vice versa. Sometimes professionals who should know better fall into the same trap, and youngsters end up being labeled as Oppositional Defiant Disorder. Such a label paralyzes rational appraisal and instead promotes a law-and-order mentality, which any halfway normal youngster will resist. The result: everyone remains aggravated while the youngster's attachment issue goes unrecognized and unmanaged.

Silent Dropping Out

At first Dyllen does not drop out, at least not physically. Years later when such silent dropouts try to recall for me their reason for leaving school, their memory is vague, a striking contrast to the typically vivid recall of angry dropouts. When angry dropouts remember, you can sense the lingering bitterness and feelings of rejection. Not so with the silent. Those years seem to be blank and empty, which not infrequently is reflected in their detached attitude and posture, as if it happened to someone else. If I inquire, they may recall panic and anxiety, sometimes little more. Sitting with them, I begin to feel as if they had been cast off, discarded, still drifting after all these years, yet sometimes engaged in heroic efforts to rescue others, as if to compensate for what they didn't receive themselves. In short, with these students, the style of their attachment issue is not potentially self-correcting because it is so colorless and unlikely to attract attention. It is vital, therefore, that we seize what may be the only opportunity to remediate such youngsters before they slip into an intractable disability.

True, Dyllen slips away, but only into the background, not out of school. I surmise that as his teachers learn to ignore him, there are fewer panic attacks, perhaps none. But his worries about panic continue; he is now afflicted with anxiety about anxiety, so to speak. At first he was only concerned about what his peers might think or say should they figure out what was troubling him. They would think he was weak, a baby. Eventually, however, his anxieties widen; now he wonders about everyone—teachers, neighbors, relatives, even complete strangers. He finds himself ruminating about what others might think about him whenever he is in public. Sometimes the thought pops into his head that they even seem to know what he is thinking. This is a crazy idea, he knows, but he can't get it out of his mind whenever he is out of the house.

In a sense, he is "rescued" by his subsequent substance abuse.

The "Solution" of Addiction

A study of more than ten thousand adolescents aged thirteen to eighteen reveals approximately 5 percent report alcohol use by age six, increasing to about 30 percent by age thirteen. Moreover, by then approximately 5 percent of kids describe regular/abusive consumption, rapidly increasing thereafter to 50 percent by age eighteen.[4]

Dyllen, however, eventually comes to prefer pot, possibly because it is cheaper, more available, less detectable than alcohol. Besides, he doesn't want to turn out like his father, whose use of alcohol made him angry and violent. With pot Dyllen is more comfortable socially; enjoys mellowing out with his few close buddies. His anxieties fade away.

And his motivation fades as well. He neglects his homework. At first this has little impact on his marks because in the early grades homework is not as important as test results. He does surprisingly well on tests because he is a good listener and has a good memory. So he can get by with just paying attention in class. His teachers recognize this and make allowances for his avoiding recitation. Eventually, however, the absent homework is more and more of a deficit. They tell him he would be getting much higher final grades if he would just do the homework. They tell him he has potential, which makes him uncomfortable. It's not that he deliberately neglects to turn in assignments. But in the back of his mind he knows this is a way of keeping the heat off. If he is not successful, after a while people will have less expectation that he behave more like a grown-up. In his experience grown-ups are unhappy, have responsibilities. He would rather remain like a kid, knowing there will always be someone to look after him if things do not work out. In short—as I summarize it for my patients—*Success DANGEROUS!! Failure Safe.*"[i]

He drifts along. In high school his teachers start to ignore him, are less forgiving. No homework or assignments, no passing grades no matter how well he does on tests. They bestow their energies on his more promising peers, in part perhaps because they can't fail to note he hangs with the burnouts, the "druggies." Before, he had a reputation as a sometimes amusing clown, but now he is seen as a pothead, which becomes the explanation for his failure to perform. It's not that he doesn't have the ability, his teachers say, it's just that he's tuned out because of the marijuana. So he is referred to the school counselor, a one-on-one trial that he approaches amid considerable trepidation.

---

i. The fear of failure is a well-known component of performance anxiety. Less well known is that there is always an associated fear of success. Both involve concerns about the loss of a dependent relationship and rejection. Success is dangerous because it might lead others to assume you no longer need help and can manage on your own, or evoke feelings of jealousy. Fears of success are characterized by a pattern of doing well followed by collapse. With students, grades unaccountably tail off, especially before a transition. In adults the signature of a "success phobia" is a cyclical employment history, one of rapid promotion, then some kind of disaster. In hospitals and residential treatment centers you see bouts of acting out just prior to transfer to an open unit or discharge. I encountered this fresh out of my residency in 1965 when I started work at Anoka (MN) State Hospital. In many settings a behavior modification approach can be helpful with success fears because it teaches the client how to negotiate change in small steps. I discuss this at greater length in the case of Jackie, chapter 4.

The Threat of Help

At the interview there is no confrontation, just a friendly interest in him, which is even scarier in a way because it excites his paranoia. He could handle being chewed out; he's had a lot of experience with that from his mother and his brother. But all this niceness! What is going on here? So he clams up, in part because he himself doesn't understand his issues—he's forgotten about the anxiety attack of years before—and in part because he's too ashamed to reveal his worries regarding what people might think about him, including the counselor. How could she not conclude that he's just a big baby? Finally, if he told her too much, he might get her worrying about him. He's already made a lot of people unhappy about him—his mother, his brother, his aunts and uncles, his gearhead neighbor; he doesn't need more guilt.

So the counselor does most of the talking. She brings up his potential, how he needs to put it to work; otherwise, at this rate, he won't graduate. She delicately refers to his using, suggests he might want to join a discussion group of students with similar problems. Finally, she tells him that she liked meeting him, thinks she can help him, invites him to return. He promises to think about it.

It is always easy to second-guess a professional's prior behavior when you know the outcome. If the interview had been more or less successful, possibly Dyllen would not be in my office, or would have come for help much sooner. Perhaps a somewhat brisker, less personal approach would have been more effective, one focused on the facts of his performance, on *what is* rather than *what should be*. This, then, might have been followed by asking Dyllen why he is bothering to attend school—in other words, *what could be*. Had he ever thought about dropping out, or attending an ALC? Things obviously are not working out for him, so how about a different approach?

In any event, afterward he completely rejects attending

the discussion group; it would mean encountering his old bug-a-boo of performance anxiety. On the other hand, for a few days Dyllen actually does indeed consider her suggestion to return for another one-on-one discussion; then the idea fades into the background. When subsequently he sees they might pass in the hallway, he turns aside or otherwise avoids eye contact. Perhaps she tries to corral him, but he mumbles an excuse, so obviously uncomfortable that she backs away. Soon it is like they are strangers and the meeting never happened. In faculty conferences when he is discussed and eyes turn to her, she shrugs helplessly. She's left messages for his mother, but there is no reply. Well, at least he is not a discipline problem. He becomes even more invisible.

The meeting actually did have an impact. Dyllen now realizes he is too far behind to graduate and comes to wonder why he is bothering to attend. He starts to be absent, becomes identified as a truant, which brings him to the attention of the authorities. He and his mother are summoned to family court, and that finally gets his mother's attention. Up to now she's been consumed with the task of keeping the household afloat since his father no longer pays support.

At his hearing the judge lectures him, tells him to attend school. Although he is not charged with breaking a law, the judge still assigns a probation officer, which makes Dyllen very uncomfortable. In some respects it's a repeat of his meeting with the school counselor: he mumbles, shrugs, lets the officer do all the talking. But now the focus is not on his presumably bright future, but more on his current abysmal performance, including his using, to which he admits. The officer strongly recommends he attend the discussion group.

The judge lectures his mother too, tells her to make him go to school. There is no discussion of an alternative learning center as an option.

Back home his mother really reads him the riot act, weeping, angry, despairing. First it was his father, then his half-brother, and now she is going to lose him if he doesn't shape up. He feels very guilty. No matter what he does, people end up unhappy. Everything is his fault. So he stops skipping school, is there every day. But his attitude has changed. He feels resentful, which is apparent in his expression and behavior. It's not that he is outright disrespectful or insubordinate, just quietly disdainful. Now at test time he doesn't even try. Teachers avoid him; he avoids them.

Interestingly, his drafting class is an exception. He likes the way he can control the black lines on the pure white paper—it is kind of exciting. He designs futuristic buildings and furniture. When his teacher says he has real talent and should experiment with drawing, he is not threatened. In fact he has already started doing so. In his bedroom he has notebooks of drawings that no one knows about except his brother.

Otherwise, he continues to fail.

The Solution of Work

Then his mother does a surprising about-face and gives him permission to drop out and go to work once he turns sixteen. Thus he can accept an offer of a part-time job at an auto parts store where his neighbor, who manages a different store, has put in a good word for him. Possibly the neighbor has been part of his life for many years and has become sort of a brother surrogate. And it is obvious from his interview behavior that Dyllen is a likeable kid.

In retrospect I can say that for Dyllen, dropping school in favor of work turned out to be an excellent decision. He moved from a world where he was viewed as a failure to one where he was treated with respect.

It's really a cool job, with both inside and outside work so he is not pinned down. Either he is in back stocking shelves, or in the truck delivering parts to garages. He gets to read all the recall bulletins and remembers most of the details. He remembers so much of this stuff that after a while the clerks up front start consulting him about customer problems; he's sort of the in-house mechanic. He likes to hang around even when he's off shift, so his boss gives him keys to the place so he can come in and open up for early deliveries. Pretty soon he's working full time. Even when he's not at work, he likes to wear his baseball cap and T-shirt with the company logo.

The Threat of Success

Then attachment issues return with a bang.

One day his boss takes him aside, says he's ready for a promotion up front behind the customer service desk. He will have more face-to-face contact with customers, take their orders, discuss their problems, make recommendations, things of that sort. His boss tells him he's ready. Better yet, it's more money, and if he does well the boss will recommend him for an assistant manager spot. Also, if he gets his GED he will be eligible in a few years for a manager's job at one of the other stores. He's got a good reputation and a good future in the company.

Dyllen listens, silently, with increasing discomfort. He's starting to feel trapped, hot, flushed, smothered, desperate. He's too ashamed and not articulate enough to reveal his anxieties about social contact. And the idea of going back into the classroom is dreadful. He finally mumbles that he'll think about it, that he's got some stuff that has to be delivered. He starts to walk away. His boss calls him back, starts to lecture him a bit about what a great opportunity this is, and that he should act more grateful. Now Dyllen is getting irritated, starts to speak up. He says no one has the right to tell him how he should feel. Now his boss, feeling rejected, really gets hot. To Dyllen it's turned into an old story: "help" means letting other people run your life. Now they are arguing. Totally disgusted by now, Dyllen pulls off his cap, tosses his keys on the counter, and walks out, saying he quits.

Back home everyone is upset: his mother, his brother, the neighbor who helped him get the job. No one can figure out what got into him. Even a few of his buddies are puzzled. When anyone tries to talk him into returning, he just gets stubborn, walks away. His mother is patient for a while, figuring he'll find another job. Instead Dyllen starts sleeping in, staying out, smoking more.

Let us imagine he knows he's blown it but can't figure out why or what got into him. A couple of times he thought about returning to the store and talking things over—he's heard that customers and coworkers miss him and want him to return—but the idea of sitting down with his boss really makes him uncomfortable: what would he say?

Finally his mother loses patience, says he either goes to work or gets out. So he finds odd jobs at garages where he used to deliver parts when they need extra help. He buys more tools, works in the street on his buddies' cars, pulls parts for them at junkyards. He hooks up with local stock car racers, starts to hang out at the races. The life is attractive and exciting, and he makes enough to get by. Finally he sets up housekeeping with a few buddies and moves out. He begins to smoke less. When a team mechanic quits, he is invited to sign on.

The Mystery of Change

Things become mysterious here. Even if I have the opportunity to develop more detail, it is likely I will never fully understand why things begin to take a turn for the better. In my experience it always seems easier to reconstruct why things fall apart versus why they improve. Let's just chalk this up as a specific example of the mystery of learning. That is, to paraphrase the old saying, non-learning has many parents; learning is an orphan.

So I will simply say that Dyllen is beginning to learn from experience. Which came first, more trust or less using, is not really that important. What counts here is changing for the better. Perhaps in the world of stock car racing, smoking pot is not forbidden but not glamorized either. Racing engines are expensive, the races dangerous, and the stakes high, so you have to be alert and focused when working in the pit.

Or let us say that at one of the races he meets a girl who isn't like the usual racetrack groupie. She just likes cars, even likes to work on them, doesn't sleep around, doesn't use, asks him why he does. No one has ever asked him before; they just tell him not to do it. She's interesting, works as a certified nurse assistant, wants to be a nurse, so why is she spending weekends hanging with this bunch? he asks. This really pisses her off. Why can't a woman like cars and be a nurse at the same time? Which intimidates him, yet makes her all the more intriguing, makes him think. Maybe he needs to use less, think more about his future. It really irritates him that she might be right, yet it is hard to stay away from her.

Eventually he stops using pot altogether. Without the marijuana his denial defenses begin to dissolve and evaporate. It turns out a world without pot is startling. Things are clearer, he can think faster, has more energy and motivation, catches on quicker. People comment on the change. Then the anxiety creeps in, for there is a down side to viewing life without the filter of alcohol or drugs. It is harder to ignore the pain of loss, whether past or anticipated. *What if* thoughts bedevil him. What if she finds someone else? What if he doesn't fit in with the team? He begins to pop panic attacks. The disability of his youth has returned. Yet the panic has significance beyond the apparent for it signals the possibility of recovery.

Dyllen is now beginning to face the possibility that he could lose what is important again. He is doing less pretending, minimizing, denying: he is more open to the pain of life … and its hurts. But without experiencing this pain, he is doomed to a life where he does not learn from experience. He would simply retrace the circle of disability, not stalled out but unlikely to move onward to a life of greater productivity and satisfaction.

Thus his misery and pain are adaptive because, now that he rejects pot, they motivate him to seek relief.

When his lady friend recognizes his panic from her nursing classes, she talks up seeing a psychiatrist, which really bugs him because he knows she's right. Finally, in part to get her off his back, in part to get some relief, he shows up on my doorstep.

Dyllen's Prognosis

Dyllen's prognosis strikes me as promising. He is owning his suffering, for example, not pretending it will go away by itself, a very important first step in recovering from any kind of disability.[ii] He does not come across as much of a blamer, either of himself or others. Moreover, he is focusing on what can be changed, although this will pose a problem because changing may mean accepting help—an old issue for him, as we have seen. In his experience "help" means surrendering independence. Indeed, he is more than a bit ashamed that he can't manage his anxieties and worries better, that he simply can't "tough it out." But he's through pretending; he knows that if spontaneous improvement were likely, it would be happening by now.

The ability to accept help is particularly a stumbling block for someone afflicted with social anxiety, an issue with Dyllen

---

ii. Recovery from disability of any sort is quite variable because it is a function of learning, the speed of which varies from person to person. Yet recovery is simultaneously invariable because it always involves the same three dynamics:
- Clarify the disability.
- Assign no blame for the disability.
- Focus on what can be changed.

The processes are not sequential. They loop back on each other. But recovery is not retracing a circle, but akin to walking a spiral where the ground is both unfamiliar yet familiar because you now have a perspective from which to view the past and anticipate the future with some equanimity. I will discuss these three management principles at greater length in chapters 11 through 13.

alongside his panic. The very act of seeking help for anxiety stirs up anxiety, a Catch-22 conundrum. Accepting support from his lady, friends, and family will hopefully be less problematic. Fortunately, his anxiety does not seem to have affected his work performance. His prognosis is somewhat better because side-by-side workplace relationships offer him the opportunity to slowly become accustomed to more threatening face-to-face personal situations.

The odds of a medication being helpful to Dyllen are about one in two. Taking a medication symbolizes not being in control, an issue for many individuals that may prove to be the case with Dyllen. Some adolescents refuse medications, not only because they either did not help or caused side effects in the past, but precisely because they *did* help. They feel medication renders them too vulnerable, too likely to cooperate, without their accustomed angry edge. Others feel there must really be something wrong if they need a medication to feel comfortable about life. Still others feel trapped by having to rely on prescription medications when you can buy relief on the street without a script.

Moreover, Dyllen's medication options are limited to those prescription drugs without an addictive potential. Theoretically a behavior modification technique known as *exposure/response prevention (E/RP)*[iii] might be very helpful. But practically, it is not feasible because it requires counseling to explain and supervise the process, which implies a certain degree of comfort in a one-on-one relationship—in other words, the very quality the treatment hopes to provide. Catch-22 again.

On the plus side, while he might slip now and then and use, I doubt he will ever return to heavy using. He knows—step one clarification at work here—he must now find a different way to manage his discomforts. It is unlikely he will attend an AA activity organized according to its traditional precepts:

---

iii Cf. chapter 13 for a discussion.

group meetings, personal disclosure, sponsorship, and so on. Again, such activities require from the get-go the possession of a certain degree of social finesse, sadly deficient here. Perhaps an alternative approach to addiction management, such as relapse management, might be more tolerable if his slips become a problem.[5]

Dyllen Returns

After a couple of years or so, much to my surprise Dyllen returns to see me. I'm really curious about how things have gone, so I start with one of my usual gambits: asking him to tell me about his "adventures." Which he politely does. He is different: more comfortable, less vague, more spontaneous, more insightful. In fact he shows up today without his girlfriend in tow.

It turns out he tried the clonidine I prescribed for a while; maybe it was helpful. In any event, he's less freaked out these days. And to his surprise, his girlfriend has stuck by him despite his "weirdness." It doesn't seem to bother her as much as it does him. In fact it doesn't seem to bug *him* as much as before; maybe knowing she's around has helped. He's starting to think of marriage, even though at times she can be a nag, just like his mother. The two of them really get along. But his older brother is cautious, tells him that women are a trap.

Then Dyllen gets to the point of this return visit. Things are going quite well at the dirt track, the crew say he's the best mechanic they've ever worked with. But they also say he should get his GED in order to go to the community college and learn computer language. He explains if you're going to race with modern engines you have to know how to tweak engine management systems. It's not that computers are a mystery; they're like engines. He has built his own computer and likes to troubleshoot his friends' systems—it's sort of a hobby. He knows hardware, has even explored writing code. It actually is not too mysterious because it is so logical, you just need a lot of practice and patience.

The classroom, that's the problem. He's checked out the GED program. Most of it is online, no sweat, he's used to it. However, he can't take the test online. He has to show up in person, sit in a room under supervision. That stirs up bad vibes. Moreover, while most of the software courses can be taken online, there is still some required one-to-one and classroom stuff. What to do? What if he tried school and it didn't work out? Would his crew give up on him? Or, worse, what would they expect if he did learn how to write code? Who would be his backup?

Cautiously, not wanting to provoke success anxieties, I acknowledge the request for help by suggesting that Dyllen explore online the idea of performance anxiety, also an anxiety management with E/RP. Using this approach, I explain, he can design his own program to "toughen his hide" without having to see a counselor on a regular basis. And his girlfriend can work with him. He's intrigued, says he will look it up.

I sense he will go ahead and find a way to overcome his performance issues, or if not, at least learn to live with them enough to proceed with his education. And I hope I won't have to wait too many years to find out how things are going.

[CASE STUDY]
Holden Caulfield: To Care Is Dangerous

Like Dyllen, Holden Caulfield is also a creation, but one assembled in imagination rather than constructed from the kaleidoscope of clinical experience. He emerges from the pages of J. D. Salinger's *The Catcher in the Rye*, which was first viewed as a vehicle for a controversial examination of postwar American society. Reviewers did not hesitate to compare it to *The Adventures of Huckleberry Finn* because both works embody similar conventions (the journey, a coming of age) while incorporating social commentary in the guise of a youth adrift in an adult world. The book was the subject of intense literary comment—praised, mocked, parodied—which reflected the intensely conservative culture of that era, when the bestseller lists were dominated by historical romances or dramatizations of World War II combat. The mining of postwar American suburban culture in New Yorker short stories by the likes of John Cheever and John Updike was yet to come.

It is now hailed as one of the hundred best twentieth-century American novels, and has the unusual distinction of being simultaneously the most recommended and most banned book in American high schools. For decades, no high school backpack was complete without a well-thumbed copy, the ultimate catechism of the true-believing rebel. Sixty-five years after publication it remains in print, selling a quarter million copies a year.

Our interest here is not to examine its literary or moral qualities but to recapture Salinger's keen insights into the adolescent spirit as presented in the person of his protagonist, the impulsive, bumbling, sensitive, horny, opinionated, compassionate, grieving Holden Caulfield. Decades of adolescent readers have come to adopt Holden as the embodiment of lost innocence, of rebellion against corrupt adult authority. But this does him and Salinger a disservice. Rather, Holden's adventures represent his struggle to cope with separation and loss as well as his ambivalence about reaching out for adult support, which is the signature conflict of today's troubled adolescent. Salinger was eerily prophetic, to my way of thinking. And therefore what we want to take away from the book is not a notion of the adolescent as rebellious but the adolescent as ambivalent, struggling to risk attachment in a world revealed to be painfully unpredictable.

The Backstory

Amid the drama of Holden's tumultuous departure from Pencey Prep—the third one he's flunked out of—Salinger only gradually introduces us to the grievous loss Holden sustained three years previously when his beloved eleven-year-old brother, Allie, died from leukemia. As the book unfolds it becomes clear that Allie, while only infrequently mentioned by the wounded Holden, remains his ideal of a loving and secure relationship, the standard by which all others are measured and found wanting, with the exception of his older brother, D. B., his younger sister, Phoebe, and his sweetheart, Jane.

And Allie certainly sounds like he was a perfect younger brother, a nifty kid: smart, worshipful of Holden, red-haired, funny, tolerant, a comfort as a sib. Almost too perfect, for one wonders if, in fact, Holden has idealized the boy. Like all the Caulfield offspring, Allie enjoyed literature. One of Holden's most poignant memories is of Allie writing poems in green ink on his baseball mitt so he would have something to read in the outfield while waiting for a batter to come to the plate. Holden assures us we would have really liked Allie—"really"—and the boy seems so charming you feel a bit of a loss yourself not to have known him. I imagine him dreaming the game away in the outfield, peering into his mitt until his teammates yell at him to pay attention. Holden later tells us he talks to Allie "sort of out loud" when he feels "depressed." He reminisces about their attendance at the Radio City Music Hall Christmas show when both were fascinated by the kettle drummer.

The night Allie died, Holden slept in the garage and broke windows. Clearly more than windows were broken that night, and not all has been repaired even three years later. Holden is being kicked out of Pencey not because he isn't smart but because he is blocked, which most likely accounts for his three prior prep school debacles. When his conceited roommate, Stradlater, asks him to ghostwrite a composition due in two days, he admonishes Holden not to look *"too* good ... That sunuvabitch Hartzell thinks you're a hot-shot in English, and he knows you're my roommate." Holden proceeds to knock off the composition in an hour, which is how we learn of Allie's tragic death: it's not dangerous to perform on behalf of the other, only on behalf of oneself. Here the idealized image of the lost relationship both comforts and paralyzes the survivor. At one point, feverish and exhausted from an incipient pneumonia, Holden calls upon Allie to sustain him as he staggers to a rendezvous with Phoebe. Holden remains gripped by what has been lost.

The same is true of his parents, but their sensibilities and personalities are vaguely drawn in contrast to Holden's vivid portrayal of his sibs (loving), peers (unflattering), and adults (insincere). To be sure, he does mention his parents in his opening paragraph: they are "nice" but "touchy" when it comes to "anything pretty personal about them." But they hover at the margins of his awareness. We learn that his father is a corporation lawyer—well off enough to invest in Broadway shows—a profession of dubious ethics in Holden's view. The father seems to be coping with Allie's death by staying active; for example, too busy to attend a play in which Phoebe is the lead. He considers Holden immature for his age. Phoebe worries their father will "kill" Holden when he discovers that Holden has again been kicked out of school.

Of his mother there is even less. Holden reports that his mother is "very nervous" and hasn't felt well since Allie's death, later states that she "still isn't over my brother Allie yet." In contrast to his father, who has maintained momentum, her life is clearly in suspension.

Each in his or her own way has withdrawn from Holden, who understands their "touchiness" because of his own misery.

So he evades them, sneaking in and out of their apartment on a midnight visit to see Phoebe.

Holden's Character

Intolerance of Insincerity

Holden is considered by some the prototype of teenage rebelliousness. True, he is forever detecting "phoniness" in his world. Few adults escape his critical eye. Culprits include professors, headmasters, alumni, heroines, performers, patrons of swank bars, perhaps his father. And as might be expected, peers—especially Stradlater, who is in Holden's fevered imagination a serious rival for the affections of Holden's girl-next-door sweetheart, Jane. Other peers who prompt his scorn include a former girlfriend, the pretty but shallow Sally, "the queen of the phonies"; Sally's Ivy League acquaintance, George; indeed, all prep school students.

However, Holden does not play the rebel, does not debate or argue or confront or otherwise engage any of these figures: the hallmark of the rebel.

Rather, he withdraws. At one point Phoebe asserts that his problem is that he doesn't like anything, and Holden is hard pressed to refute her. His critical spirit is not one of antagonism toward others but protective of himself. True, he does get into a fistfight with Stradlater, but only to defend Jane's honor. His fantasy is to go on the bum, find a job at a filling station, and pretend to be a deaf-mute: "and then I would be through with having conversation for the rest of my life." Later he would build a cabin in the woods, marry a beautiful deaf-mute, and hide their children. The idea of someone mourning him after death is repellent. He hopes someone "has sense enough to just dump me in the river or something ... Who wants flowers when you are dead?"

Yet Holden himself is not above employing insincerity and

pretentiousness, his unwitting defense against closeness. As he puts it, "I'm the most terrific liar you ever saw in your life." On the train to New York, he is recognized as a Pencey student by a "very good-looking" woman whose son, Ernest Morrow, is also a Pencey student. Does Holden know her son? Indeed he does know the boy, "the biggest bastard that ever went to Pencey." Rather than reveal the truth, Holden starts "shooting the old crap around a bit" in the process making the jerky son into a shy and sensitive soul, so noble he sacrificed a chance to be elected class president. He finishes this gambit with a flourish by inviting her to have a drink with him. She declines graciously and retreats to a magazine, perhaps sensing that the figure Holden describes cannot possibly be her son. Having boxed her out with words, Holden is safe.

Protectiveness

Holden's dream, and the theme of the novel, is his notion of protecting children from harm. As he explains to Phoebe, he would be stationed at the edge of a cliff by a field of rye in which thousands of kids play unsupervised, with "nobody big" to catch them if they run too close to the edge and fall over: "If they are running and they don't look where they are going I have to come out from somewhere and catch them … I'd be the catcher in the rye." It turns out, however, that Holden is protective of everyone, which is another function of his insincerity. His hurt is so profound he dreads anyone feeling the pain of separation and loss.

For example, Salinger has Holden being called to the study of his history teacher, the ailing and decrepit "Old Spencer," who asks to see him for a final good-bye before his eviction from Pencey. Spencer is a total phony in Holden's judgment, a façade of concern and sympathy masking a nasty and sarcastic personality. Holden had penned a footnote to his penultimate but totally inadequate examination, advising Spencer he would bear no resentment for the inevitable flunk "as I am flunking everything else except English anyway." The old hypocrite, having ostensibly invited Holden to come by for a friendly send-off, proceeds to humiliate Holden by reading word for word his wretched performance, lectures him while simultaneously asking his forgiveness for flunking him. What would Holden have done in his place? Holden sees that Spencer feels "really lousy" about the flunk and finds his hate of the ailing and feeble professor being replaced by sorrow and pity.

It develops that Holden is inclined toward feeling sad or sorry for most everyone: the uncouth Ackley, who rooms next to him at Pencey, naïve tourists, ugly girls, a girl nobody likes, a prostitute, two impoverished nuns, even Shakespeare's Mercutio. And of course, the ducks.

Holden's concern about the ducks in the Central Park lagoon is a recurring theme, obviously a symbol of the kids at unsupervised play in the field of rye. Who takes care of the ducks in the winter after the lagoon is frozen? Does someone come by and take them away? He questions taxi drivers. Are they taken care of, or do they take care of themselves and fly away south? Eventually he checks out the lagoon for himself: no ducks anywhere.

Finally Holden has a chance to exercise his protective instincts when he persuades Phoebe, who is determined to run away with him out west, to stay home. At first she angrily rejects him, refuses his offer to accompany her back to school, and runs through traffic across the street, where she stops and eyes him. Figuring she will follow him, Holden enters Central Park, where they have spent many afternoons playing. She catches up with him, and after he changes his mind and promises her he won't leave town, she relents somewhat. On their way home they pass the carousel, Phoebe's favorite, still open despite the season. He persuades her to take a ride, she agrees, and suddenly she's no longer mad at him. She kisses him, rides again.

As she rides he gets soaked in an unseasonable winter rain, but he doesn't care because she is so happy going round and round. "I was damn near bawling, I felt so damn happy." Having accepted her gift of the redemptive power of unconditional regard, he has begun to heal and with it, realizes a fundamental truth about childhood: "The thing with kids is, if they want to grab the gold ring, you have to let them do it, and not say anything. If they fall off they fall off, but it's bad if you say anything to them." He has learned that to be alive is to accept uncertainty and not be trapped by protective feelings toward others. And he is no longer threatened by feelings of joy and happiness.

And it seems he has learned another lesson. He reports he's sorry he's talked so much because he now realizes he misses everyone he's talked about, "Even old Stradlater and Ackley, for instance … It's funny. Don't ever tell anybody anything. If you do, you start missing everybody."[iv] Holden senses that his preoccupation with insincerity is a way of protecting himself, that to confide is risky because it establishes intimacy and vulnerability. Be careful, he tells us.

The Significance of Holden's Behavior

Death Paralyzes

After three years, the tragic loss of his younger brother still haunts and cripples Holden's spirit. One wonders, Whence Salinger's uncanny insights? Part of the book's artistry is the subtle manner in which Salinger introduces us to Holder's grief

---

iv. It seems Salinger followed Holden's advice. In the years after publication he became reclusive, retreating to a remote New Hampshire town, never giving an interview, publishing little. One wonders if he later felt he had revealed too much of himself as he constructed Holden's identity; hence his protectiveness.

and suffering, while precisely capturing the adolescent struggle to cope with loss. Death deflates, stuns, numbs. Kids (and adults) wander into my office distracted and diffident, not enraged; they are reluctant or even unable to reveal the shock precipitated by death of sibs or peers or parents or beloved grandparents. School performance declines and may even evaporate.

Holden is aware of his loss—this is not true of all. With some, a tangible external loss has evolved into an intangible inner loss; that is, they feel they have lost control of their thoughts or feelings or bodies. They have lost security. Only at home, sometimes only in their bedroom, do they feel safe. Their loss, whatever its content, has taken on symbolic qualities. Usually most of the familiar necessities remain—home, family, circle of friends, shelter, food, clothing. All needs appear satisfied. Yet things are different, irrevocably changed. Their tomorrows now appear less inviting.

These youngsters show up in my office with very vague explanations of why they are not attending school: they just don't want to, it is boring, they feel "depressed," and so on. Sometimes they can't sleep; other times they sleep all the time. Typically they look more anxious than "depressed."

Some youngsters, less gripped by denial, have enough insight to be able to describe the turmoil of their inner world. They talk about unwanted emotions: jealousy, anger, even love. Or distressing repetitive thoughts (obsessions) or behaviors (compulsions). They say their body feels funny or sick: their heart pounds, they can't stop sweating, they are dizzy, they feel walled off from everything, that is, dissociated. Typically, they worry that if people knew how they felt or thought, they would be judged weak or immature or helpless. The truth about their inner world would be catastrophic if known to others. *People will withdraw from you and abandon you. Or they will tease you and pick on you. Or, worse yet, they will overwhelm you with help and you will be smothered.*

Even these relatively insightful youngsters may have

difficulty relating their feeling state to a prior loss. They shrink from the obvious connection. It just feels safer to stay home, go to school online. Relationships are less dangerous at a distance. Otherwise they feel as if their identity might dissolve.

Authority Inspires Distrust

Authority has nothing more to offer; authority is bankrupt. So Holden runs away and begins his quest, his search ... for what, he's not sure. Does anyone care? Is there anyone whom it's safe to care about?

Generally youngsters on the run don't go far. Typically the running is a sign of a different kind of Attachment Disorder, which I will discuss later: Attachment Acting-out. Such kids have not given up on authority, so they end up running ... to another relationship. They are taken in by parents of peers or seek refuge with relatives or, if their parents have split, end up at the other's place. In chapter 10 I will discuss Maddie, who, after her father refused to be intimidated by her threat to run away, went on the run for all of twenty minutes before returning with the police to try another gambit: parental abuse (which neither he nor the police bought into). Here, running is an example of Winnicott's notion of acting-out as a claim on the environment to draw attention to an unmet need.

However, a run such as Holden's is a different matter. It signifies hopelessness about relationships, a giving up on the past. Youngsters simply take off, disappear, go missing for days, sometimes weeks, sometimes forever. This is a dangerous frame of mind, rendering them very vulnerable to exploitation as they search for something to provide meaning to a life without purpose.

Thanks to Salinger, Holden's quest is not completely aimless for he gives Holden a goal: his concern for the ducks. But his quest doesn't protect him from his naïveté. He is punched out by Maurice the pimp, later manages to escape a pass from a former teacher, Mr. Antolini. And not every runner is fortunate enough to be rescued by the loving concern of a Phoebe. Some are never saved.

To Care Is Dangerous

Holden is burdened by excessive sensitivity, by a crushing concern for the feelings of others. To care is dangerous because you can get swallowed up—trapped—by the emotions that encumber any human relationship but also serve to draw us into relationships. Only the ducks are safe to care about. And Phoebe. So his running is not toward something but away from something: relationships. He is quite extreme in this respect. When kids go on the run, they usually seek an exchange of relationships, hoping for one that provides more need fulfillment with less entanglement. In this respect running is a healthy adaptive response to unmet needs, but it is a risky "solution," one with potentially perilous consequences.

[CASE STUDY]
Helen: Loss of Trust

In contrast to Dyllen and Holden Caulfield, this case report is quite authentic, neither a composite nor a literary creation.

Helen is a twenty-year-old bioengineerig student I first saw while she was on a medical leave of absence from school because of "the side effects of medication changes."

Three weeks previously, Helen had been started on Zoloft (sertraline), 50 mg per day, helpful with loneliness, "depression," sadness, and anxiety. She was also on Lexapro (escitalopram), 5 mg per day, recently tapered from 30 mg per day with relief of side effects such as headache, light sensitivity, and confusion. At first the Lexapro was helpful—"it gave me an energy boost"—but then the side effects intervened. She had continuing issues with dizziness, nausea, and poor appetite, as well as reduced ability to concentrate and focus. Things were better now that she was back home while avoiding stress. However, she was afraid to exercise because of an exertional headache associated with dizziness.

By way of past history, Helen reported that twenty-one months previously, following graduation from high school, she had started the Lexapro, 10 mg per day, with benefit for a year, but eventually began to experience a return of prior symptoms such as declining productivity, increasing isolation, and oversleeping—all issues throughout high school. A progressive increase in dosage to 30 mg per day was temporarily helpful, yet her long-standing issues returned. There was no history of prior treatment with psychotropic agents. However, Helen had received grief counseling off and on since age eight, following the sudden death of her mother from an undiagnosed sepsis. Her family's support was provisional, only present when she was "happy" and attending school, making her feel like they "wanted me to be a different person."

At direct examination Helen presented as a cooperative, compliant, intelligent, articulate, well-groomed, tense, tight young woman who looked her stated age and who looked tearful as she discussed her difficulties in maintaining relationships. She was insightful regarding boundary issues: "I've learned to keep my distance … scared of abandonment."

My impression was she demonstrated an Adjustment Reaction. I recommended she continue her current medications and resume grief therapy. Later I prescribed low doses of Ativan (lorazepam), then propranolol for relief of anxiety symptoms such as chest tightness and tachycardia, but without sustained benefit. At weekly visits Helen reported other dysphoric feelings and thoughts: "I desire to be alone all the time [tearful] … I'm afraid I'll remain in a limbo of being okay as long as I'm alone versus slipping back into depression when I'm with other people." Later she reported learning of the death of an acquaintance in a motor vehicle accident: "It hit me hard ... I'm reaching out to his best friend, I know what he's been through." Nonetheless, after six weeks she felt improved enough to return to school.

At the end of the summer session, Helen reported that her two classes had gone well. She had switched psychiatrists and was now taking 100 mg of the Zoloft plus Klonopin (clonazepam) for anxiety, which was initially helpful with anxiety but less so recently. She was also seeing a therapist every week and had joined a Depression support group. Nonetheless, during the summer she had felt "mini-detached ... I take the blame for everything ... my relationships."

Helen returned during Christmas break. Things had not gone well. She had to take incompletes in three out of her four classes: "I couldn't get out of bed, think straight." Also, "I'm scared life is not going to get better ... I'm either numb or depressed ... I don't feel supported or wanted anywhere, feel alone." She had no appetite, had lost ten pounds, felt abandoned by her best friend during a visit to her. I suggested, in order to begin clarification of her emotional fog, that she learn to think of herself as "fearful" rather than "depressed."[v]

Three weeks later she returned to announce that she had applied for medical leave, packed up her belongings, and sublet her apartment. Moreover she had enrolled in an adult day treatment program and planned to obtain consultation with a very well-qualified neuropsychologist to learn anxiety management. Helen's psychotropic regimen now consisted of Luvox (fluvoxamine), 200 mg; Zoloft, 100 mg; Klonopin, 1 mg four times a day; and Adderall (detroamphetamine salts), 20 mg. Yet she continued to experience sadness, reduced appetite, low energy, low motivation, and constant fatigue—"depression" as she put it. On the other hand, she had found a second job as

---

v. See chapter 11 for a further discussion of this first principle of therapy, *clarification*.

a receptionist at a law firm, in addition to her part-time work as a lifeguard.

I wondered about the changes. "I'm angry ... I expected more." I suggested, not for the first time, that perhaps she was still dealing with her mother's death of many years before, a trauma residual. She finally did admit her mother's death remained an issue. "I don't trust people ... people are selfish, do what's best for them ... I have to bend over backward."

There followed a series of more lengthy and more frequent visits—fifteen altogether—incorporating a combination of medication management and psychotherapy. Typically I would begin by addressing the former with a goal of simplifying and tapering the regimen, which obviously was not particularly beneficial in view of Helen's continuing symptoms, both in my opinion and hers. I suggested she take the initiative in determining the sequence and rate of the tapering, that she "be your own doctor"; this would promote her sense of mastery while reducing my role to that of an advisor and co-observer.[vi] Later in the visit, announcing I was donning my therapy "hat," we segued into a discussion of intervening life events, her emotional responses to them, her decisions, clarification of her thoughts and feeling, and, particularly, owning the pain in her life without blame.[vii] Helen also continued to see the neuropsychologist to learn anxiety management.

Over the ensuing weeks, despite her suffering and sense of paralysis, she demonstrated increasing decisiveness. For example, she decided to drop out of day treatment. "In light of my mother's death, as I think about it, it is all related ... unconditional love ... abandonment ... conflict avoidance ... I don't know how to do it." Later she changed grief counselors. Helen made plans to move out of her parents' place into her own apartment. She began to connect with a coworker, arranged a

---

vi. See chapter 13 for a more detailed discussion of this management technique, focus on what can be changed.

vii. See chapter 12.

coffee date: "trusting [was] strange, to be myself." Via fits and starts she began to catch up on her incompletes.

At a subsequent visit Helen described spontaneously assisting a bus passenger who was having difficulty navigating his wheelchair while juggling his belongings: "I forgot about everything … it made me feel good I did something for someone … the happiest in months." A few weeks later she reported an insight derived from her work with the grief counselor during their first direct discussion of her mother: "It is hard to hear what others say about her … I want her memory to be mine [not what others remember] … whenever I talk about her my memories don't spill out because I don't have many." At her next visit: "at peace … it's in my relationship with her … a load off my shoulders." She then recalled how for years she had been very fussy about having perfect nails as a way of controlling obsessive tendencies, but lately she had ceded responsibility for their care to her beautician. After I noted this was a sign of increasing trust in people, "I didn't think of it that way … a lot of things are coming together … with friendships … people are not a hundred percent self-centered … they do the best they can … I'm at my best when I'm helping someone."

On later visits we discussed Helen's need to develop a different set of career goals because of her excessive feelings of empathy. Still later, she reported that with the help of her neuropsychological training, "I'm learning to stay calm and focused in the midst of chaos," also that she was learning to form her own image of her mother versus others' recollections. Subsequently she managed the thirteenth anniversary of her mother's death in conjunction with her family's celebration of Mother's Day.

The interval between visits began to lengthen as Helen continued to improve while tapering her medications via trial and error, eventually comfortable with a combination of Zoloft and Luvox, 100 mg each per day, helpful with anxiety and stress management. She decided to return to school and suffered anxieties about arranging accommodations from afar, as well as the possibility that a professor might renege on a commitment to allow her to make up an incomplete without penalty. She had a brief return of feeling unloved, wondering if she had ever been loved, even by her mother. But by the end of the summer she was back in school.

Six months later by phone she stated things were going well, she was getting along with her roommates, was considering switching to a doctorate in neuroscience: "I feel I can help more people that way." Later, at a graduation party held by her family, she summarized her recovery: "I learned to reach out to people."

The Significance of Helen's Behavior

Helen's experience is among the many cases of Attachment Disability I encountered during my fifty years as a psychiatrist. I have placed her case foremost among authentic profiles not only because of its authenticity—versus Dyllen's (a composite creation) or Holden's (literary)—but also because it clearly illustrates a number of themes that are vital to the understanding of attachment issues. I believe introducing these concepts now will enrich the reader's understanding of the two dozen or more cases I will subsequently present and discuss.

The Persistence of Attachment Disability

As discussed above, attachment issues are considered to be solely a phenomenon of early childhood. Moreover, according to *DSM-5* it is uncertain if it is evident in older children. In other words, the idea seems to be that youngsters will "get over" attachment problems. This is a serious, even tragic misconception that dooms such children to misdiagnosis and mistreatment, not to mention a lifetime of suffering and underperformance.

Obviously Helen did not "get over" the death of her mother

at age eight. Although she never described in detail her subsequent adjustment, by high school she had become isolated, withdrawn, and less productive. Her family was of little solace because of their expectations—a second loss, in other words. Her previous underperformance collapsed into disability so severe she had to take medical leave. In short, not only did Helen not "outgrow" the attachment issues precipitated by the death of her mother, but they festered throughout childhood and adolescence only to explode once she left for college.

The Dynamism of Self-Management

In the introduction I recommended that when dealing with attachment-disabled individuals, the traditional medical concept of diagnosis/treatment be replaced by the notion of understanding/management. The idea here is to maintain awareness of two basic dynamisms that energize their behavior—distrust and vulnerability. In addition, incorporating this approach brings into play a counterdynamism: the expectation that the disabled can learn to self-manage.[viii]

The traditional medical approach is hierarchical: active doctor/submissive patient. This works well when the pain is one of disease. In that case typically the history is clear cut—findings tangible at examination, and laboratory studies confirmatory. The doctors are truly the experts and can go by the book because their particular findings conform to what is in the book: it pays to do what you are told, so submit.

However, the traditional approach does not work well when the pain is one of disability, whether physical or emotional. Here it is more likely the history is vague, findings questionable, and lab studies at best suggestive. And the "book" comes cloaked with generalities. Moreover, other issues become relevant such as aging, social support, financial resources, dietary and exercise

---

viii. See chapter 7 also for a discussion of this dynamism in the management of individuals disabled by chronic pain.

habits, value systems, belief systems, and—most pertinent here—loss history. Even highly motivated and otherwise experienced doctors begin to flounder in the face of persisting disability because when their suggestions are either ignored or prove fruitless, it undermines their role.[ix] They need another hat, so to speak, one that does not read "expert": another persona, in other words. They need to assume the guise of a teacher, and to view the individuals consulting them less as patients and more as students.

A teacher/student interaction is less hierarchical. True, the teacher is also presumed to be an expert and is responsible for providing guidance. Yet the student also has responsibilities, as we all know from our experiences as students. Students must take the initiative to attend and pay attention to lectures, study assigned materials, prepare to recite in class, appear for testing, and so on. Fortunately, health care is moving in this direction as providers and insurers, public and private, are becoming increasingly aware of the disabilities presented by an aging population.[x] The growing mass of health care information disseminated via print and electronic media actually represents a much needed move toward self-management. In other words, while this approach might at first seem counterintuitive, it is actually part of a broader initiative to promote a healthier population better prepared to cope with disability.

As I listened to Helen, what I heard was that years of grief counseling and more than a year and a half of medication management had been of only temporary benefit, and not much at that. In fact, things were worse. Obviously it was time to adopt a different strategy.

While I did not define until later that a change was needed—

---

ix. See my further discussion of this point specifically with reference to the management of chronic pain in chapter 7.

x. A notable example of this trend is the idea of integrated care; that is, combining behavioral health with primary care. See my discussion in chapter 14.

I think Helen had already come to the same conclusion—and while I did not brandish a baseball cap identifying me as "coach," this was the role I decided to adopt after hearing her story. What she needed was not *treatment*, of which there had been plenty, but *management:* specifically, learning how to manage her disability herself by determining what helped and what did not. In short, she had to learn to be less accepting of what was handed down, in favor of a more open and skeptical attitude. Interestingly, months later, this produced an unexpected but critical dividend in the form of an epiphany when she realized she was ignoring her own memories of her mother in favor of what others recalled: "I want her memories to be mine."

As her history indicates, Helen responded well to an *understanding/management* strategy. She took the initiative, in essence designing her own therapy: for example, when to take or terminate medical leave. She sampled day treatment and decided it was not for her. She opted to obtain neuropsychological consultation, determining it might be helpful in learning anxiety management, which proved to be an accurate judgment. Later she decided to switch grief counselors, which provided an immediate payoff in helping her "own" her own thoughts and feelings. And she took charge of her psychotropic regimen, determining the rate and sequence of her tapering schedule, with the outcome a much more favorable benefit/side effect ratio. Notably, this process was well entrenched by the time I formally announced, some six months after her initial visit, that my plan was to teach her how to "be your own doctor."

Helen's Presumptive "Depression"

Despite the presence of what seemed like a clear-cut "depression," her treatment with Antidepressants was at first either not particularly helpful or was accompanied by troublesome side effects. Only after trials of five different psychotropics during a three-year interval via trial and error did she discover a beneficial regimen, not unusual in my experience. (Many a "depression" does not respond to Antidepressants.) Nor was it unusual that the beneficial combination helped her not by relieving "depression" but by reducing anxiety and stress. The former, actually a cognitive issue, had responded to the guidance of her new grief counselor, who had helped her own her thoughts and feelings about her mother and not be afraid of them, especially her loving memories. That is, the therapy allowed her to relieve the self-blame that had crippled her for years because she was unable to buy into the shared memories of her family and her mother's friends. She was unable to participate in the consensus, unable to be a true believer. For years she was alienated. When this began to dissolve, her need for boundaries evaporated and she began to reach out. Of course, given her now enhanced clarity of thought and emotion, she fully realized the risk in so doing: hence her persisting anxiety, which the Antidepressants helped.

In chapter 9 and in volume 2 of this series I will discuss these concepts at greater length. Here I would just like to introduce the notion that Antidepressants are beneficial to the extent that they help manage the stress of life and therefore should be more properly be viewed as "antistressants."

Another idea I would I would like to review here, briefly discussed in the introduction and in greater detail in chapter 9, is that the term "depression" be abandoned because it is so ambiguous, is without any specific content, and leads many a treatment plan astray. In particular, it is vital that a patient's self-designation as "depressed" not be uncritically accepted as valid without a careful scrutiny of its referents.[xi] If they do not take care to parse such a global statement, to identify in detail the specific behaviors and experiences it encompasses, therapists and physicians are at risk of overlooking an understanding

---

xi. See chapter 8 for my ten-year mismanagement of Rebecca because of my failure to avoid this trap.

essential to patients' effective management. Specifically, this requires an awareness of their history of abandonment and loss, as well as a constant awareness of such patients' damaged ability to trust and vulnerability to feeling rejected.

In my experience the majority of such patients are to some extent paralyzed by unrecognized anxiety and stress, while blaming themselves for their emotional disability; that is, they view themselves as "depressed." They minimize or otherwise deny the significance of lost relationships or traumatic experiences that generate their anxieties, tending to focus more on the consequent paralysis—for example, home boundedness, withdrawal from relationships, low motivation, lack of satisfaction in life, and so on. They come to believe such issues are their "fault." In other words, their behavioral paralysis is compounded by a cognitive paralysis, so to speak, a failure of adaptive learning, which is much more crippling and isolative. While they may need medication, a more vital need is their learning the three principles of effective management: *clarification, acceptance,* and *focus*.[xii]

Helen's Future

Well, as with all of us, Helen's future is not written. I suspect, however, it will include a passionate devotion to providing help to sufferers. Therein lies a risk, for it is essential she develop healthy boundaries. If she is highly motivated to love her neighbor, it is critical she remain motivated to love herself, as the Second Greatest Commandment tells us.

---

xii. Again, discussed at length in chapters 11 through 13.

3

Attachment Entanglement: Four Cases

Some youngsters who are stuck in relationship sensitivity, and thus are unable to construct boundaries, become too immobilized to escape, instead sinking into a state of emotional paralysis: Attachment Entanglement.

[CASE STUDY]
Amy: The Threat of "Help"

Unlike Holden's and Dyllen's histories in chapter 2, Amy's history is authentic, and I will present it blow-by-blow to illustrate how Attachment Disability and mistrust have the potential to invade even presumably supportive contacts. To be sure, Dyllen makes oblique reference to this problem: he found the friendliness of his school counselor threatening. And this is also true of Holden, given his avoidance behavior. But some youngsters and young adults are quite forthright in this regard: if they have trust issues, you will hear about it, no detecting required.

Amy was a college student referred from an emergency room where she had been seen three days earlier because of suicidal talk. Along with the referral for a psychiatric evaluation came a recommendation that she start attending day treatment. She had been taking an Antidepressant in therapeutic doses for the last four months without either side effects or benefits. I saw her with her mother.

> Dr. C: What brings you here today?
> Amy: "They made me go ... I don't know ..."
> Dr. C: Silent, waits for her to proceed.
> Amy: Sits defensively, with her legs curled up against her. Grooming is good, she's alert, there is no evidence of psychomotor retardation. Yet she remains silent, then engages a bit with a smile, then withdraws.
> Dr. C, deciding to provide some structure: "Any other treatment?"
> Amy, a bit more forthcoming: Yes, she has a therapist whom she's been seeing three times a week for the last three weeks: "I don't why." Before that, once a week. Good chemistry between them.
> Dr. C: Prompts a bit to elicit more information.
> Amy: Gets angry, looks tearful, gives up easily.
> Dr. C, wondering: Is she afraid of responsibility, of growing up?
> Amy, disgusted: "My medicine does not work." She becomes openly tearful.
> Mother intervenes: Agrees there has not been much improvement since starting the medication. Her daughter is not smiling, not happy, is "depressed ... just getting through the day ..."
> Amy: Remains huddled, withdrawn, unhappy.
> Mother again intervenes by providing background information. She attends a small college visited by a double tragedy the year before. First a student suicided via an overdose; two months later another died from bone cancer. "Since then the whole school

is shook up ... everybody ended the year numb, came back this year angry." Moreover, she recently broke up with her boyfriend of two years, and a small clique of students is badmouthing her. Formerly an excellent student and athlete, she's now angry, rebellious, "depressed," and anxious.

Dr. C: *Wondering, what is going on here?*

Amy: *Remains huddled, unengaged, close to tears.*

Dr. C: *Begins to realize he has misinterpreted her resistiveness and withdrawal, that they are not signs of immaturity, given her previous record of performance. And that is why the interview is going nowhere—not making any headway. Is entanglement the issue? Figures a different approach is needed. Decides to create some distance by going into lecture mode.*

Dr. C, *utilizing some stagecraft,[i] removes glasses, dramatically rubs his eyes:* "I'm tired ... besides we are not getting anywhere ... so let's try a different approach."

Dr. C: *Dons his lecture persona and discourses at length about "antistressants": how people avoid intimacy by building barriers through behavior rather than words, how vulnerability and fears of trusting might signal entanglement issues, and so forth.*

Amy: *much more engaged, smiling, sits forward, listening attentively.*

Dr. C: "Do you think the cliquish girls are jealous of you?"

Amy: *Ignores him.*

Dr. C: *Discusses her vulnerability to sudden self-destructive impulses. Her behavior says she's isolated, guilty, beginning to feel hopeless.*

Amy: *Nods.*

Dr. C: "And that's why they recommended you start

---

i. See chapter 10 for a discussion of this technique.

a day treatment program, to provide a support system until things are better. It's important that you attend."

Amy: Nods again.

Dr. C: Recommends adding a second "antistressant" since the first one doesn't seem to be helpful.

Amy: Agrees.

Dr. C: Makes a recommendation, writes a script. Then, "You know, your behavior is really different now than it was when you first sat down, right?"

Amy: Agrees.

Dr. C: "Why is that?"

Amy: Smiles, shrugs. She doesn't know.

Dr. C: "Let me guess. You were afraid to let me get too close—then you would have someone else to worry about. You already feel a lot of responsibility for everyone."

Amy: "Yes." *Leaves with mother, script in hand, with instructions to return in two weeks to see if* "you have experienced any stress relief or not."

The Significance of Amy's Behavior

Amy's behavior at examination is a fine illustration of a long-standing psychiatric dictum: "You watch what patients say and listen to what they do."[ii] Her case also demonstrates the value of including sponsors[iii] in the evaluation process, both to flesh out the interviewee's history and to have the opportunity to observe the sponsor/interviewee interaction. As Amy's situation unfolded, it began to shout entanglement and a need for a less

---

ii. See also the case of Renée, chapter 7, for a more extended discussion of this maxim.

iii. Another interview technique, also discussed in chapter 7.

personal relationship, which I created by assuming the guise of a pedant.

Pretending Ignorance

Pretending ignorance is a form of *resistiveness*, which I discuss at greater length in chapter 10. It represents a surrender of responsibility, a silent plea to be treated as a kid, a child in need of protection: *Don't expect too much of me.* This is why, even if the reason for the consultation has been well documented in advance by report or phone call, I always begin the interview with an open-ended, unstructured question of this sort: "What brings you here today?" It gives me an immediate global assessment of the maturity of the individual before me.

Except for the infrequent situation when I am dealing with an obviously angry individual (see Mr. POP in chapter 10), I generally do not directly challenge such a pretense of ignorance. Instead I prod a bit and provide structure in the form of cues that might offer a relatively safe topic for discussion. This approach brought no luck with Amy, however.

Defensive Posture

Youngsters present in a variety of ways. Some are elaborately groomed and coiffed, with an attentive posture and expression. Some are Goth, with black makeup and multiple piercings (not as frequent these days versus two decades ago). Others slouch, or play with a cell phone, or bicker with the adult who accompanies them, or sit rigidly with a defiant expression, or—especially younger ones—roam the office. Amy's posture is unusual; it clearly signifies she requires careful management.

The Mother's Intervention

Typically the adults or sponsors in the room do not intervene, unless things have begun with an argument or confrontation, until I signal for their input. But here, the mother sees that her daughter is foundering and comes to her rescue. She provides critical information that the daughter could not bear to reveal herself. This suggests Attachment Entanglement guilt and provides an understanding of her resistiveness to engagement.

Greater Comfort with an Impersonal Approach

In chapter 10 on management of Attachment Disability I will discuss at greater length what I call "stagecraft": designing the setting and style of the interview to retain and promote the interviewee's attentiveness. That is, there is no one-style-fits-all mode of interview technique. The thrust of this book is that the attachment-disabled child, adolescent, or adult has difficulty learning because they are experiencing "emotional interference."[iv] In other words, fear and distrust erode their attentiveness and ability to learn from experience. Stagecraft is simply the manipulation of the learning venue to retain the learner's attention. Good teachers are performers ... as are good therapists. As a therapist I am always titrating the degree of distance/intimacy required to enhance attentiveness without smothering it. So with Amy, I both announce and signal a change in the interview transaction with a bit of stagecraft designed to create distance by reverting to a format familiar to her student persona: the lecture. The idea is to address the notions of trust

---

iv. I was introduced to the term by Dr. Frederick Sheridan, principal of the Work Opportunities Center (WOC), a Minneapolis Public Schools program for high school dropouts. In his view, emotional interference was a silent factor contributing to what he called the "dropout equation." I will discuss his insights and their influence on the evolution of my psychiatric career in volume 2 of this series.

and entanglement in a very general fashion, without specifically stating that these might be her personal issues. This leaves it up to her to decide whether they fit or not.

Vulnerability to Suicide

Amy's change in posture and smiling attentiveness are signals that these ideas are a fit. So it seems safe to personalize things a bit by addressing what her behavior is saying: she's isolated, guilty, feeling hopeless. In short, her support system is shaky and attending day treatment is important. Her silent agreement means that death thoughts, perhaps even suicidal ruminations, have been on her mind, so there is no need to have her confirm this with a direct inquiry. For the same reason, adding another "antistressant" makes sense to her.

Entanglement Confirmed

This is an excellent example of how an entangled youngster's overprotectiveness can extend to relative strangers. Her concern is that if she tells me what she truly feels—for example, her guilt and feelings of hopelessness—I will be upset, which means she will have more to feel guilty about. She doesn't need another soul to feel responsible for. Hence her initial resistiveness and seeming immaturity.

What is important here, however, is not *why* she is the way she is, but confirmation of the *way* she is: entangled. What she needs in order to learn how to manage the anxieties of relationships is an *understanding* of her predicament, not an *explanation*. Hopefully Amy's individual and day treatment therapies will provide this clarification.

[Case Study]
Charlotte: Shark Attack

Entanglement Disability has the potential to persist into young adulthood and beyond, creating a lifetime risk of employment underperformance and social avoidance.

Charlotte is a thirty-three-year-old single mother of two, returning to my office after an absence of seven months with complaints of anxiety, a change from her former concerns about attention issues. There are three obvious stresses: she is applying for a position as an attendant at a facility for the disabled, she is moving, and her abusive/assaultive partner is due to be released from prison. I recommend propranolol for the anxiety.

She returns two months later. The propranolol has helped. "I don't feel like a fish in a pool of sharks."

Two months later she reports that not only has the propranolol stopped working, but she has also developed panic attacks so intense she had to quit her job at the facility two days after being hired. The feeling of being trapped in a "pool of sharks" had returned. Her mother had instructed her to request an Antidepressant.

We turn to the subject of her mother. "She controls everything I do ... we talk every day ... we have an intense connection." In fact, one reason for the move was to put more distance between the two of them. Now Charlotte hopes to return to school. On a hunch I ask if brief work at the facility had felt like every client wanted a "piece" of her? Yes! Had she ever felt way that before? Yes! As a kid she had to care for her meth-head mother.

We review her chart, which refers to at least five failed

trials of psychoactive medications. At a visit three years earlier, she had reported witnessing the physical abuse of her mother, describing a "love/hate" relationship. In a later visit accompanied by her mother, Charlotte was agitated and frustrated by her, and the two of them interrupted each other. Her therapist noted she was protective of her mother, playing the role of caretaker. But in these visits nowhere does Charlotte refer to her mother as an addict.

I decide to postpone addressing the significance of this missing piece, instead focusing on the matter at hand: her panic. I recommend a trial of clonidine. I also say that next visit I plan "to put on my 'therapist hat' since medication alone is not going to be the answer—we have to fill in some of the blanks." She agrees.

Once again she does not follow up.

The Significance of Charlotte's Behavior

I assume that the revelation about her mother's addiction is authentic. Its belated appearance I attribute to her persisting need to protect "Mom," which binds her to her mother and will continue to do so indefinitely. Charlotte senses her mother would experience her independence as abandonment—a symbolic death—and thus continues to endure her mother's hectoring and fussing in order to provide her mother with a feeling of being needed. She is unable to escape the persisting clutch of her youthful caretaker persona. She is "entangled."

This perspective provides an understanding of her resignation after only two days on the job. Charlotte's entangling experiences have sensitized her to suffering and promoted highly developed empathic feelings. In this respect, her choice of work was not uncommon for someone raised in an abusive environment. But once on the job, she was overwhelmed by the needs of her disabled clients, feeling consumed by them. And it seemed there would be no end to the calls for help. She was trapped. She panicked. She had to get away. More entanglement would be the death of her!

Conclusion

To be sure, the conflicts Amy and Charlotte encounter are extreme examples of the ambiguities of attachment. But the fact is that all of us already encounter to some degree the energizing dilemma that is the very core of attachment: the risk/reward of reaching out. We can't live without relationships, but this means living with the risk of relationship trauma, however manifested. And this means that life is never threat free. However, accepting the pains of attachment is a highly adaptive move because attachment has survival value.

Entangled Parents

In the last decade or so the media has drawn attention to "helicopter parents," referring to a tendency of some parents to hover over and scrutinize their youngsters' activities in excess of reasonable safety precautions. The temptation to closely track youngsters has no doubt been prompted by the advent of the cell phone, magnified by the anxieties of parenting in the midst of an "other-directed" environment, as sociologist Riesman describes it in *The Lonely Crowd*.[v] This overinvolvement may even extend beyond high school: for example, to the choice of a college roommates or intervening with professors in grading issues. Indeed, college orientation now includes both first-year students and their parents, especially mothers, to sooth adult attachment distress.

Sometimes the hovering of parental involvement becomes

---

v. See volume 2 for an extended discussion of this book.

so intense that an entanglement dynamic of reversed polarity is generated—the *parent* remains entangled long after the child is ready for independence. Occasionally the intensity of an entanglement by a needy parent will trap and emotionally suffocate youngsters as graduation from high school looms.

[CASE STUDY]
Georgina: The Danger of Graduation

Georgina was a seventeen-year-old high school senior I saw for "depression … and suicidal thoughts." She had been charged with misdemeanor consumption of alcohol twice since the start of school two months previously. Also, she was using marijuana. Two weeks earlier she had been evaluated at a walk-in clinic, started on an Antidepressant, and referred for both counseling and psychiatric follow-up.

Georgina reports five years of self-injurious thoughts, with one overdose one year previously, without complications and no further attempts. "What's the point?" she asks.

In other words, she is a failure even at suicide.

Her parents had divorced when she was eleven. There is a stepfather who she describes as bossy and strict but not the sort of person who could inspire suicidal feelings, although he can stir up rage. She has a history of performance anxiety in the middle and early grades. Her GPA to date in high school is 3.25, but recent grades are close to failing. On the other hand, there apparently are no discipline issues. Money has been set aside for her to attend college, which her mother strongly advocates. There is an older brother away at college; I gather the two sibs are fairly close. She has a driver's license, works fifteen hours per week, and gets along with her supervisor and coworkers. She has a few friends her parents do not approve of because they also smoke weed.

At examination in the presence of her mother, she presents as a good-looking, mature young woman who is remote, detached, undemonstrative, compliant, composed, impassive, waiting for cues. Occasionally she engages me, then lapses back into her withdrawn mode. She tends to minimize while stoically enduring her mother's hectoring about the dramatic decline in her school performance, her pot smoking, her friends. In the midst of these exhortations, the mother glances at me, hoping to solicit my support. At one point, when describing her strict stepfather, Georgina is a bit more animated. She reports no improvement from the Antidepressant but a good connection with her therapist.

Although she is clearly "depressed," more striking is the hopelessness she radiates. But I judge her as not acutely suicidal because, despite her alienation from her parents, she does have a support network of a sib, peers, coworkers, and teachers.

Deciding it would not be helpful to get sucked into this parent–young adult power struggle, I opt to match Georgina's disengaged style. So in a rather distant and pedantic fashion I discourse on how the paralysis of severe and prolonged stress could appear disguised as "depression." Possibly the Antidepressant she is taking would be helpful because of its stress-reducing potential. In fact, it could be thought of as an "antistressant," but it is too soon to determine its effectiveness, if any. Not wanting to excite her resistiveness, I delay making a recommendation until the very end, at which time I casually suggest she might want to continue the medication. She agrees. On the other hand, I strongly endorse continuing the counseling: "You need to figure out your stresses."

At follow-up, again in the company of her mother, she is the same—impassive, undemonstrative, terse, tight, minimizing, denying problems: "Nothing, really." She had continued the

Antidepressant and the counseling. She reports no change, but her mother describes her as "somewhat better ... more interactive." Again I take charge of the proceedings, this time focusing more on Georgina rather than the two of them, droning on about abandonment issues, hopelessness, and the importance of therapy. I deliberately refrain from endorsing either the mother's report of improvement or her lecture on the perils of marijuana. Then I spring a very pointed question: Does Georgina ever feel her mother doesn't want her to grow up? Georgina's reserve briefly crumbles as she glares at her parent. Yes!! Moreover, Mom's lectures are annoying, she is impossible to please, nothing is ever good enough. Interestingly, Mom doesn't even blink, giving me the impression she is simply waiting for her girl to finish so she can continue her admonitions. I also wonder if some of the mother's behavior is a performance to demonstrate to me what a good parent she is, but I don't comment on this. Instead I instruct the girl: rather than stoically enduring her mother's lectures, she needs to learn how to signal her that she has done her parental duty, that she is a good-enough mother.

Over the next year, there are five follow-up visits. Her therapist writes that things are looking a bit better. Georgina herself reports continuing the Antidepressant, says her suicidal thinking had disappeared, that she is less remote and more responsive. The mother agrees she is improving but continues to fuss about the marijuana, also that she needs to "straighten up ... go to college." To this, Georgina expresses skepticism that it will ever happen. Her grades continue to slide, but she does graduate and enroll in college, where she plans to join the ROTC. She now has a boyfriend. Eventually she discontinues therapy. That summer she spends a month abroad.

That fall she remains terse and undemonstrative, reporting she is in college, studying "a lot" of engineering and accounting. In the interim she had been diagnosed with and begun treatment for a chronic inflammatory illness. The mother reports that at first Georgina struggled but now is more attentive to her studies, "pretty happy." I renew the Antidepressant then and again four months later.

The next summer she returns to have the Antidepressant renewed. In the waiting room I notice two striking changes: she gives me a bright, welcoming smile, and she is accompanied by her stepfather, not her mother. At the interview she returns to her taciturn, undemonstrative ways, waiting for questions. So I mirror her distance with a structured interview, beginning with the usual questions. Medication still helpful? Yes. Working? Yes. School? Going okay, but she has dropped the engineering—too demanding. Substances? Very little marijuana, but some alcohol. Then I switch to questions with more of an emotional valence. How are things with her stepfather? Getting along better. Then the critical question: Is her mom starting to let go? Yes.

I renew her prescription, reminding her to reschedule in four months.

Twelve years later, she has yet to return.

The Significance of Georgina's Behavior

Entangled Parent

Note that in this case it was the parent, not the child, who could not let go. Georgina was keenly aware that behind her mother's exhortations to grow up were intense feelings of abandonment, that she would experience as a death Georgina becoming a responsible adult. But Georgina was unable to discuss this issue because of her mother's vulnerability.

Her report of long-standing suicidal ruminations clearly indicates that for many years Georgina felt trapped by her mother's dependence. The abortive overdose, which sounded like a plea for help, seems to have backfired and confirmed her sense of utter helplessness. Hence her comment about the pointlessness of further attempts. Her "solution" of alcohol and marijuana helped distance her from her mother's unexpressed but powerful pleas for her to remain a kid.

The Abyss of Graduation

Even under ordinary circumstances, graduation from high school is a time of ambivalence for both parent and student, a mixture of joy and dread. *Now what?* both parties feel and think. For perhaps the first time, their relationship encounters an unquestionable point of no return, no going back to the old way of adult leading, child following. Now there is a new way: adult negotiating with adult. If the relationship is buttressed by a reasonable degree of trust—a "good enough" relationship in Winnicott's terminology—parent and student will bridge the transition more or less smoothly.

But there was a trust deficiency in Georgina's world, a world dominated by her mother's entangling dependent personality that left little room for Georgina to mature. Perhaps it would be more accurate to state that the mother's personality prevented her from recognizing her child's maturation; that is, finding work, getting along well with her teachers and coworkers, and so on.

Thus as graduation approached, Georgina, perceiving the transition as an abyss rather than a bridge, began to flounder. Her use of alcohol and marijuana did not protect her from freezing up under the stress of her mother's mixed message: *I expect you to succeed—although it will kill me.*

Fortunately Georgina's capacity to trust is not completely obliterated. She is able to accept the support provided by her counselor, her work, and a boyfriend, and she navigates the gulf without crashing.

My Relationship Style

Because of the entanglement issue, it was critical to avoid duplicating it during treatment. That is, through my behavior I had to make it clear to Georgina that my esteem would in no way be dependent on her performance as a patient or student or family member. My behavior had to say I was a resource, not a cheerleader; not an enforcer of conventional values but a consultant to be called on only for information and recommendations as she struggled to establish a life path and value set. In other words, it was essential that I define a clear boundary. Even two years later when it became apparent that she had become more trusting—the welcoming smile, her stepfather's presence—it remained imperative that I remain cautious and distant, and not co-opt her improvement.

Her failure to return I interpret as further evidence of progress—as a graduation of sorts.

[CASE STUDY]
The Punker

Anxious hovering is not the only way entangled parents can undermine their children's maturation.

In my role as a consultant at a private mental health clinic I am asked to see the Punker because of his problems with concentration, declining school performance, trouble sleeping, temper outbursts, and "unusual" dress. At staffing his counselor reports that he just can't seem to reach him despite very intense work. Pointing out to him how his behavior probably elicits the scapegoating and rejection he is experiencing seems to have no impact. Could he be "depressed"? Could be, I say, although to me he sounds more provocative and rebellious than "depressed."

Despite the forewarning of "unusual dress" I'm not prepared for the vision of soignée punk that materializes for the evaluation: black jeans and shirt, black leather jacket, spiked hair, with enough pierced jewelry, ornaments, chains, and medallions to short out metal detectors. Only missing is black makeup—which is to appear at subsequent visits.

Such attire would occasion comment even in relatively blasé Minneapolis, but we are not in Minneapolis; we're in redneck country, a hotbed of blue-collar, conservative, pickup-truck virtue. I'm tempted to smile. *What on earth,* I ask myself, *is this youngster attempting to accomplish in a place like this?*

But I control myself and solicit his story. He proves to be respectful and compliant, perhaps somewhat sad and discouraged as he describes how he doesn't get along with his teachers, parents, and most of his peers, who scapegoat him and his clique. Interestingly, he describes no problems getting along with supervisors, customers, and coworkers at a gaming arcade.

I prescribe some medication that affords marginal symptom relief but he eventually discontinues it. Yet along the way I find it impossible to just focus only on medications. Given his strenuous efforts to provoke his teachers and peers, I can't resist the obvious question: Why doesn't he just drop out or enroll in an alternative program?

His response is immediate and plausible. If he drops out his parents would take away his phone and his car. Later he reveals a greater ambition: he wants to open a business, a goth clothing store, and for that he needs an education.

I also ask another obvious question: Has he ever been rejected or abandoned? His response to this inquiry is less forthcoming, but eventually he reveals concerns about attachment: "It fits … I had two friends move away … it's like when I get a good friend, something happens … they aren't there."

Eventually he also reports it is satisfying if he can get people pissed at him.

However, despite what strikes me as satisfactory progress, his case is again reviewed at a staff conference (which I can't attend due to scheduling conflicts) because of his anger outbursts and provocative remarks. When I have a chance to review the conference summary, I discover the consensus recommendation is that he switch to an adolescent psychiatrist. Was it felt he needed a more law-and-order approach to psychotropic management? If so, it was an ill-considered suggestion since, mind you, this was someone who routinely questioned authority.

He nonetheless appears as scheduled for his next appointment. As might be expected, he refuses to switch to another psychiatrist.

Thereafter he continues with monthly "med checks," although he had long ago discontinued his medication. He enrolls in an alternative school. Feeling discriminated against by a teacher, he complains to the principal, then negotiates with them to resolve the issue. He reveals that he takes the scapegoat role to protect his more vulnerable buddies. His garb—at least during his visits to me—becomes less outlandish. He reports he is now on schedule to graduate with his class.

His begins to mention his parents, especially his father; they are still not satisfied despite his dramatic progress. Are they somehow afraid of him growing up? His grades improve, and eventually he makes the honor roll, which his father ignores. He rather sorrowfully concludes that his father recognizes him only when he is not doing well. He drops out of treatment.

The Significance of the Punker's Behavior

Provocative Behavior

The Punker's fear of attaching is a glaring illustration of what fuels a good deal of adolescent provocative and rebellious behavior. Now, there can be no doubt that the Punker was rebelling, as his dress glaringly and consistently proclaimed. And he had a temper. But there was never any evidence of him being dangerous. It was his way, albeit a somewhat self-defeating one, of establishing a boundary, of creating a barrier behind which he could feel safe, free from the possibility of further abandonments. If he did not feel close, how could he feel hurt when someone left—as experience showed they invariably would? And if he could provoke anger, so much the better. He would feel powerful for a change, liberated from his parents' pessimism.

Work Behavior

So why did he get along at work? After all, the workplace is rule oriented, authoritative, and supervised, utterly toxic for the rebel spirit, you might think. But these very qualities actually melded well with the Punker's personality for they provided structure and predictability in relationships without too much closeness. Of course, as we all know, enduring, sometimes lifetime relationships spring from workplace experiences nourished by the formal structure of work.[vi] This environment provides limits that can be invoked to ensure privacy and prevent too much intimacy—so you don't have to provoke an argument to establish a boundary. Hence the Punker flourished in this environment, as did Dyllen (chapter 2).

Behavior in Therapy

The Punker was originally referred to me because of his failure to improve despite "intense" therapy. Later he was asked to seek another psychiatrist because of his continuing anger and provocativeness. Ostensibly he failed to improve, this despite

---

vi. In volume 2 I will present the testimony of social activist Elijah Anderson in this respect.

his doing well at work: no problems there with authority, or accepting supervision, or treating customers and coworkers disrespectfully. Moreover, he was a good worker. And his ambitions were not out of the mainstream; he wanted to be a businessman.

In my view the proper professional role in circumstances like this would be to help the Punker take responsibility for his rebelliousness—whether he could control himself or not—and its consequences. The goal here is evaluation, not judgment. For example, not *Why do you dress like this?* but *Dressing like this in a town like this makes me wonder what you are trying to accomplish.* This addresses the first rule of management: *clarification*.[vii] Had this been adroitly accomplished by his counselor, it is likely no subsequent psychiatric consultation would have been necessary. The Punker would begin to reveal his abandonment issues, as he did with me promptly on the occasion of our initial contact. And this would have led quite naturally to the third step of management: *focusing on what can be changed.*[viii] Here, as with so many provocative youngsters, the goal is learning to create boundaries through negotiation, not through angry or provocative behavior.

So why did the therapist and clinic staff discreetly recommend a change of psychiatrists?

The primary reason was his therapist's failure to establish a proper boundary, one that respected the Punker's autonomy. The Punker had the power to refuse and prevent engagement, which is true of all patients.[ix] Moreover, his therapist and the staff had been seduced into believing that their role was to defend society's authority, not to teach the Punker how to live with authority, something all of us must learn lest we become hermits or outlaws.

---

vii. Discussed at length in chapter 11.
viii. See chapter 13.
ix. See chapter 10.

4

Attachment Acting-out: Three Cases

As I mentioned earlier in the book, Acting-out Attachment Disability can be thought of as one corner of a disability triangle, the other apexes of which are the desperate clinging of entanglement and the isolation of avoidance. It partakes of both yet remains unique because its basic dynamism is ambivalence. In other words, acting-out youngsters are deeply attached but *ambivalently* so.

Ambivalence is a simultaneous attraction toward and repulsion from an object, person, or action. This is an excellent characterization of the minds of acting-out youngsters and young adults. They long to attach yet are terrified by the impulse. Their "solution" is to establish a perimeter of angry behavior behind which they connect to authority via rebellious manipulation, which is the gist of Winnicott's notion of antisocial behavior as a "claim" on the environment. Management of this issue consists of teaching them how to *set boundaries with words rather than behavior*. I briefly discussed this notion in the case of the Punker, but his ambivalence was circumscribed: confined to home and school but absent in the workplace. And it had a highly symbolic quality.

This most definitely was not true of Jackie, a patient I

met forty years ago while working as a staff psychiatrist at Anoka State Hospital. My work with her introduced me to the ambivalent variety of attachment dysfunction, although I did not recognize it as such at the time. Her ambivalence was profound, as was her influence in the development of my subsequent deeper understanding of Attachment Disability, as well as her reaction to a "token economy" treatment program that our team had developed and installed on the female admission unit in the interval prior to her rehospitalization.[i] If you are not familiar with it, a token economy program is one in which physical tokens such as suitably modified poker chips or metal washers are handed out to patients whenever they exhibit specific desired behavior: for example, being on time, grooming appropriately, or completing work assignments correctly. Patients can exchange the tokens they earn for such things as food, personal items, or special privileges. Studies at the time indicated that this system has several potential benefits, including giving patients a sense of control over their own circumstances.

Now, four-plus decades later, I see that the token economy also functioned as a security blanket of sorts as we weaned patients away from the predictability of the locked unit, to which they clung in a hostile-dependent fashion. And it is now quite clear that their highly disruptive acting-out was a function of *powerful ambivalent attachment* dynamics. As an illustration I will now present here—both abridged and expanded—Jackie's case history from our paper describing the program.

---

i. See chapter 5 for program details, also the paper we later published: Curran J, Jorud S, Whitman N. "Unconventional Treatment of Treatment-Resistant Hospitalized Patients." *Psychiatric Quarterly*. 1971; 45(2), 188.

Attachment Acting-out: Three Cases

[CASE STUDY]
Jackie Encounters a Token Economy

Twenty years old, Jackie had been readmitted to the unit because of the return of suicidal threats and an extensive history of cutting. I characterized her as a "notorious Personality Disorder," in view of a four-year history of multiple admissions not only to Anoka but to community hospitals as well. Psychiatrists sighed when they heard her name. Now, in the midst of the token economy we had installed in her absence, she expressed unmistakable disgust regarding the program. She then assiduously began to work the program, steadily amassing tokens as a quasi-technician per program procedures. None of the acting-out behavior of previous admissions ever appeared, but she did not hesitate to provide a running critique of the program and our lack of empathy. After thirteen days on the unit she plunked down the price of a direct discharge—fifteen thousand tokens—and left.

Thereafter she called me off and on, ostensibly to threaten to expose our "inhumane" program. She sent a well-written complaint to the governor's office. On occasion she seemed depressed, but according to reports from the county welfare department, there was no evidence of acting-out. She was admitted to the county hospital but only to medical units for ill-defined somatic complaints. Later she became pregnant and elected to raise the baby (girl) herself. Her calls became less frequent and began to include inquiries about how things were going with patients she had helped, also about staff who had worked with her. Sometimes she commented on parenting problems. Two years after discharge, during several brief unscheduled encounters at the county hospital, she impressed me as composed, sad, and, for her, quite formal.

In the commentary section of the paper we noted that this remarkable change in her lifestyle—from acting-out scourge of the psychiatric community to social critic to medical patient to welfare mother—could be due to the persistence of adaptive behaviors learned during her exposure to the reinforcing nature of the token economy. We suggested that the program, by allowing her to manage her own treatment step by step, provided her with the opportunity to learn impulse control (versus being lectured or hectored to do so). We predicted that ultimately she would marry, and do well as a mother and wife, but eventually begin to demonstrate Depression and anxiety.

In hindsight I also suggest that the program allowed her the opportunity to learn how to modulate and revise her attachment issues. From using self-destructive behavior to keep people at a distance while maintaining a claim on them, she progressed to verbal and written criticism, then to a balance of comfort and distance in her authority relationships. Next to emerge was an attachment style much more familiar to physicians and psychiatrists: *somatization*—a state of emotional excitation being experienced as physical discomforts. Becoming a welfare mother represented Jackie's mature attachment configuration; that is, connecting with other adults via her child. Her child came to serve multiple roles: a social conversation piece, a protective barrier during one-on-one encounters, a ploy for the opportunity to covertly solicit information and assistance, and so on. In short, Jackie developed a personality style familiar to any parent.

Decades after we published our paper, I can now present an epilogue.

Attachment Acting-out: Three Cases

Jackie: Epilogue

Shortly after I entered private practice in 1970, Jackie applied for a consultation. She had, indeed, developed problems with anxiety and "depression," for which she had been followed by the county. Would I take her on as a private patient? Since our relationship was now less contentious, I agreed.

Thereafter I see her off and on for the better part of twenty years, less often after I relocate my office to the suburbs. Occasionally she is a bit cocky, presenting a façade of toughness and independence. She by now has a second child by the same man, who, it turns out, remains her lifelong companion and partner. She disdains the idea of marriage and sometimes mocks his commitment and loyalty, at other times wonders why he puts up with her. Occasionally, she drops her guard and speaks of what sounds like years of extreme childhood and adolescence sexual abuse by relatives; then she clams up. It becomes clear, as is the case with so many other trauma victims, that this was the source of the protective behaviors with patients we observed while she was on the unit years earlier. It also underlay her bitter complaints about the other patients' ostensible neglect, the letter to the governor, and her ferocious protection of her girls, whose rambunctious behaviors are the occasion of much of her anxiety. Adolescents now, they sound like pretty good kids, as smart as she but enough on the wild side to drive her nuts as a parent.

After I moved my office I saw less and less of her; transportation was a problem, plus her issues became more medical than psychiatric. Perhaps her last visit was about twenty years ago, yet every year on my birthday she would send me a card with a wistful inscription saying that she was thinking of me, wondering how I was. Only when her obituary appeared in the paper eleven years ago or so did I realize I had stopped receiving her annual card. She was remembered as a loving companion, mother, and grandmother. It's sad to think of her as no longer in this world. I hope some of her protective spirit lives on in her children and grandchildren.

I could write a separate book with Jackie in mind for those who wish a deeper understanding of the vicissitudes of adolescent (and adult) attachment issues. Her life offers many lessons. Here I will comment on several of the most important: briefly but with enough detail to provide the interested reader the opportunity to investigate further.

The Significance of Jackie's Behavior

The Impact of the Token Economy

The thirteen days Jackie spent in our program completely and permanently transformed her.

In that era the city-county-state hospital treatment community was not fragmented. By law, every committed patient was assigned a county social worker who attended discharge planning and helped construct follow-up treatment. I was a member of the county psychiatric society and later resigned from Anoka to take a position in the outpatient department of the county hospital. Our community of psychiatrists, psychiatric nurses, and psychiatric social workers was tightly knit. Everyone knew everybody, and above all, everyone knew of Jackie—she had scorched four years of community treatment planning. She was a slender, attractive, engaging, and intelligent young woman whose charm sucked you in. Then, without warning, charm gave way to scorn, sarcasm, and angry outbursts that typically ended with her stalking away. The very mention of her name elicited a shudder, and any acting-out or psychiatric hospitalization would promptly be posted on the therapeutic grapevine of that day.

So why did the token economy program work for such a challenging case?

Attachment Acting-out: Three Cases

Under ordinary circumstances, learning involves observing the consequences of behavior, whether experienced or witnessed. If there is no significant lag in the maturation of the prefrontal lobe, only a few trials of behavior are required to promote learning; hence the gold stars and smiley faces primary school teachers affix to the papers of their students. And the consequence of learning is twofold: a skill and a strengthened attachment. But apart from issues of prefrontal development and innate ability, stars and faces are not effective for all children, one cause of which is the appearance of attachment issues. Youngsters stall out or fall behind.

Jackie dreaded attachment, and the venue in this case was not the classroom but life itself. In her experience, to attach or to trust meant exploitation and abuse. Any relationship was hazardous and risky. And successful treatment, if not abusive or exploitative in itself, signified a return to the very environment in which she previously had been abused. She had learned that to get "well" was dangerous.

Abuse—in fact any kind of trauma, say the loss of a dearly loved—creates distrust, which lingers. To be well in her case meant to lose the angry wall behind which she felt safe from exploitation, betrayal, or loss. Yet once ensconced behind that wall, she yearned for solace and comfort, which attracted attention. Thus she cycled in and out of treatment arrangements and exhibited disruptive behaviors while within.

A token economy seeks to correct maladaptive learning by creating a special learning situation. In fact, a token economy is nothing more that the tangible manifestation of the recommendation so often appended to psychological testing, for example, "This client will likely benefit from a structured, step-by-step treatment plan designed to acquire mastery of identified life skills." Specifically, a token arrangement undermines the dread of attachment by carefully defining the limits of performing. Recognition—a token—for performing an identified behavior carries no implication or expectation of further performance.

Nowadays acting-out kids who end up in day or residential treatment program are managed by a modern version of the 1960s token economy, loosely conceptualized as "consequences." However, if the program does not carefully take into account the attachment dynamics provoking the acting-out behavior, kids are at risk of flunking out or experiencing a return of acting-out once released, because in either case they have learned no adaptive skills. When such kids end up in my office, it is apparent that while deviant behaviors were carefully defined for them, reinforcing strategies were not. Such children are very slow to attach, and when they do they are reluctant to relinquish attachments once secured. In short, it is vital that the consequences in response to acting-out *not include a revocation of previously earned reinforcements.* And likewise, a consequence in response to a demonstration of adaptive behavior must never—*never!*—embody the implication that such behavior is expected thereafter. Furthermore, recognition of performance must be carefully and rigorously managed step by step. Remember: these are kids for whom recognition has a toxic potential. *Recognition dangerous; failure safe* is how their midbrain is programmed.

Jackie's Complaints

At first we took Jackie's complaints and letter about the program's "inhumanity" as sour grapes. That is, in the depths of a seemingly benign program—power to the patient!—she detected a more sinister, manipulative intent. Its rules were not negotiable. Or, from another point of view, the only way to change the rules was to escape them by working the program. And her perception was accurate. The program was fundamentally manipulative.

However, this is also true of learning where parents, teachers, mentors, or coaches expect to promote skill acquisition in a child subject to their authority. So we coax, wheedle, encourage, guilt, and challenge kids to try harder, practice longer, rehearse, and stretch themselves—only we call it motivating, not manipulating. We use bonds of attachment, and sometimes the threat of the loss of thereof, to help children move beyond what they view as possible or necessary.

I now realize that Jackie's criticism was founded on a deeper concern. Her distress was not that of a manipulator who had the tables turned on her. It was her abuse background—concealed beneath a veneer of toughness, which served as a boundary—that came into play here. She who had been so exploited by the powerful was not going to let it happen to other patients if she had anything to say about it; her protective instincts were aroused. In my experience this is the more frequent, indeed much more frequent, abuse fallout. The abused are (fortunately) much more likely to become protectors than exploiters of the vulnerable. Many express an interest in returning to school to pursue a career in health care, social work, or law enforcement.

On the other hand, victims frequently suffer an excess of empathy, which puts them at risk of further exploitation, especially if the perpetrator is a relative and the family guilts the victim into participating in a "code of silence." Or they become gripped by a dimly perceived rescue fantasy that sucks them into attachments with partners who are dependent, if not substance abusing or violent. In the world of Al-Anon or Alateen, they are categorized as "enablers." I will leave Jackie's story for a moment now to offer an example of this enabling behavior.

[CASE STUDY]
Amanda: A Familiar Scenario

Amanda returns for an appointment after an absence of some months. Our previous contact had been lengthy and strenuous because it was difficult for her to work the three steps of managing Attachment Disability. Not that she was disabled physically or economically; she was a good worker and regularly employed, supporting her slacker partner, Pete. It was obvious, however, that she was trapped in a relationship that was no longer gratifying but from which she was unable to extricate herself. I had struggled to clarify (note the first management principle here) that her many issues with "depression" were actually fears of abandonment ignited whenever Pete threatened to leave or demonstrated behavior that made Amanda consider giving up the relationship. As we discussed this, she eventually revealed a history of abuse and abandonment that left her extremely sensitive to and sympathetic for others with the same background, even animals.

I worked at length to persuade her to accept this personality dimension, without blaming (the second principle) herself for being "weak" by letting Pete take advantage of her "weakness." I explained that this was a trait that now was "wired in," that had to be "owned" rather than ignored or suppressed. Otherwise, "it will come out of nowhere and trip you up again."

At the same time we discussed what could be changed (the third principle). I observed, based on my professional experience, that it was not wise to continue a relationship with the expectation that the other would change. "Certainly Pete can change and will change … sometime … but it is a mistake to think that you could or should promote it. It will just frustrate the two of you. You need to think about what *you* can do differently."

We went around and around, discussing, debating, clarifying. Gradually complaints of "depression" evaporated as she began to focus on the specifics of her unhappy situation. With some trepidation she initiated a more pointed dialogue with Pete regarding her dissatisfactions, specifically that she was thinking of moving on. Eventually they agreed to split up and he moved out. At follow-up visits she was happy, pleased with the change in her life, and we decided to continue only as needed. My only somewhat facetious parting comment at her last visit was something like "Remember to abstain from men." She laughed.

Now, months later, she was back, looking quite flustered. I ventured, "Let me guess. There's a new man in your life."

Now her laugh was a bit rueful. "Yes."

So we went back to work. Her "relapse" was understandable. Anyone who has been involved in Al-Anon or Alateen will tell you that the grip of enabling personality traits is powerful indeed. You are always vulnerable to pleas for help. The trick is to find a productive and creative way to manage the itch, so to speak, without compromising yourself or fostering dependency in the other. As Amanda's experience demonstrates, this does not happen overnight.

Returning to Jackie now, in comparison she seems to have avoided this trap. Writing to the governor's office about her concerns was certainly a constructive use of her energies. And her lifelong commitment to her partner was devoid of exploitation on either side, although on occasion she expressed frustration over his unwavering loyalty, wondering how he could put up with her.

And she recognized that her girls had inherited too much of her grit and energy to simply comply with her admonitions without some experimentation of their own. While she complained to me about their stunts and sometimes reckless behavior, I could see she realized she would have to tolerate some erratic behavior as long as it did not lead to abusive relationships.

Jackie's Cutting: A Sign of Entanglement

In certain clinical situations, patients deliberately and repetitively self-inflict pain—for example, scratching their wrists or burning themselves with cigarettes—where it is obvious their intent is not to harm themselves. Or they tattoo or pierce. For many years psychiatrists assumed that patients who engaged in such minor self-injurious but not life-threatening behaviors were trying to evoke more stimulation from their surroundings, a payoff in the form of attention. This was a serious misconception—frequently the result was the opposite. Such patients were rejected, even abused by emergency room personnel and shunned by therapists who felt exploited and coerced. The hidden plea for help and the attempt to make a "claim" on the environment were overlooked because the message was packaged in such an unattractive and immature manner. The truth is that mutilations, particularly cutting, are often concealed and not revealed unless discovered by accident.

Now we understand that such behaviors are driven by *negative reinforcement*.[ii] Such patients, upon careful examination, frequently report "feeling better" despite, say, burning themselves with a cigarette or having their ears or eyebrows pierced. It seems that a sharply localized somatic discomfort externalized to the skin is preferable to the prior diffuse, unfocused indescribable state of internal misery. The intolerable becomes tolerable.

In the 1960s self-mutilating behavior (SMB)[iii] was much less frequent than today.

Now no workup is complete unless one inquires about "cutting," and no explanation is needed because everyone, male and female, knows what is meant. One also has to inquire about things like self-inflicted burns, abrasions, gouging, picking at

---

ii. Also to be defined and discussed in volume 2.

iii. To be distinguished from SIB, self-injurious behavior; that is, behavior accompanied by suicidal intent.

open sores, things of that sort, even compulsive tattooing. Obviously SMB has become a routine feature of today's adolescent and young adult environment.[iv]

If self-mutilation is present, I have learned to make a follow-up inquiry: "Do you worry a lot about other people being unhappy, that somehow if someone is unhappy it is your fault, either because you caused it or have not fixed it?" If the response is affirmative, I continue with a question our professors frowned on because it might "encourage" the behavior: "What does it feel like?" Self-mutilators respond variously. Some say they don't feel a thing, no pain or discomfort. Others say they feel pain, but prefer an external, focused discomfort to a previously internal, unfocused ache or misery; in effect, the pain is a welcome distraction. And some are more perceptive, realizing that it relieves guilt or anxiety.

It seems pretty clear that the cutting or burning or abrading or gouging or (sometimes) tattooing is a way of stabilizing a shaky identity. Unhappiness and suffering confuse these youngsters because they have difficulty determining who owns the pain. Physical pain helps to establish a boundary. They often come from an abuse background, but one where the abuse

---

iv. Another routine inquiry these days is eating disorders. While now also very common, bulimia and anorexia are not amenable to the three-step attachment disability management approach I advocate because eating disorders are too complex. They require diagnosis and treatment by a team including an internist, a dietician, and a therapist trained in both individual and family therapy. On the other hand, eating-disordered individuals abound with attachment issues. Why attachment problems more commonly appear these days in the guise of SMB and eating disorders is most likely due to the evolution of society amplified by the bourgeoning social media. I will discuss the power of these trends in volume 2 of this series when I address David Riesman's notion of "other-directedness" as described by him in *The Lonely Crowd*. Riesman D, Glazer N, Denny R (New Haven, CT: Yale University Press), 1961 abridged paperback edition.

more likely was witnessed, where the victim was someone else, usually a parent or sibling. In such situations youngsters adapt by assuming a role: protector, enabler, scapegoat, or nurse, for example. Whatever the guise, the final pathway is an exclusive focus on the needs and feelings of the victim to the exclusion of their own needs and feelings, which are submerged and ignored—in a word, "dissociated." They become strangers to themselves. Thus, should they then encounter a needy individual, they are unprepared to address and clarify the discomfort stirred within by the impulse to rescue and protect. They do not know how to "own" the misery of witnessing suffering without becoming disabled by it. They do not know how to establish boundaries; many times are not even aware of the need to do so.

By the time I started to follow Jackie in my office, she had stopped cutting, so addressing that was not a treatment goal. We focused more on the here and now, with only an occasional reference to her upbringing and her abuse, obviously painful to consider. It was in the past, she had survived; now the issue was to protect others, which I now realize she had learned to do without getting sucked in. She could help without having to damage or sacrifice herself because she had established boundaries. I can only surmise that there was more victimization in her past than just her own.

Understanding Jackie's Diagnosis

At the time we published our findings, our focus was on therapeutics, not diagnostics. Hence in our report we simply utilized our patients' admission diagnosis of record, some of which had been developed years previously, and analyzed the program results accordingly. As we noted in our paper, much to our surprise, we found that improvement was a function of total months of prior hospitalization, not diagnosis. Hence our discussion was so focused.

But now, after decades of APA tinkering with our diagnostic nomenclature (see chapter 14), it is an interesting exercise to examine Jackie's diagnosis according to contemporary standards. I will leave it to the reader to determine which, if any, of the following diagnostic considerations apply to Jackie.

Borderline Personality Disorder?

In our report we described Jackie as a "notorious Personality Disorder." *DSM-5* describes ten different types of personality disorders. All have one quality in common: failure to learn from experience. Today a panel of psychiatrists and psychologists reviewing her prior history would most likely diagnose Borderline Personality Disorder (BPD). Of the nine criteria required to qualify for this diagnosis, in my opinion the most important is an inability to maintain stable relationships. Such individuals adore and flatter you now, only to instantly and without warning become angry, rejecting, hostile, and critical. This is what makes treating them such a challenge—you never know who is going to walk through the door.

Earlier I wrote that youngsters "solve" ambivalent attachments by erecting a barrier of resistive and angry behavior behind which they connect to authority at a distance and manipulate the fulfillment of their need for love and support. Disruptive and self-defeating as it might appear to others, such a technique feels less risky when it comes to establishing—as Winnicott puts it—a "claim" on the environment. In my view, therefore, the critical element in BPD is not the behavioral instability but the personality dynamic that drives it: extreme attachment ambivalence. BPD patients thirst for love but are terrified that they will be consumed and destroyed by it and then abandoned. Therefore, when you as a parent or teacher or nurse practitioner are confronted by such erratic behavior, the first thing to pop into your mind should be entanglement awareness. You must ask yourself: How much distance do I need to establish here? If the three rules of real estate are *location, location, location, t*he three rules of emotional instability are *boundaries, boundaries, boundaries!* I will discuss this notion at greater length later in chapter 10.

Bipolar Disorder?

In the many years that have passed since Jackie's encounter with our token economy, diagnostic styles have changed. Manic-Depressive illness has become Bipolar Disorder (BD) and its many variants. Accordingly, our panel of experts might well so diagnose Jackie in view of her many hospitalizations and lack of response to treatment—a frequent error, in my opinion. In the course of my consulting work, I frequently encounter victims of severe abuse with similar histories misdiagnosed as BD rather than trauma residuals.

Some years ago, for example, I had the opportunity to review the discharge summary of a twenty-seven-year-old mother referred for medication follow-up. The summary was extensive—five plus pages—and quite well done. It revealed that the hospitalization was precipitated by a housing crisis: the woman and her three children were facing eviction by the end of the month. There was a history of at least four prior psychiatric hospitalizations as well as trials of twenty-five different Antidepressants, Mood Stabilizers, and Antipsychotics— carefully enumerated by the attending psychiatrist—without any sustained benefit. Reading between the lines, I suspected noncompliance was a huge issue, judging from the tone of the discharge instructions, which seemed a desperate plea for the mother to follow through with very extensive discharge planning. There was a brief reference to abuse by her father. No surprise that her discharge diagnosis was Bipolar II Disorder.

No surprise either that she did not keep her appointment with me.

Hers was a typical misdiagnosis. First of all, in such instances the mood changes, while profound and dramatic, are abrupt, of sudden onset and remission, typically hour to hour and not infrequently minute to minute. This is quite uncharacteristic of the gradual onset and persistence of authentic BD mood fluctuations, which evolve and remit over a period of days or weeks. Second, Mood Stabilizers are effective if the diagnosis is accurate. Also, compliance is at least, and sometimes better than, average. Mood-disordered individuals, once recovered, are not burdened by the lingering trust issues that afflict trauma victims and undermine compliance.[v] Physicians and medication represent power and authority, soothing to those who have had happy encounters with such figures and agents, threatening to those who have experienced exploitation and abuse in their power encounters.

Oppositional Defiant Disorder?

A diagnosis that our panel of experts might also confer on Jackie, other than BPD or BD, is Oppositional Defiant Disorder (ODD), defined as persisting defiant, vindictive, and hostile attitude toward authority. I think of this as the "empty calorie diagnosis" because it is a tautology without any therapeutic or management content. What is defiant, vindictive, and hostile behavior? Why, ODD, of course. What is ODD? Well, defiant, vindictive, and hostile behavior, most certainly. In short, the label creates the illusion of knowledge. Of the many fatuous diagnostic categories in *DSM-5*, this is one of the worst. *DSM-5* devotes two hundred lines of fine print to defining ODD diagnostic criteria and features, but only in passing mentions that "Harsh, inconsistent, or neglectful child-rearing practices are common in families ... [and] play an important role in many

---

v. I will also discuss this topic at greater length in chapter 10.

causal theories of the disorder ..."[1] The most relevant information is buried in a thicket of pontification.

In my view, besides adding nothing to the understanding and management of troubled kids, the label reinforces the myth that the essence of the adolescent spirit is anger and rebellion. Thus you see the label applied to many a kid who is just an unruly, argumentative, rebellious spirit at home or at school but who otherwise gets along with adults and at work. This is utter nonsense. As I will describe at length in volume 2, the emotion that grips the mass of adolescents these days is anxiety, not anger. The violence of gang behavior is driven not by establishment resentment but by a need to "pass for bad" on the street. I recall a dedicated inner-city high school instructor once remarking that his students would jump off a third-floor balcony if that was what it took to fit in, to gain "street cred."

A similar dynamic is present in crowd participation in bullying. Twemlow and Sacco, reviewing bystander behavior, comment, "It is a well-known fact that children, especially during their adolescent years, tend to look to their peers for clues about how to respond to everything in their social environment."[2] Adolescents, en masse, in fact prefer life in which authority is stable, predictable, and reasonable—that is, safe to bitch about. This engenders a sense of security as they go about exploring their widening world. It is when adult authority collapses in the face of adolescent crankiness that complaining begins to mutate into anger. Deeply rebellious kids are those who have lost the confidence that predictable authority inspires.

Finally, when an angry youngster is labeled ODD, the term is a distraction, misdirecting attention to the anger and away from the underlying fears and insecurities that are driving it. When we encounter such a kid, our first thought must be *What is he/she afraid of?* Our assumption must be that we are dealing with an attachment issue unless subsequent events conclusively prove otherwise. Our next thought must be to consider the degree of distance to create in the transaction; that is, where the boundary is to be established to protect both ourselves and the youngster from provocation. I will discuss this at greater length in chapter 10.

In short, avoiding the "empty calorie diagnosis" when dealing with an angry youngster will more reliably point you in the direction of a management plan. To be sure, Jackie's acting-out behaviors were so deeply entrenched by the time she encountered the token economy program, with spectacular and persisting disability, that her underlying attachment issues were neither readily accessible nor easily recognized as such. Therefore I will present here a more representative case, also authentic, of what a teacher or parent might encounter when acting-out behavior pops up seemingly from nowhere. Fortunately, her mother was perceptive and avoided the "empty calorie" dead end.

[CASE STUDY]
Maya and the Absent Father

Maya is a thirteen-year-old referred by her mother, a former patient, for follow-up of Antidepressant therapy begun several months earlier. I interview the two of them.

According to the mother, the first sign of trouble was her daughter complaining of headaches. Then she began to cut. Eventually other problems emerged, such as talking back to her mother, acting-out at home, talking back to teachers, drinking, threatening to get tattooed. Finally the mother realized that the girl's problems began when her father, an extreme sports enthusiast, went on an extended climbing vacation. Later, after a fight with her mother—the worst ever—the girl admitted she was quite fearful about her dad.

By the time I start to see her, she reports feeling less angry and less headachy, which she attributes to the Antidepressant she is taking. At a second visit she remains improved, describing feeling more energetic, happier, less angry. She also admits to worries about the mother. The two seem supportive of each other.

I discuss the "antistressant"[vi] properties of her Antidepressant, suggesting she continue it under the auspices of her pediatrician. I also suggest she start seeing a therapist to "work on your worries," briefly reviewing the three stages of recovery from disability. Finally, I recommend no follow-up for now.

The Significance of Maya's Behavior

I have not presented Maya's history in detail because by the time she arrived on my doorstep, the healing of her trust issues was progressing nicely; hence little was required of me other than to endorse the process. On the other hand, her history, telescoped as it is, is a fine illustration of the dynamics of acting-out behavior: fears of abandonment masked by anger. Again, among the central concepts of this book, one of the foremost is: *when dealing with an angry adolescent, always look for the abandonment fear behind the anger*. It is fear that invigorates all of Maya's decisive experiences and behavior.

Maya's Disguised Response to Loss

Secure attachments promote trust and strengthen stress resistance, which are undermined when these attachments are lost or weakening. Maya clearly had a powerful reaction to her father's junket—there seems to have been more here than just the loss of a supportive relationship. Perhaps she also experienced it as a sign of immaturity and impulsivity. Adolescents, as much as they might decry the burdens of adult supervision, still expect the adults in their life to act grown-up. Ordinarily adult juvenility is not particularly problematic for their kids, just an

---

vi. See chapter 9, also the chapter, "Are Antidepressants Effective?," forthcoming in volume 2.

embarrassment. But Maya developed substantial fears. Would Dad engage in risky climbs, get hurt, even killed?

Maya's Hidden Awareness

Maya's awareness of her fear and anxiety is suppressed. Now, note how I formulate her neuropsychological state. To say, "She suppressed awareness of the fears" would imply this was a conscious activity on her part. Perhaps it was and perhaps it wasn't; we'll never know. In fact, were I to have a follow-up opportunity to inquire, it's highly probable that she herself would admit she doesn't know. Recall that Dyllen also did not seem to be aware of the connection between loss—his brother entering the army—and subsequent panic attacks and use of marijuana and alcohol.

But whether the suppression is conscious, preconscious, or nonconscious, she remains energized by her fear and anxiety. Her stress mounts, the first manifestation of which is a headache, later followed by cutting.

Maya's Cutting

As discussed earlier, SMB such as cutting and tattooing or burning does not necessarily signal Depression or suicidal preoccupation or intent. Rather, it provides a way of substituting an external localized discomfort for an internal diffuse but intolerable misery. In my experience cutting is always—*always!*—a sign of entanglement. On the other hand, if the psychological burdens of entanglement are not relieved, the persisting misery can lead to death ruminations. Rather than fearfulness, the notion of death generates a sense of peacefulness; that is, release from suffering. I will discuss at greater length later in chapter 11 the notion of death ruminations as consolation.

Maya's Entanglement

Eventually Maya reveals that she also worries about Mom. Recall that her mother was my patient with undoubtedly—I don't recall—her own set of worries and concerns. Youngsters are sensitive to their sponsors' troubles; no exception here. Moreover, youngsters worry that their own struggles will be a source of additional stress for their sponsors. This sets the stage for an escalating, exhausting struggle during which each party tries to "fix" the other while resisting efforts to be "fixed."

Maya's Anger and Acting-out Protect Against Entanglement

Maya's acting-out behaviors offer a compromise "solution." On the one hand, she does not completely withdraw into isolation, yet neither does she wish to get too close to the adult figures in her life, Mom or others. She does not want to get entangled. Her behavior tends to keep people at a distance, especially adults, therefore making closeness less likely. By provoking irritation and anger, she protects herself from feeling hurt and rejected by subsequent abandonments—which, in her experience, are now inevitable. When the other shoe finally drops, she can think *I don't care—I didn't like her/him/them anyhow.* If you are not close to someone, how can you be hurt if they leave you? Yet the anger and disruptive behavior, as Winnicott suggests, signal distress. Fortunately, her perceptive mother reads the behavioral subtext, and the truth finally emerges. No doubt the Antidepressant helps by reducing the stress and anxiety attached to the possibility of loss. Now there is a greater likelihood that Maya can negotiate supportive bonding without feeling her independence compromised, a compromise solution between avoidance and entanglement.

Maya's Mother Resists Rejection

Demonstrating admirable resolve, Maya's mother does not give up, suspecting there is more to the story. She keeps boring in, finally convincing Maya that her mother—her nagging and demanding mother—is tough enough to be trusted with the truth, that she won't collapse when Maya finally reveals her concerns. This is terrific leadership, the very quality that adolescents need most of all.

A Final Comment About Diagnosis

I have developed this lengthy discussion of diagnostic conventions to amplify the vital distinction I made in the introduction: *diagnosis/treatment* versus *understanding/management.* Which is this: when it comes to Attachment Disability, understanding leads to management with its possibility of trust enhancement, but diagnosis tends toward obfuscation with an attendant risk of making things worse by pathologizing distrust. Some may question the validity of this dichotomy. But the more relevant issue, to my way of thinking, is the validity of the concept of Attachment Disability to begin with. And what are its origins? These are legitimate concerns that I will review in chapters 5 through 7. It seems to me that should the concept prove valid, then the dichotomy follows.

Part 3

Origins of the Theory of Attachment Disability

5

Early Origins

The Validity of the Theory

Alert readers may wonder by now about the validity of the concept of Attachment Disability. Why not make use of a more traditional *DSM-5* category? It is my view that using the standard approach to categorization is both deficient and misleading for the following reasons:

While *DSM-5* contains the category of Reactive Attachment Disorder, it specifies that the disturbance must be evident before age five. Because it is "unclear" if it occurs in older children, we are cautioned to be careful in making the diagnosis in that group. The former category of Reactive Attachment Disorder, Disinhibited Type—now retitled Disinhibited Social Engagement Disorder—is deemed applicable even in situations where there is no evidence of neglect or disordered attachment. It is not believed to be present in adults. Nowhere in *DSM-5* is acting-out behavior—designated there "externalizing behavior"—considered to represent an attachment problem.

On the other hand, Posttraumatic Stress Disorder would by its very nomenclature seem apropos. But there are problems here as well: it is not inclusive enough. Death of a relative or friend due to natural causes does not qualify; e.g., the deaths of Holden Caulfield's brother from leukemia or Helen's mother from an undiagnosed overwhelming sepsis. And, even if the diagnosis is correct, it does not go far enough. It does not penetrate to the essence of the disorder—damaged trust, of others and self. You lose confidence in your thoughts, feelings, and emotions: they now seem threatening. The previously reliable becomes unreliable.

Moreover, too shallow an assessment risks the distrust becoming pathologized: an abnormality to be overcome with treatment rather than accepted as a normal, albeit intensely painful, very human response to a catastrophic loss of security, whether real or symbolic.

I cannot say when I fully developed the idea of extending the notion of early childhood attachment issues to later childhood, adolescence, and adult disabilities. Looking at my office charts now, I find that the term does not appear in my own records or in accompanying medical and psychiatric records until sometime in the early 2000s when I had been in private practice for more than three decades. Once, perhaps in 2005 or thereabouts, while I was evaluating a young woman who had, as I recall, just been discharged from an intensive residential treatment center, she happened to remark, "My therapist said I had attachment issues."

However, deficiencies in diagnosis do not necessarily demonstrate the validity of a proposed alternative. The power of the concept of Attachment Disability remains to be established, which I hope to do in this section of the book.

Origins

Where, then, did my ideas come from?

Reviewing the many adventures of my career, I can identify at least eight sources:

My specialty training at the New York State Psychiatric Institute (PI) 1962–65, especially my supervision by its director, Dr. Laurence Kolb, who firmly believed that all anxiety is related to separation.

My clinical and research experiences at Anoka State Hospital, 1965–68. As noted earlier, our team established a "token economy" treatment program to manage acting-out behaviors, which we interpreted per Winnicott as a call on the environment for relief of unmet needs. Here also my research mentor, Dr. Bertrum Schiele, introduced me to the idea that treatment should be directed toward relief of symptom/disability rather than diagnosis. And I fell away from true belief in the efficacy of Antipsychotic medications to relieve all manifestations of psychotic decompensation. More was needed.

Partnering with Frederick Sheridan PhD, 1982, to design a grant application to take national his alternative learning center (ALC) program of voluntary attendance and continuous education to combat "Affective Interference," his term for what I years later identified as "Attachment Disability."

Consulting experiences 1985–88 at the Lakeland Mental Health Clinic, Fergus Falls, Minnesota, with behaviorally oriented PhD psychologists Ed and Mary Schmidt. Rather than a total reliance on psychotropic medications, Dr. Ed taught the staff of area group homes to turn to behavioral analysis for management of their developmentally disabled residents. In her office work Dr. Mary practiced a very active intervention style of restructuring and redirection techniques to teach similarly disabled clients how to assess the consequences of their behaviors.

Research for a manuscript on separation and loss, 1984, portions of which are included in this book. For example, my interpretation of Salinger's *The Catcher in the Rye* (death of the beloved sunders the possibility to relate, chapter 2), my analysis of Mann's *The Magic Mountain* (death gives meaning to life, chapter 9), and my synopsis of the history of education (volume 2).

Office practice 1990–2012 teaching pain management to adults disabled by chronic pain. Eventually I realized that my therapy—indeed perhaps all therapy—could be summarized by three principles; clarification, acceptance, and focus. Later I began to incorporate these principles into my management of Attachment Disability. Most of the cases I include in this book come from the later years of this era and are derived from my office notes.

Consultation work with Focus Program, a K–12 ALC administered by the Elk River, Minnesota, School District. The great majority of Focus students were in the middle and later grades, as well as few young adults in aftercare. This work showed me that attachment issues were not an early childhood phenomenon. They were potentially lifelong because of a persistently wounded capacity to trust, the management of which, the Focus staff emphasized, begins with avoiding pathologizing mistrust.

Learning from my patients.

My conclusion: my concept of Attachment Disability emerged by osmosis from these sources, and no doubt others. It is up to the reader to judge its validity. To assist you in making your judgment, I will now provide more detail about each "clinical adventure."

Origin #1: I Learn That All Anxiety Is Related to Separation

Dr. Kolb uttered this idea in a rather memorable way, not only because of the locale but also because for once he was not exasperated by my obtuseness; as a psychiatric resident, to use a sports analogy, I was a "project." To preserve the structure of this book, however, I will postpone revealing this adventure until chapter 8 and include it in the context of a more complete discussion of the notion of anxiety.

Origin #2: Anoka State Hospital (Mis)Adventures

At the end of my training at PI, I lined up a half-time research position with the Department of Psychiatry, University of Minnesota, working under the supervision of an eminent professor of psychiatry, Dr. Bertrum Schiele. The idea was that I would be stationed at the nearby Anoka (MN) State Hospital, the locale of the research. Dr. Schiele then suggested that I apply for a half-time position at the hospital as a staff psychiatrist, referring me to its medical director, Dr. John Docherty. We hit it off, so he took me on.

I will review in great detail my clinical experience at Anoka, for my service there shaped my professional career as profoundly as my six summers as a ditchdigger for the Saint Paul Water Department shaped my personal life.

My Limited State Hospital Experience
True, PI was a state hospital, but it was primarily devoted to teaching and research. Most inpatients therefore were young, attractive, verbal, intelligent, more or less acute, and voluntary. And also true that I had served for three months as a first-year resident at the Manhattan State Hospital located on Ward's

Island in the East River, whose wards served the chronically mentally ill for the most part, in effect the mirror image of the PI inpatients.

My assigned duties and clinical responsibilities there were restricted to working up one newly admitted patient per day. So each day I would report to the admissions unit, interview and evaluate my assigned patient according to approved PI protocol and dictate a report, and then eat lunch with the staff. Never were my reports critiqued by one of the senior staff, nor were any afternoon assignments ever forthcoming. So after lunch I would admire the view of the New York skyline or the bustling river traffic from my office, then go home early.

Apart from vague recollections of the pleasures of a three-month respite from the stresses of a first-year residency, I have only two memories of those months that might have served me at Anoka.

One is definitely idiosyncratic, evoked on occasion by, of all things, contemplation of cooked rice. A regular lunchgoer was an older, slightly shriveled psychologist who brought his own meal, always carefully wrapped in foil, always consisting of one item: unseasoned, unadorned cooked rice. Every day he quietly seated himself, solemnly unwrapped his humble package, and religiously consumed its contents, occasioning no comment from his tablemates. The ritual attracted my surreptitious attention. It was obviously not a matter of poverty given his dress and state of employment. Was it a compulsion?

He eventually noticed my scrutiny and explained. He had hypertension and was practicing a novel therapy—a low-salt diet—just recently recommended by a recognized expert in the field, Dr. Louis Tobian, Jr., and rice was notably low in salt. So we bonded via a discussion of the intricacies of diagnosing and treating illness—medical illness, that is, not mental. Was it working? I can't recall his verdict, but my recollection of him hunched over his rice expounding on Dr. Tobian's theories is still vivid.

Another time I was asked by the director of resident training to interview a patient before the assembled residents, which I proceeded to do in approved PI style: detailed mental status, detailed history, *this-is-what-I'm-feeling feedback*,[i] psychodynamic formulation, and so on. After my presentation there was a pause. Then the director remarked, "Yes, that's how they do it at the Psychiatric Institute," and immediately changed the subject. Even the insensitive dolt that I was then could recognize the subtext: *that's not the way to do things here.* I suppose if I had shown more initiative—asking to work on one of the units, run a group, do consults, things of that sort—he might have been more favorably disposed toward me. But I don't think his opinion of my lackluster performance had much of an impact back at PI. As I mentioned earlier, my professors there were already aware of what they were dealing with.

Thus I arrived at Anoka a state-hospital greenhorn, my expertise limited to novel antihypertensive diets and how *not* to interview the chronically mentally ill.

The Research Setting

Dr. Schiele proved to be a valuable mentor. He was a full professor of psychiatry at the University of Minnesota and had trained at Cornell Payne-Whitney in the late thirties. By the time I met him, he was one of the leading clinical researchers in the country. His research team, one of several nationally, participated in the ECDEU (Early Clinical Drug Evaluation Unit) research initiative organized, as I recall, by the psychopharmacology branch of the National Institutes of Mental Health. The various teams participated in regular conferences to share research studies of newly developed, presumptively nontoxic agents thought to possess psychotropic efficacy. His team was split into two units; the Anoka unit evaluated candidate compounds

---

i. For an expert demonstration of this technique, see the interview of Mr. Resistive, chapter 10, by Dr. Harold Searles.

for antipsychotic activity, and the university unit evaluated candidates for antidepressant or anti-anxiety activity. Although his office was at the university, Dr. Schiele drove out to Anoka at least once a week, sometimes more frequently. Moreover, every week all researchers from both units assembled at the university for progress reviews, updates, and, of course, gossip. He ran a happy, effective, and productive ship.

My duties as a research associate were not especially taxing. The research format was well established, and I will not describe it in detail here except to say it involved studying the antipsychotic potential of novel compounds on Anoka inpatients. Plodding, potboiler stuff indeed, but to strike pharmaceutical gold someday, you first have to do the plodding. Which I did by simply following the territory traversed by so many similar past studies: introduction regarding need, presumptive antipsychotic potential of the new compound, its toxic potential, and so on.

Dr. Schiele's Perspective

On the other hand Dr. Schiele's perspective on things psychiatric was hardly plodding. He was more astute than I realized at the time.

He was not a diagnostic devotee. Of course, our research protocols by necessity required a certain amount of, shall I say, diagnostic purity. After all, if the goal of a research investigation is to determine whether an agent demonstrates therapeutic properties, you must specify the condition in need of therapy. If the agent is deemed to have potential as an Antidepressant, you recruit Depressed subjects; if anti-anxiety properties, anxious subjects, and so on. At Anoka, it was inpatients with a chronic psychosis that was poorly responsive to standard Antipsychotic medication. Dr. Schiele did not rely on the prevailing *DSM-II* diagnostic criteria; rather, he specified that I employ what he called "physician's global judgment," both for selection and subsequent research assessments, as well as rating scales. His attitude about chronic psychosis was a bit like the Supreme Court's position on pornography: you know it when you see it. And when discussing psychiatric treatment in general, he never referred to patients by diagnosis—for example, as a "case of Depression." Instead he typically referred to individuals in terms of their misery or suffering, and how treatment needed to address "target symptoms or target behaviors."

I imagine Dr. Schiele would not have found congenial the diagnostic format later embodied in *DSM-III*, with its five axes and lists of inclusion and exclusion criteria. He never impressed me as a picky diagnostician. I now see that his diagnostic style remained a persisting influence throughout my subsequent psychiatric career. At first it took the guise of designing treatment to address symptom rather than diagnostic category. Of course, to satisfy professional and insurance standards, it was necessary to specify a formal diagnosis, so I duly filled in the blanks per protocol—not that I firmly believed in the validity of the words so set forth. Some of Skinner's credo had rubbed off on me because I had witnessed the power of his principles in action: behavior and symptoms captured the issue better than diagnosis. That is, eventually I became what might be termed a "diagnostic agnostic," although I did not advertise myself as such, of course.

The Clinical Setting: Anoka State Hospital Circa 1965

Anoka State Hospital was designed and built in the early 1900s, a time when the optimistic nineteenth-century belief in "moral therapy" treatment of severe mental illness had collapsed under the weight of increasing populations of "chronic" treatment-resistant patients. This was the unhappy story in Minnesota until the late 1950s when a progressive legislature funded the creation of a community mental health center in every county throughout the state. Moreover, the Department of Welfare director of medical services, Dr. David Vail, initiated changes to mitigate certain "dehumanizing" state hospital practices. By the time I started in 1965, the impact of these and other therapeutic concepts was obvious: the hospital census was now 850 versus 1,150 just three years before. The more passive patients were now being discharged into the community because resources were now available for placement and follow-up.

For example, I recall making discharge plans for an elderly woman whose chart number was in the 900s as opposed to contemporary chart numbers in the 15,000s, implying she had probably been admitted in the 1920s. She had been a resident of her cottage for decades and had become a de facto member of the cottage staff, with her own nook in the basement where she laundered the linens. As I listened to our discharge planning, I noticed some of the senior nursing and assistant staff looking quite sad. I realized she was their pet and now they were losing her; the cottage had been her "home" for decades. But citing the therapeutic zeitgeist of the times, I explained we had to discharge her to a group home in Minneapolis as planned. So she left, still hallucinating despite years of treatment with Antipsychotics, amid tearful good-byes, puzzled by all the fuss, not really understanding what was happening.

Nor did I. Only later, after I developed some understanding of state hospital dynamics, did I realize that it was not a lack of community resources that had blocked her discharge. Rather, much of her "treatment" consisted of the selective reinforcement of her more passive and obliging behavior. Perhaps in the early years of her stay she had been more rambunctious—records from those decades were long lost—but by now all of her assertive energies had been trained out of her.

Initially I was assigned to Cottage Five, a "mess" according to Dr. Docherty; it was the only remaining locked female unit at Anoka except for two geriatric units. His goal for me: unlock and eventually close the unit.

What constituted the "mess" was soon apparent: the rapid

downsizing of the census had sifted the more passive patients out into the community. Left behind was a cadre of more aggressive, disruptive patients who, as the hospital census shrank, constituted a growing, largely female fraction of the hospital population. What happens to such patients when they proved unmanageable on open units, as anyone who has ever worked in a state mental institution knows, is exile to locked units and the seclusion rooms therein.

My task was to stabilize things enough to unlock the unit and discharge or transfer its residents.[ii] Fortunately, I had inherited a highly motivated team as part of the "mess." By teaching team members how to accept delegated authority for treatment decisions, and with everyone working hard, within one year we were able to discharge or transfer to open units fifty-nine of the seventy patients who were present on the unit when I started in July 1965. Dr. Docherty deemed our results successful enough to permit a transfer of staff and patients to a smaller, also secure unit in a newer building. But we remained short of his ideal goal of closing the unit altogether.

By this time we realized we had exhausted the potential of our former tactics. Hard work was no longer the answer; it was time for a change. To quote from our paper:

> It was apparent that not only would the hard core [of eleven] patients prevent the unit from closing, but that the prospects of reducing the census any further were small since the [eighteen] newcomers formed a pool which had approximately equal rates of entry and exit. Furthermore, we feared that a number of the newcomers had hard core potential.[1]

---

ii. To learn more about the unit and the early teamwork required to manage it, I suggest reading our subsequent publication, noted above. Curran J, Jorud S, and Whitman N. "Unconventional Treatment of Treatment-Resistant Hospitalized Patients."

Eventually we came up with three conclusions:

1. Out-of-control (OOC) behavior, rather than "mental illness" as such, was now a problem shared by all patients
2. The very prospect of transfer or discharge tended to provoke OOC. That is, the unstable behavior was caused by separation anxiety,[iii] more specifically by Attachment Acting-out, although in our paper we did not label it as such.
3. Therefore we needed to develop a program that specifically targeted separation anxiety.

Accordingly we initiated two changes. First, we introduced a paradox. We advised newcomers that we would allow them to stay indefinitely, hoping this might undermine their acting-out ("externalizing" is the current terminology) behaviors while promoting either faster discharge or less disruptiveness. Second, we started looking for a therapeutic program specifically devoted to teaching behavioral stability.

Enter Serendipity

During the year I resumed contact with a few of my college buddies, one of whom was Fred Sheridan. In college we had played basketball together and then had gone our separate ways, he into education, I into medicine and psychiatry. Fred taught and coached at a large suburban high school for some years, then accepted an assistant principal position at North High in Minneapolis. So it happened that about the time I was struggling with program development at Anoka, he was similarly preoccupied at North.

We met after work now and then at a local watering hole, The Point, to recall over a beer or two our college and basketball adventures and to share our professional concerns. It was eerie

---

iii. See chapter 8.

to hear him describe his problems. When he talked of two groups of problem students, the withdrawn/uninvolved versus the rebellious/defiant, I found myself thinking of my problem groups: regressed/undersocialized versus impulsive/assaultive.

Now and then Fred was joined by another North High assistant principal, Richard Green, also a rising star in the Minneapolis Public School System. I recognized him from our basketball days when he played for Augsburg, another college in our conference. He was agile and fast, the sort of pesky guard who bedeviled me throughout my basketball career, lurking ready to snatch the ball away from me after a rebound. He was just as imposing now because of his intellectual rather than athletic skills. The contrast between the two of them was striking: Fred tall and boisterous and outspoken, Richard short and deliberate and intense. But it was obvious they were the best of friends.

One day, after listening to yet another account of our programmatic impasse, Richard mentioned that while researching programs to manage classroom behavior, he had come across one to mobilize and augment social behavior in chronic state hospital patients: the "token economy." He explained that the therapy was based on principles of *operant conditioning* and *contingent reinforcement* derived from the work of behavioral psychologist B. F. Skinner. He suggested I look into it.

As I listened, I remembered hearing the name "Skinner" during my college general psychology class, but nothing more—I had no recall whatsoever of his learning theory. And in retrospect from a distance of five decades, I remain convinced that nobody mentioned him during my psychiatric training at PI, which is understandable since most of my professors at that time were true believers in the existence and power of intrapsychic forces in the genesis of behavior. Or, if they recognized the influence of social forces, they did not understand them via the terminology of reinforcement theory.

True, they differed about the exact nature of the forces. A

few remained strictly Freudian. Many were in the neo-Freudian camp, as I discussed above. They recognized that the expression of intrapsychic energies was modulated by the world of extrapsychic (that is, developmental) events.[iv] Then there was the *interpersonal* concept of human behavior, espoused by the medical director of PI, Dr. Lawrence Kolb (chapter 8) and by Dr. Harold Searles (chapter 10), the amateurish demonstration of which I ignominiously displayed during my brief tenure at Manhattan State Hospital. Other professors lectured us on games theory of human interactions, while still others demonstrated family and group therapy techniques.

Moreover, in the background were a number of figures destined to completely revise the structure of American psychiatry. There was the psychoanalyst cum psychopharmacologist Dr. Ronald Fieve, who was to open the first outpatient clinic devoted to treatment of mood disorders. Also roaming the PI hallways were Drs. Robert Spitzer and Jean Endicott, who later presided at the birth of descriptive psychiatry in the form of *DSM-III;* Dr. Howard Roffwarg at brown bag seminars giving us the scoop on the new discipline of EEG sleep physiology; group therapist Dr. Jack Sheps; pediatric psychiatrist and eating disorder theorist Hilde Bruch; epidemiologists; community psychiatrists; and a host of others. And knocking on its doors was Dr. Donald Klein, destined to become emeritus professor of psychiatry at Columbia, who had just published a revolutionary paper on

---

iv. An outstanding example is the concept of "Adaptational Psychodynamics" proposed by the Hungarian psychiatrist Sandor Rado. In his view intrapsychic energy rested not in the internal interplay of Ego/Id/Superego, but in the interaction of emotion with external events. Interestingly, he revised the Aristotelian/Scholastic division of emotion from concupiscible/irascible to welfare/emergency. I was then—and remain—fascinated by his conception of emotion as an organizing principle of human behavior rather than a disorganizing one. This runs contrary to most psychological speculation, which places cognitive function in the driver's seat.

the treatment of panic with the Antidepressant imipramine.[v]

In this sense our training was truly eclectic. We residents passed the hours debating the virtues of one discipline versus another when it came to promoting mental health, such as community psychiatry versus psychopharmacology. And offstage were our professors trolling for acolytes and recruits to enlist in their respective disciplines. But regardless of theory, our professors insisted that every patient workup be grounded on three legs: *history, mental status/testing findings,* and *psychodynamic formulation* incorporating data from the first two. They insisted that no scrutiny of patients was meaningful if it was not based on an assessment of the interaction of the intrapsychic (energies and conflicts) and extrapsychic (life events). Only then could we incorporate, say, family or social or psychopharmacological considerations.

On the other hand, no one was singing the praises of Dr. Skinner, which was understandable considering his position regarding intrapsychic phenomena: not knowable, therefore not susceptible to scientific scrutiny. The organism was a "black box" that emitted behavior in response to external stimulus configurations. Thus the proper object of psychology was measurement of behaviors demonstrated by the organism and its response to a stimulus array presented to it.

So it was that Richard's suggestion fell on a blank mind—but not on deaf ears. I went to my staff with his idea and, in the absence of obvious alternatives, we investigated token-economy treatment programs for chronically hospitalized patients. We found that the literature reported such programs effective in mobilizing social skills in withdrawn and passive patients. However, by implication it seemed that even disruptive behaviors, which in our experience tended to flare up as discharge or

---

v. Klein D and Fink M. "Psychiatric Reaction Patterns to Imipramine." *American Journal of Psychiatry.* 1962 Nov; 119: 432–38. I will present in volume 2 a detailed discussion of the profound significance of his discovery.

transfer neared, might undergo socialization as well if exposed to targeted reinforcement. In other words, give patients a tool to titrate their degree of freedom by earning and spending tokens (ordinary metal washers)[vi] to ease transitions. So, after discussing the idea among ourselves and with Dr. Docherty, we designed and implemented a token economy on our closed unit.[vii]

Ways of earning tokens included working on or off the ward, neat grooming and bedding, attending activities, supervising other patients, and so on. Tokens could be spent on a private room, privileges, release from restrains or seclusion, transfer or discharge, home passes, individual therapy, candy—things of that sort. The wage or price of every activity was posted. We managed acting-out or otherwise unstable behavior by placing the miscreant on *time-out;* that is, by temporarily removing the opportunity to earn tokens, although patients could spend previously earned tokens.

The program proved to be very effective in reducing unstable, acting-out behavior. The need for seclusion rooms declined so rapidly that eventually we had the locks removed so patients could go to a seclusion room voluntarily if they wished more privacy, always in short supply on our crowded ward. After six months we closed the unit.

In our paper we presented a description and analysis of our results, including the surprising finding that response to the program was not at all related to diagnosis. On the other hand it was clear that response was directly but inversely related to

---

vi. Purchased at hardware stores in the vicinity of the hospital. After we closed the program, I turned over to the hospital's maintenance department what must have been several decades' supply of washers. Later I enjoyed a fantasy about the local association of hardware store managers at their monthly golf outing puzzling over the mysterious case of the hospital washer boom-and-bust.

vii. See also volume 2 of this series for a more extended discussion of reinforcement theory and practice.

the total months of current and prior hospitalization. Chronic hospitalization, by undermining the social repertoire, promoted chronicity. In short, a good deal of what we labeled "Chronic Schizophrenia" was actually iatrogenic; that is, the result of treatment. In our publication we included some comments on the social and cognitive dimensions of what, on the face of it, appeared to be a strictly behavioral process.[viii]

In the article we also drew attention to Winnicott's idea that acting-out behavior potentially carries within it the seeds of a reparative process by making a "claim" on the environment that, hopefully, will draw attention to the unmet needs of the disruptive party. Frequently, however, the disguised call for help backfires, accentuating the defective environmental relationship and increasing the risk that the troubled individual will become identified as a criminal or mental patient in need of institutionalization. On the other hand, we found that acting-out behavior in a token environment, muffled as it is by the "time-out" contingency, went unreinforced and tended to extinguish. Troubled patients in effect "earned" a socially sanctioned vacation, often remarking that they might as well relax since there was no opportunity to earn tokens that day. So they sloughed off, some spending what they had earned.

We also speculated that the use of seclusion previously had the paradoxical effect of actually reinforcing and encouraging unstable behavior in hallucinating patients bedeviled by the perceptual uncertainties and sensory noise generated by their psychotic experience. A seclusion room offered both privacy and

---

viii. To be fair, I must say that back then a good portion of the hospital's catchment area (the geographical area it served) was rural. On occasion a first admission might arrive already "chronic" despite no past history of hospitalization, having lived for years in farm outbuildings (the equivalent of a back ward) under the supervision of parents or relatives. Typically the admission was precipitated by the death of a parent or sale of the farmland.

a reduced environmental stimulus load. So you soon learned that if you wanted peace and quiet—or to avoid transfer—you need only provoke a fight or make a threat.

We also found that the tokens protected boundaries. The unexpressed needs that motivate acting-out behavior typically elicit burgeoning anxiety in caregivers, as any therapist or teacher or parent knows, creating risk of a reciprocal acting-out, or staff splitting. But our staffers were protected from impulsively punishing or forgiving proscribed behaviors by an established, highly visible schedule that clearly defined corrective procedures. In addition, we concluded,

> It becomes difficult for patients to coerce (via guilt) staff members into inappropriate dyadic relationships. Given the abundant and explicit opportunities for need fulfillment (freedom, privacy, predictability, and social intercourse are patient needs particularly well satisfied by a token economy), staff members are more resistant to the otherwise seductive message, "I hurt ... love me."[2]

Anoka State Hospital: Aftermath

Before moving on to a discussion of the validity of applying attachment concepts to adolescents and young adults, I will first review the lasting impact of my Anoka experiences on my professional and personal life.

Research

After eighteen months or so, Dr. Schiele let me go. Our parting was friendly. He was kind enough to arrange an interview with another research program, and several years later sent me a congratulatory note when I published a paper on the side effects of Antipsychotic medications. And later when he was asked to comment on the token economy, he was simply quoted as saying that I had not followed traditional procedure. True enough. At the time I was not offended by his decision not to keep me on. Possibly I felt it was coming.

In retrospect, I think a number of factors played a role in his decision.

For example, I clearly recall his startled surprise, the significance of which I have come to appreciate only recently, when I submitted a complete research protocol for his review. It was my initial assignment as his newbie assistant, yet here I was dropping it on his desk one week after starting. Without bragging I can say the assignment was a no-brainer, definitely a fill-in-the-blanks exercise. The design of our research strategy had been standardized years before by ECDEU, very apparent in copies of research reports published under its auspices and among the materials Dr. Schiele gave me.

I now surmise Dr. Schiele was expecting some evidence of a struggle, a rough draft perhaps accompanied by gestures of frustration, at least a silent appeal for guidance. Instead I just sat there as he reviewed the protocol, gave me a very peculiar glance, and after a short silence nodded in approval. I think things subsequently would have gone better if I had, say, first delayed a few weeks before presenting it to him, in the meantime consulting him for tips on language, things of that sort. But I didn't, and we plodded ahead and completed the study per protocol, which was eventually published.

Another factor, I now believe, was my failure to consult him as our staff struggled to manage the Cottage Five "mess." Think about it: present on campus every week was a nationally recognized clinical psychopharmacologist, known for his expertise on the research and treatment of Chronic Schizophrenia, who was not called on for help by his research associate struggling to manage such cases by the dozens. True, I had often asked other staff psychiatrists for advice because they were much more informed on community resources than I or Dr. Schiele, who had more of an academic orientation. And from time to time I discussed our unit problems, as noted above, with Fred and Richard. But never Dr. Schiele: a professional slap in the face, although I never intended it as such.

I now see that my neglect of Dr. Schiele did not reflect a low regard for his expertise but rather the expectation that the Antipsychotics of that era had little to offer in the management of chronic mental illness. By the time I arrived at Anoka, the revolution in patient care precipitated by the introduction of Thorazine ten years previously had expended its momentum. Responders had been discharged—hence the sharp decline of the hospital census—but nonresponders remained. And all of the remaining had been thoroughly exposed to one or more Antipsychotics, sometimes in horrendous doses. For example, the young woman described in our paper as Case One had not responded to 7,000 mg of Thorazine per day; that is, ten times the usual maximum therapeutic dose. Seven thousand mg per day is almost half a pound a month! And this was not considered an extreme or exceptional management technique at Anoka.

This accounts for the ECDEU research initiative and Dr. Schiele's presence at Anoka: more effective Antipsychotics were needed to treat the nonresponder pool. But my research activities had done little to revive my declining faith in the effectiveness of Antipsychotics, whether conventional or novel. No or little improvement was our usual verdict for the Anoka patients I enrolled per our research protocol. Moreover, researchers at the ECDEU conferences I attended were of the same opinion regarding their own investigations. It was clear that there was no magic bullet in the pipeline. In fact, nothing of the sort would appear until the late 1980s when the first of the "second-generation" Antipsychotics, clozapine, was marketed.

In short, both my clinical work at Cottage Five and my research work contributed to my growing belief that much of chronic mental illness was not soluble in elixir of antipsychotica. Another vehicle was needed. In this respect I guess I was prepared to listen to what Richard Green had to say about Dr.

Skinner. No doubt Dr. Schiele became aware of my apostasy as mentee began to ignore mentor; now my agnosticism was both diagnostic and therapeutic. Thus he let me go, my separation package an introduction to one of his associates in a distant state.

Clinical

However, I decided to stay at Anoka, not only because Dr. Docherty offered me a full-time position but also because I enjoyed the challenge presented by the "mess." In addition, he also arranged a Saturday consulting position at the Five County Mental Health Center in Braham, Minnesota, about seventy miles north of Anoka. This was the first of my many subsequent outpatient consulting appointments.

As an outpatient psychiatrist I enjoyed returning to the one-to-one doctor-patient format of my residency. At Anoka my professional interactions were mostly one-to-staff at conferences or one-to-group during patient meetings. Because of time constraints my one-to-one patient contacts were extremely limited: six minutes each, scheduled via a signup sheet posted every morning. It was hard to do much counseling or therapy in six minutes, although more enterprising souls were free to sign for successive unclaimed intervals. Measured against such a restriction, the one-hour appointments at an outpatient mental health clinic seemed to me a bonanza of freedom, a luxury of opportunity to observe and explore.

In particular I had an opportunity to witness the before and after of chronic mental and emotional disability and the importance of social support in its prevention and treatment. This lesson can be summarized this way: medication is helpful, social support is helpful, the combination is more helpful. Although this sharpened my awareness of the role of distrust in the genesis of mental and emotional problems, it was not until years later that I began to appreciate the connection between distrust and trauma.

I also began to suspect that the potential of conditioning to shape behavior extended beyond just our unit.

For example, as I had more time to listen to individuals struggling with addictive behaviors, the concept of selective reinforcement provided me with a clearer understanding of the role of conditioning in addiction relapse. As I will discuss more fully in volume 2, it seemed that relapse is prompted by obscure but powerful drive states ("craving") that overwhelm the option of maintaining sobriety. But relapsers frequently do not recognize that the option to resist a "slip" is absent because they have been conditioned. Their thinking is *if I did it I must have wanted to do it* rather than *I did it because I could not resist*. Which is why the first step—admission of powerlessness—is so difficult to accept and practice, and why addiction is a disease.

Relief of craving by using a substance "grooves" the neurons that support seeking and substance using, thus increasing the probability of relapse when craving returns. Relapse behavior is, in operant conditioning terminology, highly conditioned due to *negative reinforcement*.[ix] The goal of relapse prevention treatment is to teach relapsers how to recognize the drive states that signal impending loss of control and to develop habits of craving relief other than substance use. The idea is to "regroove" neurons of addicts by enlarging their "bag of tricks," so to speak.

The Publication

In the meantime, as I discussed earlier, we established the token program, the results of which we presented in our publication. One of our conclusions was that institutional chronicity—that is, Chronic Schizophrenia—was in part due to the unwitting but systematic reinforcement of acting-out as well as passive behavior. As we wrote, "Mental hospitals have made relatively normal people deviant. Correctly understood and administered, mental hospitals should be able to make deviant people nor-

---

ix. Discussed in detail in volume 2.

mal."[3] We also noted that a token program regulated acting-out behavior on the part of *both* staff and patients—on "both sides of the token" is how we put it—via its carefully designed reinforcement schedules. To use contemporary terminology, we would now say that a token economy establishes a boundary that protects both staff and patients from entangling relationships.

Finally, we drew attention to Winnicott's concept of acting-out behavior as a claim on the environment signifying unmet security needs.

In this way the defective relationship with the environment—Winnicott's notion of what causes the "bent "ego commonly seen in personality disorders—will hopefully be corrected by the environment taking notice of the individual and responding to his needs. Too often, however, this repair process backfires, the defective relationship is magnified, and the individual incurs greater risk of assuming the role of a mental patient or criminal in an institution.[4]

Our paper attracted zero interest. Some years ago I did a citation search and found only six. In large part this was due to its obscure title—"Unconventional Treatment of Treatment-Resistant Hospitalized Patients"—an obscurity for which I alone take credit. I did not realize the importance of including key search items in a publication title no matter how inelegant the phrasing: for example, "Antipsychotic Resistance Responds to Token Economy" or "Token Economy Mitigates Acting-out Issues" or even "Attachment Issues? Think of a Token Economy!" This was a serious miscue on my part for I believe some of the insights therein were—and still are—highly relevant to the management of individuals confined to treatment, residential, and correction facilities.

Moreover, there was little interest in the notion that the treatment of chronic mental illness was in need of an "unconventional" approach. The conventional approach—that is, Antipsychotic medication—was working just fine. All that was needed was a variant more effective with nonresponders or partial responders, the psychiatric equivalent of Ehrlich's "magic bullet"; thus the ECDEU initiative and Dr. Schiele. Psychopharmacologists chased this phantom for decades with merely marginal success. Only in the last ten years or so have researchers come to appreciate that the impoverished social repertoire that is part of chronic mental disability can be ameliorated with therapeutic strategies specifically designed to build social and cognitive skills in first-episode psychosis.[5] This is precisely what we discovered some forty years ago.

Personal

If the report of our experiences evoked no response, the opposite was true for me. Witnessing the power of selective reinforcement to modify behavior had a profound and lasting personal impact. It led me to question the idea of freedom, something I had never seriously examined before. Whereas I had always felt like I was a free agent, in control of my choices, now I began to consider if what seemed like a free choice was actually under the control of external, unperceived—but not necessarily malevolent—agencies. I wondered if it is when we feel most free that we are likely to be the most influenced.

I see now that I began to question my politics, unthinkingly liberal until I started working at the hospital. Although I cannot recall any discussion of politics at home during my childhood, there was no misunderstanding of Dad's pro-union sentiments. He was treasurer of the Saint Paul Firefighters Relief Association. As a kid I remember him sitting in the dining room typing out pension checks to widows and retirees. When the legislature was in session, he was always lobbying at the state capital on behalf of firefighters. At Christmas he would load a couple of cases of whiskey into the backseat of our beat-up Chevy, plump me up front, and then, consulting a list of legislators, drive house to house with me running up to deliver a bottle at each front door. My introduction to politics.

My older brother alleges that during World War II Hubert Humphrey, then a rising figure in the Democratic-Farmer-Labor party, once came to our house asking Dad to sign on to a campaign to promote the war effort by addressing unions, urging them not to strike war plants. During my ditchdigger summers with the Saint Paul Water Department, although I was not required to join the union, I benefitted from union wage contrasts. In college I was thoroughly scandalized when my political science professor mentored *both* the Young Democratic and the Young Republican clubs. How could he?

But observing the devastating effects of the selective reinforcement of passive and compliant got me rethinking the consequences of the Great Society and similar social welfare programs of the 1960s, especially those that did not expect an exchange for benefits rendered.

In contrast, pension and retirement programs provide benefits for services previously rendered. The Civilian Conservation Corps (CCC) program of the 1930s exchanged a salary for work, a large portion of which was directly remitted to worker families. Several years ago I toured Bandelier National Monument in New Mexico, which featured Ancestral Pueblo Period habitat and customs. Also featured was a well-preserved, sturdy auditorium built eight decades before by CCC laborers, in effect a cultural monument as well. As might be expected, the gift shop displayed reproductions of Pueblo artifacts and books about Pueblo society. Also on prominent display were pictures, tools, journals, and histories about the young men who built the park structures and trails. Obviously they had taken great pride and care in their work, as no doubt had the Pueblo centuries before in theirs. I can imagine contemporary fathers and grandfathers later touring the park with their families, announcing with pride, "I built that."

But if there is no exchange, can there be any self-respect? Bowery missionaries are said to have their down-and-out clientele first partake of spiritual nourishment before caloric. Here were immortal souls to be saved. Do our social programs convey similar respect for the humanity and self-esteem of those they serve? Might they even create a sense of entitlement?

I now realize my witnessing the power of selective reinforcement changed more than my political orientation. I developed a greater respect for patient autonomy—perhaps not really surprising in retrospect, since autonomy is a bedrock principle of conservative theory. I now understand more clearly how I instinctively managed certain involuntarily hospitalized patients after I entered private practice in the 1970s.

In that era the county probate court, in response to a petition alleging mental illness, might issue an order permitting the involuntary hospitalization and examination of the alleged mentally ill individual. The order would also appoint a county attorney to represent the petitioner, a public defender to represent the proposed patient, a hospital willing to accept him or her for examination only, and a hearing date usually six or seven days hence. Occasionally the hospital where I had attending privileges accepted such patients and assigned their care to me since I was then the most junior psychiatrist. My role, as well as that of the psychiatric unit staff, was simply to observe and record behavior. Other than necessary medical interventions, no treatment was authorized except in the case of an emergency, for which I was to make a separate petition.

However, the court order did not specifically preclude my giving advice or instruction to the involuntarily detained. Now what is most interesting to me, as I recall this minor clinical adventure some forty years later, is that from the very first I instructed the detainees in how to game the system. I told them they were in the hospital because "people" though they were "crazy." Also, since everything they said or did would be charted, and the chart would be part of the evidence at their hearing, it would be to their advantage not to look or talk "crazy." In other words *be nice, follow the rules, cooperate with your attorney, be courteous to the judge, don't say anything at your hearing unless in response to a question from the judge or one of the attorneys, agree with follow-up treatment recommendations,* and so on. I think I was just replaying the stance we had previously originated at Anoka. That is, if a patient was able to accumulate, legitimately or otherwise, a stash of tokens sufficient to purchase discharge, this was tangible clinical evidence of enough impulse control and foresight to qualify for discharge. Similarly, if a detainee was able to follow, remember, and cooperate after such a limited exposure to instruction, this would likely mitigate and perhaps even remove any need for involuntary treatment.

Now some readers might object to the idea of teaching someone, perhaps anyone, how to game the system. Well, readers, let's get real here. This is how society flourishes: by cooperation. So you learn the rules. Eventually you learn that the rules always change. Then hopefully you will discover (exploit? game?) the nooks and crevices that permit autonomy without injuring society: for example, writing a book that ponders the past while expressing hope for the future, or volunteering for a service organization, or, as I did above and with Mr. POP (chapter 10), manipulating (educating) individuals in such a manner that they are able to escape being trapped by society. In fact, as I review the case studies I present in this book, I now realize that the notion of learning adaptive skills is one of the threads that stitches the book together.

My advocacy did precipitate some negative feedback, but not from the probate court as you might expect. I was investigated by a hospital committee in response to a complaint by the nursing staff that I did not make final visits to those patients who had been committed to Anoka. I went before the committee to review my management tactics, noting that a finding of commitment signaled a learning failure; therefore a follow-up was pointless. At the end of my discourse the committee chair, his eyes glazed, said they would take the matter under advisement. I never heard from the committee again.

My days at Anoka ended ingloriously when I was suspended for insubordination.

In later 1967, Dr. Docherty resigned to enter private practice. Dr. Guido Schynoll, a highly qualified board certified psychiatrist, took his place as medical director. When he learned of my Saturday work at the Five County Mental Health Center, he ordered me to resign my consulting position there, which I did. I gathered he viewed it as double-dipping, something that apparently had not troubled Dr. Docherty. Perhaps Dr. Schynoll wanted me to save my energies for the hospital, for he later asked if I would fill the vacant position of assistant medical director. I declined. I think the stress and pressure of inpatient psychiatry were starting to burn me out. More responsibility was unthinkable.

Nonetheless we got along well enough until that September when my nemesis arrived at the hospital in the person of "Winston."

I recall Winston with great clarity these decades later, first of all because of the unique circumstances of his admission, secondly because of his equally unique behavior after admission. He was an engineer by education, an executive by profession. His dress and demeanor reflected his former status: white shirt, dark tie, suit, well-shined shoes, grave, deliberate, impeccably polite, but quietly delusional. He preferred solitude, and even in the midst of the full sunshine and oppressive humidity of a Minnesota summer would sit in full fig for hours on a garden bench, hands folded over his cane, quietly muttering the while.

He had been employed by a California defense contractor and had been let go, possibly because of mental/emotional disability: it was never clear. Now in his forties, single and retired, he had returned to Minneapolis and rented an apartment opposite St. Olaf's, a downtown church, the site of the forthcoming wedding of a relative of Vice-President Humphrey, who was planning to attend, Secret Service in tow. Observing from his window all of the ensuring celebrity and security fussing, Winston concluded it was a cover-up for a stakeout by foreign agents after his defense know-how. He called the police to report that he was under a threat and asked for protection. When the officers heard his story, they took him to Minneapolis General Hospital, where he was detained, observed, and committed.

We quickly concluded he was harmless. The plan was to start him on a low dose of Antipsychotics, have him stay until the wedding furor had passed, and then discharge him back to his apartment with follow-up at MGH's outpatient psychiatry clinic. He represented no danger, so we soon advanced his privilege status to off-campus.

One fine day, dressed in his usual garb he went for a stroll into Anoka. On the way he was picked up by two local teenage girls who, no doubt, were bored and seeking diversion. I imagine they quickly realized what a strange bird they had on their hands and took him to the police, who returned him to the campus. In the meantime Dr. Schynoll received a call from the civic authorities alleging that Winston had threatened the girls. He then relayed the call to me, recommending I increase Winston's Antipsychotic medication.

Based on my extensive knowledge of both Winston and the Anoka community's adolescent females' social norms and behavior—derived from my prior locked unit experiences—I demurred, suggesting the young ladies posed a more likely threat scenario than he did, and that if anyone needed treatment, it was they, not him. Dr. Schynoll repeated his statement, now more an order than a recommendation. Again I refused, suggesting the proper protocol would be for him to come to the cottage himself, perform a consultation, and make recommendations, if any. A few hours later his secretary, Pat Voss, delivered a notice of suspension for three weeks without pay because of insubordination. Upon my return to duty I was to report to Dr. Schynoll for further instructions.

To be frank, a three-week vacation in the midst of a glorious Minnesota autumn, whether enforced or voluntary, is delightful. So I built a patio fence, played golf, was present at the birth of my youngest daughter ... and one morning noted that my hair was turning gray.

Then, having done my time, I duly reported as directed. Pat Voss, who knew me well, seemed surprised when I announced I was there for my "appointment." There was no appointment on Dr. Schynoll's calendar. In fact he was not even in the office, and, indeed, she was not even sure he was on campus. Now this was strange stuff, for she had typed his reprimand and delivered it herself. I had entered a Twilight Zone in which my suspension had never happened. I left his office and drove home. Whether I ever returned to my office to retrieve my goods I can't recall. I'm not even sure I ever submitted a formal letter of resignation.

My next clear recollection—days or weeks later, I'm not sure—is of MGH director of psychiatry Dr. William Jepson asking me, "What took you so long?" I must have wrangled a job interview because soon I was working as a staff psychiatrist in the outpatient department at the hospital. I think his comment meant what had taken me so long to accept: that Anoka was grinding me down and that I was not going to change things at the hospital but vice versa. It's not that I had collapsed into a fugue state; rather, the shock of my phantom "appointment" collapsed my denial about the stress of working at Anoka and served to mobilize escape planning. I think Dr. Jepson was commenting on my denial defenses.

Yet, stress of work or not, I dearly wish now I had done things differently with Dr. Schynoll, but that would have required me not to have been so self-righteous and stubborn. I should have been more deferential, more "political." I should have listened, said I would look into it, and then investigated

Early Origins

and dictated a note. If there had been no notable change in Winston's adjustment, as I had suspected, nonetheless I should have fiddled with his medications and management planning; for example, perhaps ordering more observation before commencing a discharge plan. Moreover, the chances were Dr. Schynoll would promptly forget about the incident because he knew I was reliable. And, if he inquired later, that would have been the time to relate my findings and my surmise about what had actually happened. Perhaps at the time I had been seduced by Dr. Schiele's admonition to treat symptom rather than diagnosis, but what symptom? Submitting to the beguiling patter of two bored delinquents?

I think I did learn something from the experience because, while at MGH and later in private practice, and still later when I returned to state hospital work (see Mr. POP, chapter 10), I was more adept in dealing with authority. For example, about six months after I was hired at General we all received a lengthy survey soliciting our opinion of hospital management. At first I was annoyed, even furious about what seemed like a gratuitous imposition. *Didn't they understand how busy I was, what a waste of my precious time and energy?* Then I reconsidered. In contrast to Anoka, this was an organization that cared about what its employees thought, and really wanted feedback about its performance. So I thoughtfully completed the questionnaire. Four-plus decades later I'm happy to say that this enlightened administrative attitude is still reflected in the performance and standing of Minneapolis General's successor, Hennepin County Medical Center.

And it was reflected in the quality, dedication, and energy of my coworkers. Not that we didn't gripe and complain, but everyone for the most part worked hard and didn't slough off in the midst of the inevitable deluge of patients that will flood any inner-city public hospital. I was stationed in the emergency room, my "office" a poorly ventilated cubicle about twenty feet away from the decrepit sliding doors of the entrance through which strolled, staggered, and rolled a wash of patients to be sorted and referred on. I had no formal schedule and was sometimes overwhelmed by patients waiting to be seen and evaluated. At all times my cubicle was open to the draft that the groaning sliding door slowly but unsuccessfully labored to contain, so we sweltered or froze with the seasons. Standard garb in the winter included overshoes, coats, and gloves. In a strange sort of way it was hilarious, but how else could we have coped?

There were other responsibilities. I was on call for psychiatry consultations on inpatient neurology, an excellent preparation for my forthcoming psychiatry board exams. Also, twice a week I worked in the outpatient psychiatry medication clinic on the seventh floor of nearby Harrington Hall, a former nurses' dormitory. I saw fifteen or twenty patients each time with the able assistance of an experienced psychiatric nurse who knew them quite well and vetted their problems in advance. And each morning the unit director led the staff in a review of new cases to evaluate psychological test results, diagnosis, and treatment. On occasion I was assigned a patient to follow, one of which was Rebecca, whom I will discuss in chapter 8.

6

Later Origins

Origin #3: The Return of Dr. Sheridan and His Idea of "Affective Interference"

In 1970 I resigned from MGH to join a small private-practice group of psychiatrists and neurologists as well as the staff of Abbott-Northwestern Hospital, also in Minneapolis. The great majority of our clientele was adult, occasionally young adult. I saw very few adolescents because the health maintenance organizations (HMOs) of that era dominated referral patterns, shunting youngsters to credentialed adolescent psychiatrists and therapists. My interest in Winnicott slipped into storage as I struggled to assimilate the culture of private practice, a world not especially receptive to innovation. So I trod the standard byways of psychiatric diagnosis and treatment, with particularly decreasing enthusiasm when it came to the management of Depression, which I will discuss in chapter 9. Then in 1983 a phone call changed my path and I began my return to the world of adolescent disability.

It was Fred Sheridan calling, not only as lifelong and amusing friend but also as one professional to another. And it was now Fred Sheridan, PhD, principal of Work Opportunities

Center (WOC), the largest of several Minneapolis high school dropout programs. Under the four years of his leadership it had gained national recognition and served as a model for similar programs in Texas and Oregon. Moreover, he had the full support of Richard, now Richard Green, PhD, Harvard graduate and superintendent of Minneapolis Public Schools.[i]

As we chatted it became clear he was a natural fit in his position; he had a warm spot for the distrustful, challenging adolescents who ended up on the WOC doorstep. In such argumentative goof-offs he recognized a spirit akin to his own younger self. I think he intuitively responded to their unmet needs, an instinctive practitioner of Winnicott's notion of acting-out behavior as a claim on the environment.

Eventually he came to the reason for his call. Would I assist him in the further development of WOC's program of dropout remediation? I was intrigued and wanted to hear more, so after fifteen years we again convened at The Point, where I learned about his reformulation of the "dropout equation."

The Dropout Equation: A Third Component

He explained that the education literature presumed the student who was learning was unlikely to leave school except for a clear, self-evident reason such as physical illness, financial necessity, or fear of gangs. Otherwise the accepted cause of dropping out was academic underperformance—"cognitive interference." Emotional factors such as low self-esteem and powerlessness were either ignored or dismissed as an "attitude problem." Hence the traditional "dropout equation":

$$\text{Cognitive interference} \rightarrow \text{Dropping out}$$

---

[i]. In 1988 Dr. Green was appointed Chancellor of New York City Public Schools. Sadly, he died of asthma in May 1989, a tragic loss for his family, New York City, and all education.

But his WOC experience did not support tradition. The WOC program of voluntary learning contracts, mastery teaching, peer support groups, frequent student staffing, and individual student assessment and instruction was not enough. Some youngsters continued to fail despite good effort, and eventually would give up and drop out. Yes, they did indeed demonstrate interference, but he had become convinced the interference was not only cognitive but "affective" as well. To describe his insight, he had coined the label "Affective Interference."

As (I now surmise) he saw it, hyperactive emotions—fear or anger or anxiety, he wasn't sure—short circuit cognitive processing. Learning fizzles out. Briefly:

Affective interference →
Cognitive interference →
Dropping out

He had a hunch that certain youngsters could not learn because of anxiety and fear, sometimes apparent, sometimes quite disguised. He wondered if at times the emotional turmoil of some students would be so hidden that they themselves would not be at all aware of its existence. Youngsters with such hidden conflict would be likely to lack insight into the motives for their behavior. Therefore, they would have difficulty explaining their actions if their affective disability caused them to drop out. This would account for the high percentage of "don't know" responders in surveys studying the motivation of dropouts. Recalling my discussion of Winnicott years earlier, he wondered whether other kids might express their conflicts via acting-out behavior—what did I think?

It was well known that in the early grades some youngsters will be visibly emotionally activated. Fear or anger is apparent, sometimes disruptive. Experienced teachers are prepared to recognize and adjust the task to the student, or solicit assistance from the child's sponsors, or refer for counseling, or some combination thereof depending on the circumstances. But in his view, not all emotional activation was overt. Some remains underground behind a mask of withdrawal and underperformance, and is misdiagnosed as a cognitive or "attitude" issue (e.g., Dyllen). Fred speculated the dropping out starts at this point. Only later does what began as emotional dropping out become tangible, visible dropout behavior. Kids have learned to hate learning.

He summarized the situation with the dictum that will serve as an aphorism for volume 2: "The question is never *are they learning?* The question is always *what are they learning?*"[ii]

Now a rising star within the system, Fred was encouraged to present his reforms, together with a more fully developed theory of Affective Interference, in a grant application to the U.S. Department of Education. Would I sign on as a consultant to provide the theory to buttress the practice? His request was impossible to resist. So I signed on.

My adventures as an education consultant and coauthor of an unsuccessful federal grant application more properly belong in volume 2 of this series, which focuses on the preven-

---

ii. Fred, of course, had in mind primarily the adolescent brain when he formulated this dictum. However, some fifty years later we now realize it is likely that learning begins prepartum as the fetal brain is activated through exposure to maternal neurohormones and neurotransmitters, most certainly postpartum. Researchers now find evidence that the quality of maternal care in the earliest weeks of life influences the child's subsequent attachment and behavior style. Porcerilli JH et al. "Defensive Mechanisms of Pregnant Mothers Predicts Attachment Security, Social-Emotional Competence, and Behavior Problems in Their Toddlers." *American Journal of Psychiatry*. 2016;173 (2): 138–46. Cf. also related editorials: Perry J. "Maternal Defense Mechanisms Influence Infant Development." *American Journal of Psychiatry*. 2016;173 (2): 99–100; Chaudron L. "Mothers, Babies, Depression, and Medications: Understanding the Complex Interplay of Illness and Treatment on Neonatal Symptoms." *American Journal of Psychiatry*. 2016;173 (2): 102.

tion of Attachment Disability, rather than its identification and remediation, the concerns of this volume. Here I can say, however, that the experience heightened my awareness of a problem then bedeviling education, one that continues to date: the high rates of adolescent dropping out. And I became intrigued by Dr. Sheridan's notion of "Affective Interference." What did it involve?

Origin #4: I Learn Active Intervention Therapy Techniques

I should place "private practice" in quotes since mine was beginning to vanish. I had left my group to open a solo private practice in 1978, but by the mid-1980s referrals were dwindling. I recall on one occasion returning from a vacation to find only three appointments booked for the entire week. Only occasionally would a patient arrive having been re-referred by my former partners. And the iron grip of HMO treatment authorization was even tighter, especially for psychiatrists, and most especially for psychiatrists utilizing psychotherapy. Our role in the HMO world was to prescribe. If therapy was needed, an abundance of (less expensive) therapists was available in every neighborhood, suburb, town, hamlet—in fact, every rural crossroads, it seemed. To survive I had to widen my scope.

One option was to close my office and work full time at an HMO, not an appetizing prospect in view of my prior encounters with the ways of bureaucracy, even when adroitly managed at Minneapolis General years before. I was too independent, too given to snap decisions, too accustomed to running my own show to comfortably survive in an organization. Besides, the HMO as a strategy of cost control was merely an idea, a model without a proven technology. As costs continued to escalate, so did mission changes and reorganizations and restructurings and layoffs. Unless you were part of upper-level management, the prospect of sustained employment was iffy.

Moreover, at the age of fifty I still lacked the patience and political skill to survive while working within the system. For better or (usually) for worse, I was too outspoken or not serious enough. Better to enjoy the system at a distance, with only a peripheral connection. Now I must say that such wisdom is only recently realized, cognitively speaking. Back then it was strictly an intuitive—but quite accurate—assessment. I had gotten along quite well with Fred because we were both tall, uncomfortably perceptive loudmouths, although he was by far the better politician.

Consequently I interviewed for part-time consulting positions at community mental health centers both in Minnesota and Wisconsin. Eventually I began working at the Lakeland Mental Health Center in Fergus Falls, Minnesota, some 180 miles northwest of the Twin Cities. This was a very well-run organization with a cadre of experienced psychiatrists, therapists, and psychologists.

I enjoyed the work and even the drive because the geography and vistas of Northwestern Minnesota are both restful and intriguing, giving you time to ponder the history of the region, the state, and your place in them. For example, just outside of Fergus Falls is the southern margin of Glacial Lake Agassiz formed, twelve thousand years ago from glacier melt. The ancient lakebed is absolutely flat. Drive to a crossroads in the midst of it, and you can see to the horizon in all directions. Perspective vanishes. On a muggy, silent hot July noon, the occasional farm building or tree in the far distance seems to hang suspended on a vast stage between cloudless sky and endless field. Or visit the shuttered small country churches that dot the area with their adjacent cemeteries, all carefully maintained, and examine the pioneer graves, still occasionally remembered with fresh bouquets, a connection to the past.

I gather my name began to circulate on the mental health network because eventually I received unsolicited offers to consult at other facilities, some closer to home, two of which I accepted. I had successfully developed a second part-time career, one that enabled me to maintain my private practice. To date, some twenty-nine years later, I have consulted at more than fifteen private and community mental health clinics, plus two hospitals: St. Peter Regional Treatment Center, St. Peter, Minnesota (1988–91), and Mayo Clinic Health Systems, Austin, Minnesota (2000–2002, 2005–14).

In the meantime I got to know well a Lakeland husband and wife PhD couple, Ed and Mary Schmidt, both experienced therapists and behavior analysts. In addition to testing and working with the usual mental health center clientele, both had a special interest in the assessment and management of developmentally disabled (DD) individuals. We frequently served the same clients and therefore needed to share information and observations, mine from my office consultations, theirs from both their office and outreach consultations to the staff of area DD group homes. It was a new experience.

To backtrack a bit to my residency training, as I mentioned earlier, among the professors roaming the PI halls trolling for acolytes to sign on to their specialty interest were a few community psychiatry advocates. Perhaps I sat in on a few lectures or conferences; I can't remember. For sure, however, I did not go on field trips as did one or two of my peers. But at Anoka I actually tiptoed cautiously into the community psychiatry mainstream of that era by making a few home visits to discharged patients. I soon realized I had nothing to offer. One-to-one psychotherapy, the only arrow in my therapeutic quiver, was not what these struggling dischargees needed. They needed community support, the mobilization of which was the proper task of community psychiatry, an insight that escaped me for years until I began to work with the Schmidts. Then I had the pleasure of observing community support in action.

This was Ed's specialty. It took the form of on-site group home consultations with staff who called to report difficulty managing resident problem behaviors: for example, unprovoked aggressiveness, poor compliance with staff directives and rules, things of that sort. At a typical visit he would interview the staff, inventory the problem behaviors, and then have the staff start a day-by-day—sometimes even shift-by-shift—frequency count of each item on the inventory. After a few weeks he would return to inspect the tallies, looking for patterns that suggested occult reinforcement at work, perhaps subtle provocations by bored or troubled residents seeking an opportunity to beef to the staff, escape from participating in an activity, or manage a boundary violation. If he spotted a pattern, he might interview either resident or staff to get some idea of the dynamics involved—not infrequently a variation of my old Anoka nemesis, separation anxiety—and then devise a behavior change strategy for staff and resident to modify the presumptive *reinforcing stimuli* (see volume 2 for a more detailed discussion of reinforcement theory).

One of the more remarkable features of this routine was that on occasion the very charting of problem behaviors seemed to evaporate them. The tally would slope off and eventually disappear. Ed's hunch was that staff responding to a problem simply by recording it interrupted a prior staff behavior that was ostensibly designed to manage the problem but that, in fact, possessed hidden reinforcing qualities. This was an intriguing concept. On another level it seem to revive Winnicott's notion of acting-out as a disguised plea for help.

I have found Ed's analysis helpful in my work with adolescents troubled by obsessive thoughts. I suggest they begin a day-by-day frequency count, then return in a few weeks to review it with me. Typically the obsession count tails off, or if the thoughts are still present to a certain degree they are less troublesome. What is happening here? I suspect that an emotionally charged self-critical mental assessment—*Why can't I stop thinking this way?*—has been replaced by an emotionally neutral physical act devoid of reinforcing properties. And the obsessive thinking withers away.

Mary's work with DD and other clients was more office based. During the years we worked together, I gradually realized that effective therapy consisted of more than just attentive listening occasionally leavened with a timely interpretation. If indicated, she could change her therapeutic style from passive processing to active intervention. Let me explain why this came as a bit of a (revitalizing) shock.

As I mentioned before, as residents we were taught that a competent patient assessment rested on three legs: *historical data,* either directly elicited or collateral, *mental status/testing,* and *psychodynamic formulation.* Three legs to support a base, upon which was to be erected the structure of treatment. Now, the unexamined assumption amid this therapeutic apparatus was that "treatment" = psychodynamic psychotherapy. Which made a lot of sense to us—well, most of us, since among us there lurked fledging community psychiatrists, psychopharmacologists, and other skeptics or visionaries, depending how you look at it. At least I bought it, as I think did most of my colleagues, since I recall that we all labored to learn psychotherapy skills.

Although subject to increasing questions of its relevance, psychoanalysis remained the dominant therapeutic model of early 1960s psychiatry: active patient, passive inward analyst. In fact it was part of the popular culture, a favorite subject of *New Yorker* cartoonists. Indeed, from time to time the magazine ran a contest inviting readers to submit a caption for a stereotyped rendering of patient on couch, bearded therapist behind, pen and notebook in hand, presumably awake. Thus it is really no surprise that our psychotherapeutic training was based on the psychoanalytic model of therapy, since most of our professors were graduates of recognized psychoanalytic institutes. So we learned to practice a more or less passive, listening style, most certainly one devoid of assertive intervention except for emergent situations. It was startling, therefore, when during a lecture Dr. Bruch firmly advised us not to tolerate verbal abuse from adolescents or their parents. It was even more startling to see and hear her model how she vigorously admonished them to be more respectful. "You must not tolerate disrespect, otherwise you lose credibility ... it is just common sense!" We were not to be unreactive robots.

Well, Dr. Mary was certainly not an unreactive robot. Her clients and patients, although not notably abusive, needed intervention because of other issues such as blaming, not listening to feedback, endless complaints, rambling, and so on. In short they needed instruction on how to make use of the interview process, how to learn from the experience, and how to generalize it to other interpersonal situations. Some of the intervention techniques I learned from her, and from other therapists during subsequent consulting gigs, include at a minimum:

- Requesting that content-impoverished terms such as "depression" or "upset" be replaced by specifics
- Replacing "should" thinking with "need" thinking
- Interrupting monologues by requesting a summary statement of six words or fewer
- Requesting that my answer to a question be repeated
- Not allowing apologies for—and insisting on ownership of—"not nice" thoughts and feelings
- Redirecting "victim" thinking and speech

I will discuss these and others at greater length in subsequent chapters. The point here is that I began to incorporate such interventions into my office practice. I believe I used them first during my work with injured workers in the later 1980s, certainly during the 1990s, and definitely in the subsequent decade when adolescent referrals resumed.

A final word about Dr. Mary. While she did come across as no-nonsense and direct, certainly not given to enveloping her patients with a spurious hand-holding benevolence, she yet was warm and humorous and flexible and patient. And she was a realist, which I can best portray with a vignette.

Dr. Ed was third generation of a family entertainment business that regularly traveled a summer circuit of county fairs, small-town celebrations, and farm festivals across Minnesota and the Dakotas. Ed's family had taken pains to run an honest, inexpensive, and well-supervised operation; hence they were welcomed by local businessmen, police, and sheriffs because of their good reputation. By the time I met the Dr. Schmidts, they were taking summer leave to run the business, Ed supervising the rides, Mary the concessions.

After I left Lakeland, I tracked their schedule and visited them if I was consulting at a nearby clinic. One summer my wife and I and her sister decided to spend a few days driving around southeastern Minnesota to enjoy its driftless geography, so-called because it had not been scourged of features during the most recent glacial epoch. Rather than an unending vista of table farmland, the area features winding roads snaking from ridge to ridge and valley to valley, a feast for the eye but unsettling to the sensitive stomach, very reminiscent of West Virginia. As it happened the Schmidts were working a local county fair in the region, so we decided to visit.

It was a weekday afternoon and business was slow. Ed was working on a ride, so we passed the time chatting with Mary. After a while my sister-in-law wandered away to examine the deserted concession booths, one of which was a kiddie attraction of plastic ducks bobbing around a flowing water trough. Since each duck contained a hidden prize, the attraction was that every tyke would be a winner. Somewhat bored, after a few minutes she decided to run the booth—my sister-in-law is of the adventurous sort—barking out, "DUCKY, DUCKY, DUCKY, EVERYONE A WINNAH, EVERYONE A WINNAH, DUCKY, DUCKY, DUCKY," and so on. Well, she began to attract an audience of mothers with little kids who wanted to play and selected little duckies to claim a prize. My sister-in-law, now panicking, came running over to Mary: what were the rules for awarding prizes? Mary just laughed: "It's like life. There are no rules."

In other words, you can live by the rules, but that does not always mean you will achieve commensurate success. This is not unlike the gospel parable of the laborers in the vineyard,[iii] which had always impressed me as a tough message. So then and for years later I had to wonder what insights motivated Dr. Mary to make it a part of her therapeutic strategy, given the likelihood that a majority of her patients no doubt felt defeated by a lack of satisfaction in their lives despite trying to play by the rules as best they could. Wasn't this a cruelty?

But as I subsequently worked with my patients I came to understand her posture: if you live by the rules, at some point you must take ownership of the life the rules dictate. Unless you accept responsibility, sooner or later it will feel like you are living just to make someone else happy—a parent or wife or employer or friends, or the IRS, or even the Almighty. Eventually you end up feeling burned out at best, perhaps even "depressed," at risk of becoming a user/abuser of substances. So you seek "help." And "help," while it might include caressing your fevered brow and wiping away your tears, *must* also lead you to reconsider an unarticulated super-rule that dominates your life: *if I follow the rules I will be happy.* In short "help" includes a frank, not always comfortable assessment of the consequences of rule following, what in this book I call *clarification* (see chapter 11).[iv]

With the help of her realism I began to develop a repertoire

---

iii. Matthew 20:1–16.

iv. More recently I have begun to wonder if she was responding to changes in our culture's social character, one that relies less on rituals and rules than on crowd sentiments, the gist of which is an anxious preoccupation with social conformity. See volume 2.

of more active therapeutic interventions. This was to be very helpful when, later in my career as referral patterns changed, I once again treated adolescents, many of whom arrived in my office quite preoccupied with and ambivalent about rules: they longed for the lost security of childhood rules, yet felt ignored and demeaned when expected to live by them. It was always interesting to encounter a youngster who, typically in the presence of a parent, would announce, "I don't want to be here!" To which I would respond, "Well, why did you come? Do you always do what you are told?" Then the fun would begin (to be continued in chapter 10).

To be sure, this change was gradual, not immediately realized. In the meanwhile I tracked Fred's idea of "Affective Interference."

Origin #5: "Affective Interference" Pursued

Despite our failed grant initiative of 1983, I remained intrigued by Fred's idea of Affective Interference. Presumably the promise of certain youngsters of otherwise adequate intellectual skills was endangered by emotional/psychological dysfunction of some sort. If so, what was it?

I could not rely on data from direct observation of troubled students because so few of my patients, whether in private practice or consulting, were adolescents. It was not until 1993 that I began to see even a few adolescents again, and not in any number until 2000 or so. After years of unsuccessful attempts to be credentialed by local health care insurers as a provider of adolescent services, the winds shifted. Parents and sponsors started calling for appointments. The official reason for my previous rebuffs was usually something like "We have sufficient adolescent provider services in your community." I suspected the actual reason was that I was not boarded in adolescent psychiatry. But now not only was I squeaky clean, but even national insurers were calling on me to sign on to their provider roster.

Happy to finally be among the elect, I decided to attend a lecture on adolescent issues to reconnect with local psychiatrists and therapists. Surveying the attendees I recognized a number of nurses and therapists from my Abbott-Northwestern days. Afterward we enjoyed a lively conversation, recalling some of our clinical adventures, particularly "Bob."[v] I then noted I had recognized only one other adolescent psychiatrist. Where were the others? Their answer was interesting. The HMOs again were at work, now clamping down on lengthy adolescent inpatient hospitalizations, which—no surprise here—certain doctors had been exploiting to maximize income, forcing them to focus more on outpatient treatment. Consequently a few had moved to states with less stringent HMO supervision, or to escape the demands of evening and weekend hours that are part of treating adolescents and their families in the office. Others had stopped seeing adolescents because they were too difficult and unruly to

---

v. He was a fellow in his twenties, unquestionably Schizoaffective, who had cycled through our inpatient unit a number of times, especially memorable because of his massive build, his intense delusions, and his clinging widowed mother. She would call the nurses several times at night worried about how he was doing. She proved impossible to reassure, exhausting the patience and consuming the energy of the night staff. Finally at conference one day I suggested that we reverse the dialogue by calling her every hour throughout the night to give her an update. After two nights of this she finally said, "I get the message," and her calls stopped. Interestingly, he never again was hospitalized. At follow-up he finally accepted the need to stay on his medications, also to move out. Years later, one of the nurses reported, she happened to meet him while shopping. Totally charming and off medications, he was chagrined and amazed to recall how real his paranoid thinking had seemed. Thinking about Bob now, it is obvious in retrospect that he was deeply entangled with his mother and that she was literally "driving him nuts." By accident we had stumbled upon the definitive treatment.

manage outside of the hospital. In brief there was now a local shortage of credentialed child and adolescent psychiatrists.[vi]

Only when I had the benefit of this additional clinical experience did I begin to realize the role of loss *complicated by abandonment* in the development of Attachment Disability. Moreover, up to that point I was blinded by the traditional but narrow view of attachment dysfunction as a feature of early childhood only. Of course, as I hope I have illustrated with numerous examples, the truth of the matter is that attachment disability can strike at any time in life because the possibility of trauma is ever present. Moreover, because it wounds the capacity to trust, it can promote lifetime vulnerability to dysfunctional personal and workplace relationships and maladaptive learning.

But this insight escaped me until later. In the meantime, given the absence of clinical material, I returned to a project that had gripped me for years: constructing a master theory of human behavior, a general field theory, so to speak. My college abnormal psychology professor, Brother Julius, inspired this ambition, as I described in the preface, starting me on the road to becoming a psychiatrist—a journey of detours and blind ends but never boredom—that I am still traveling today. I think this book represents a destination of sorts.[vii]

Given Fred's hunch, I decided to rehabilitate my lifetime project by focusing on the phenomenon of *loss*, not only in relation to adolescence, but as a common human experience. Briefly browsing the (somewhat chaotic) manuscript I produced,

---

vi. In fact the shortage was statewide. On one occasion, while interviewing for an adolescent consulting position at a county mental health center some eighty miles south of Minneapolis, I concluded the meeting by clarifying I was not boarded in adolescent psychiatry. The response: "When can you start?"

vii. For any reader who has aspirations of this sort, I would recommend emotion as an organizing principle of human behavior, providing a sort of neuropsychological "gravity" uniting body, brain, and mind.

I see I have chapters entitled *Loss and Society, Loss and Chronic Pain, Loss and Aging, Loss and Addiction, Loss and Education, Loss and Abandonment,* and so on. But as things turned out, this effort was not without a clinical payoff. Two of the vignettes I present here—the Punker (chapter 3) and Darrell (chapter 13), both of whom I managed from the perspective of loss—date from this era.

Further, some of my commentary on loss invigorates this book: for example, the opening paragraphs of chapter 1 regarding John Bowlby. Also included herein is my research and reading on related topics. For example, directly relevant to loss is the most famous dropout of all, Holden Caulfield. I had, of course, performed an obligatory if cursory reading of *The Catcher in the Rye* during the third year of my training when I was chief resident for six months on the Adolescent Service. All of the kids were reading it, so I figured I should. It didn't make much of an impression then, but now, given a relative absence of actual dropouts in my practice and consulting work, I decided I could at least explore the motivation of a virtual one. What a surprise! Not the rebellious figure of dim recall, but an aching youngster riven by loss in the midst of an ambivalent search for a relationship.

Another, briefer, but nonetheless equally striking literary depiction of loss is from Jon Hassler's *Staggerford,* quoted and discussed in chapter 11. I might have overlooked the passage except for my interest in the topic. It bears repeating because of its relevancy:

> Losing. That was the melancholy strain running through dozens of papers every year. Parents lost in death and divorce, fingers lost in corn pickers, innocence lost behind barns and in back seats, brothers and uncles lost in Vietnam, friends lost in drug-induced hallucinations, and football games lost to Owl Brook and Berrington.[1]

During this interval I also passed many hours parsing another notable record of loss, William Styron's *Darkness Visible*, which I review at length in chapter 9. At first sight it is a profound albeit sparse account of a devastating Endogenous Depression, but Pulitzer Prize–winning novelist Styron, true to his craft, closes with a surprising revelation. Not only did the death of his mother at age thirteen set the stage for his later "depression," but the loss also molded his life's work.

Finally, some portions of the manuscript I wrote then I have excerpted at length herein. These include my discussion of the meaning of death, as exemplified in the experiences of Hans Castorp, the protagonist of Thomas Mann's *The Magic Mountain* (chapter 11). Also, a good deal of the history of education, volume 2, is taken from the manuscript.

However, despite the years of investigation into the various manifestations of loss, I finally put the manuscript aside, realizing I was no closer to an understanding of "Affective Interference." Moreover, both my peripatetic consulting schedule and my private practice were imposing a growing energy and time demand. There was no space for scholarly work.

7

More Recent Origins

Origin #6: Chronic Pain Disability

It may seem a bit of a stretch to consider that Attachment Disability has anything in common with disability from chronic pain, but in fact they share very significant similarities. First of all, gene expression in mouse brains demonstrates similar molecular changes in mouse models of both chronic pain and chronic stress, which simulates human Depression.[1] And there are clinical similarities. Both evoke distrust. Moreover, they require similar management techniques.

I only realized recently that while I thought I originated a number of techniques to manage adolescent attachment, I actually evolved them years earlier while treating adults disabled by chronic pain. While pondering the "origins" question, I remembered I had discussed the issue of mistrust in an unpublished 2004 manuscript on chronic pain: "Is Chronic Pain Organic? Unrecognized Brain Damage as a Source of Excess Disability." Rereading the manuscript ten years later jogged my memory.

I will summarize and discuss the manuscript at length here because adolescents experience the same kinds of abandonment, rejection, and occasional verbal abuse that chronic pain patients sustain when their pain cannot be explained or resolved by conventional treatment techniques. This is why much of what I learned from working with chronic pain sufferers later proved to be quite helpful in understanding the chronic suffering of attachment-disabled children, adolescents, and adults. Both types are crippled by similar miseries: distrust of others and distrust of emotions and feelings, even including joy and happiness. And the same is true when it comes to understanding and managing the emotional turmoil that erupts as we age—typically misdiagnosed as Depression—and experience a loss of independence as our health declines, precipitating the return of life issues previously solved by productive activity (see chapter 14). My point is that I have come to believe that all disability regardless of cause—chronic pain, aging, trauma, injury and so on—involves loss, abandonment, and the potential for attachment conflict. In my paper I first reviewed the traditional—misguided in my opinion—theory of chronic pain. Then I proposed corrective tactics.

Theory

During my years in group private practice, I developed an interest in chronic pain, somewhat by accident. One of the services for which our group was known was a willingness to perform independent neurological or psychiatric examinations, so-called "medical-legal" evaluations. Most physicians avoided such work or performed it only reluctantly because generally these patients—typically referred by attorneys or insurance companies—were only minimally cooperative. Furthermore, the referral usually was accompanied by piles of medical records that necessitated hours of detailed review and summary, an arduous process congenial to only a somewhat obsessive mind, a turn-off for the average overwhelmed practicing physician. Then we were expected to produce a report detailing the history we obtained from the patient, our examination, our review of the records, and a diagnosis and recommendations along with a summary supported by what attorneys term a "reasoned medical judgment." Finally there was implicit in all of this an understanding that we might be called upon in court or at a hearing to defend the latter on cross-examination.

This was a side of private practice for which I was totally unprepared. At one point I asked my senior partner for advice on how to manage cross-examination—which was *always tell the truth, be prepared to say that anything is possible, and then repeat your opinion.* I shouldered my burden and began to evaluate the medical-legal patients he referred to me.

Many turned out to be workers disabled by either injury—frequently work related—or disease with a common complication: pain out of proportion to findings. In other words, despite apparently adequate treatment and rehabilitation, such patients still reported continued pain and limited functioning. Repetitive examinations, testing, and retesting had not been successful in isolating an "objective" cause of their complaints and disability, much to the consternation of doctors, attorneys, insurance companies, and—let us not forget—the workers themselves.

In the early seventies traditional psychiatry offered two explanations for disproportional *disability:* Malingering and Hysteria. Then as now, both entities were relatively rare. On the other hand, referrals for disproportional *pain* were a different matter indeed. At one point I was seeing one or two per week.

As a medical student and intern I had, of course, been taught that pain is a sign of tissue damage; therefore, the rule was *when there is pain look for the tissue damage.* But with disproportionate pain the traditional rule did not work. Either there was no evidence of tissue damage, or, if there was, the damage was not sufficient to explain the pain, particularly continuing pain, and, most particularly, pain that did not respond to traditionally effective treatments. *Chronic pain,* in other words.

I could not recall any formal training or lectures on chronic pain evaluation and management other than brief references to the notion of *psychogenic pain*. This was a theory proposed by an eminent internist and psychiatrist of the 1950s, Dr. George Engel, published in the influential *American Journal of Medicine*.[2] Looking for guidance, I studied the article closely.

According to him, "pain-proneness" is a pain experience in which there is no damage to tissues or organs, therefore no irritated nerves to send messages to the brain. In other words, he suggested that you can have pain without any peripheral organic tissue damage. It is thus "psychogenic" and can be thought of as a hallucination.

He went on to say that "psychogenic" pain was most likely to be found in certain individuals with a history of:

- Relief of guilt through pain
- History of suffering and defeat
- Intolerance of success
- A large number of painful operations and treatments
- Conflicts about being assertive
- Development of pain as a replacement for a real or threatened loss
- A history of a psychiatric diagnosis

In short, in his view, chronic pain was more likely to occur where there was a history of hardship and deprivation—what today we would call abuse and abandonment. He illustrated his concepts with case studies of nineteen patients.

Although his ideas were stimulating, I did not find his thinking especially persuasive based on my own experiences with chronic suffers. For example, while there is a category of chronic pain that is unquestionably hallucinated—phantom pain—it is easily distinguished as such by the patient.

Moreover, in my experience a background history of pain or prior psychiatric diagnosis is present in only a small percentage of chronic pain sufferers. In fact my careful review of his nineteen cases revealed that Dr. Engel's formulations were biased because only two of the nineteen had sustained trauma, and none were incapable of working despite their pain.

On the contrary, my evaluations of chronic sufferers revealed that many had little or no prior experience of pain. They did not seem to have a history of "pain-proneness." True, some had a background of hardship and deprivation, but they had escaped from it, sometimes early in their teens, through hard work and initiative. Hard work was the way—for some the only way—to deal with obstacles. They enjoyed the companionship of the workplace and took pride in their success, relishing the economic and personal freedom it provided. Moreover, prior to their injury most had been in excellent health or, if they had sustained obvious trauma or acute illnesses, had recovered promptly. Indeed, they tended to avoid doctors and prescription medications, preferring home remedies or over-the-counter preparations. And a history of psychiatric diagnosis was very rare, although many were uninsightful and unimaginative. Their strong suit was energy and a strong back.[i]

However, individuals with this otherwise winning combination of good health and industriousness are not prepared for an encounter with pain that persists despite otherwise adequate treatment, especially if repeated examinations and testing are essentially negative. Previously, their occasional encounters with the medical system were brief and effective. But now encounters are neither brief nor effective. Everyone becomes frustrated: patients, doctors, family members, therapists, claims managers. If the pain is not rectified, patients find themselves

---

i. A somewhat similar dynamic seems to be true of Vietnam-era veterans who are now beginning to flood VA hospitals seeking help for emerging posttraumatic symptoms. Their aging bodies limit their ability to suppress symptoms such as sleeplessness, "depression," and flashbacks via constant activity. Here, of course, the trauma is not a childhood of deprivation and hardship, but combat and the death of comrades and civilians. "Rising Numbers of Veterans See Help Decades After War." *The Wall Street Journal*. November 29–30, 2014, 1A.

plunging into the equivalent of a childhood they fought hard to overcome, and escaping the misery through hard work is no longer an option.

In part their pain is amplified by a tendency for others to blame them for the pain. Sometimes this is rather subtle, such as doctors not being careful when they comment on the absence of test results. It is one thing to say *I can't find anything wrong*, another thing to say *I cannot find an explanation.* Patients are liable to walk away from the former thinking *He says it is all in my head.* Sometimes blaming is not so subtle. Examiners and attorneys may strongly imply deception or even directly accuse patients of "faking" or "making it up" or "exaggerating," typically without any evidence to support these allegations. No matter how strongly patients resist "buying" the blame, at some level it sticks and the belief begins to percolate, *Maybe all this is my fault after all*.

Not infrequently, the blaming is accompanied by abandonment, again sometimes subtle, sometimes overt. Doctors become abrupt and impatient, eager to cut off discussion and end the appointment, while suggesting a longer follow-up interval or even no follow-up at all. Or they refer for psychiatric evaluation and treatment, which frequently is interpreted as a rejection and, in fact, sometimes may well be. Partners and friends hesitate to inquire how things are going, change the subject, walk away. Coworkers, mostly likely because the sight of an injured buddy stirs up their own insecurities, are more direct, telling patients they are not welcome at union meetings, parties, company functions, and so on. Perhaps jealousy is a factor. In any event, this is a replay of a painful youth.[ii]

---

ii. Those suffering the torments of physical pain elicit a different response from professionals than do sufferers crippled by the fear and distrust of emotional pain. Typically we nurture and protect the former, and do not question the legitimacy of their misery. In other words, their pain is not an illness but a sign of illness. But when physical pain persists without an obvious cause—"chronic pain"—it risks being transformed

In my view the blaming and abandonment stem from multiple causes, one of which is the pernicious but persisting influence of Dr. Engel's theories, while another is the very misunderstanding of chronic pain itself.[iii]

Briefly, my years of listening to pain-disabled patients and their families, and my meticulous reviews of their records, had convinced me that for them pain, which at first signaled tissue damage, had now come to also signal loss and abandonment. The experience of pain itself has become stressful. Even if the objective tissue damage, of which the pain is a signal, is not catastrophic or disfiguring or tangible, it comes to symbolize the possibility of loss: loss of salary, loss of workplace relationships, loss of self-esteem.

Some injured workers manage these possibilities well. Despite the anxieties that such possibilities inevitably generate, they tolerate them with relatively little anticipation of rejection. Their ability to turn to others for support is not crippled. They work cooperatively with health care professionals, comply with treatment and rehabilitation formulations, learn pain management, and so on. They begin to heal, pain is reduced, and they experience hope. True, pain may continue, perhaps indefinitely, but they have learned to identify and accept their physical boundaries, which can be exceeded but at the price of pain. When contemplating exertion, they learn to perform a mental cost/benefit analysis, perhaps a novel way of operating compared to their prior "pedal-to-the-metal" approach to life,

---

from a sign of illness to illness itself.

iii. For the readers who are intrigued by technical aspects of the dilemma of chronic pain I recommend you review the entry in recommended reading section of volume 2. Although Dr. Engel's observations are both archaic as well as highly speculative, I sense they still influence contemporary diagnosis and treatment of chronic pain, therefore are worthy of review for their historical perspective. *DSM-III* was a reaction to psychodynamic conjectures of this sort.

but one that restores to them a sense of control. Thus with its customary and familiar stresses, life goes forward. These injured workers, certainly the majority, never cross my threshold. For them the "system" works.

But should blaming erupt, either via scapegoating (by health care professionals, independent examiners, coworkers, family, employer, claims adjustors) or via a negative self-assessment, abandonment enters the picture. Either the abandonment is tangible—the scapegoaters criticize and withdraw support from the injured workers—or it is intangible as the latter, projecting their self-disgust onto others and anticipating they will be rejected, adopt a defensive posture and withdraw, frustrating offers of support and assistance. In either case healing is undermined and stress is aggravated. Eventually pain, initially a signal of tissue damage, comes to signal *abandonment* and *loss* as well. It comes as no surprise to me that recent neuroimaging studies of the somatosensory representations of social rejection and physical pain reveal they share similar features.[3] A downward, mutually reinforcing spiral of pain issues and abandonment issues ensues. Pain and stress become chronic. Brain damage ensues.

In short, no matter its origin, if not relieved their pain eventually becomes baked into their neurons. Their brain and peripheral nervous system are damaged. Moreover, this is accompanied by a second, more pernicious, "baking": They have come to believe that "treatment" means more frustration and eventual abandonment. They have lost trust. *They have become conditioned to expect rejection.*

Management: Three Principles

Strictly speaking, the goal of chronic pain management is not so much relief of pain, although this is certainly welcome, but *relief of excess disability,* especially the disability of *distrust*. It is one thing if the distrust is overt because it is potentially more accessible via a cognitive, sometimes gamey contest of verbal thrust and counterthrust; for example, Mr. POP, chapter 10. But oftentimes the work is arduous because the distrust lurks behind a smiling and compliant façade, a barrier that may require months and years of work before patients risk lowering their guard. Eventually I found it helpful to provide in advance an outline of what we were hoping to accomplish, which went more or less as follows:

> *You are here because your pain and disability continue despite the best efforts of all the doctors, specialists, and therapists working with you. You still hurt. Moreover, it is rather unlikely that further evaluations will uncover a cause of your pain that everyone overlooked. The experts have nothing more to offer. So, you have to learn to manage your chronic pain by yourself—"to be your own doctor," in other words, which I hope to teach you how to do. This will be based on three ideas:*

- *Clarification:* paying attention to your pain and learning to describe it clearly, especially what makes it better, what makes it worse
- *Acceptance:* owning your pain without blame
- *Focus:* putting your energies into what can be changed

With permission I would invite family members and relatives to sit in. My intent was to create a role for them, not only to protect them from the loss of morale that comes from being helpless in the face of the suffering of those they care for, but to enlist them as co-therapists to reiterate and reinforce these ideas between visits.

Self-Management

This is a very reasonable therapeutic posture in chronic pain situations where all the usual evaluations and treatments have not helped. By the time this develops, patients either have given up—with no faith that anything more can be done—or their doctors have and are reluctant to order more testing or treatment despite their patients' earnest pleas. But the practical effect of self-management is either patients becoming less dependent on traditional medicine, or becoming "better" patients, so to speak, because they are better historians. Just as psychiatry rests on a three-legged platform of history, examination, and testing, so does all of medicine. And the history leg is crucial when it comes to chronic pain. If patients bedeviled by chronic pain become more skilled at noting what makes it better, or worse, they or their doctors are likely to become better at managing it.

Detecting Hidden Distrust

In "Is Chronic Pain Organic?" I noted that the expectation of rejection may be quite apparent in patient behaviors such as overt anger or frustration, or it may be buried. Many disabled workers become secretly convinced their spouse will leave them, which accounts for their irritability. Otherwise innocuous gestures or changes in routine by their partner ignite abandonment concerns that can explode into corrosive arguments.

Other signs include:

- Blaming (either themselves or others)
- Not listening to feedback to the questions they pose
- Minimizing positive feedback

To be sure, all of us have moments of anger, frustration, blaming, rambling, inattentiveness, and discounting. However, because our conditioning is not so lopsided and because our hippocampal function is not damaged—we have access to recent facts and events—we are able to process both the circumstances and our reactions and make an adjustment if called for. We are flexible and adaptive in our interaction. Sufferers are inflexible and unable to adapt.

With these demoralized patients I gradually realized that my customary, classic therapeutic strategy of listening, with an occasional (hopefully) insightful comment, was not working. Nothing changed. I was too passive. Moreover, the longer the behaviors continued unchecked, the greater the risk that I would tune out, lose interest, and withdraw, setting up the patient for another rejection. Eventually—this took years, in fact—I began to put into practice the more active and engaged techniques that I learned from the Schmidts and others. The idea was to not allow patients to display the behaviors driven by their conditioning, of which in great part they were unaware. I had to be more active in order to neutralize their conditioned distrust with its anticipation of rejection.

Neutralizing Hidden Distrust

Distrust is rarely liquidated by the direct approach of earnestly soliciting trust. Only the gullible respond. And I can assure you that by the time a patient with chronic pain walks into your office, all gullibility has been leached away.

Conceivably a more effective gambit is to meet distrust head-on. That is, if my patient greets me with the challenge, "Why should I trust you?" I might riposte with something like a forthright "Well, why should you? You hardly know me." Or "That makes two of us." Interviews that start like this often turn out to be very interesting and entertaining, because I am actually, as our professors used to say, *talking to the unconscious*. Patients like this wish to have a relationship but are afraid of one, so this introductory palaver helps establish a comfortable boundary.

Anger

The thing to remember about anger is that it is fear with a different face. Anger and fear are twins—they always go together. But they differ in this respect: Generally it is easy to help patients tap into the fear behind anger, but the reverse is much more difficult. It is easy for the fearful to recognize how they are intimidated by the prospect of others' scorn or anger, much more difficult for them to accept that their fears serve to keep their own furies in check.

An angry person is someone who expects to be rejected, discounted, rebuffed, ignored, perhaps even abused. In their experience "help" is a noise that people make when they are about to exploit or betray you. Occasionally I deal with this directly by saying, "Okay, I know what you are angry about—now tell me what you are afraid of," or, "I get the impression you figure I am going to be like the other doctors and give you the brush-off." Sometimes this pays off and we go directly to the distrust and abandonment concerns.

More often, however, after allowing patients to ventilate for a while, perhaps an interview or two, I will coach them as follows: "Let's see if you can repeat what you have just said but in a more conversational, quieter tone." Then I might model the same words or phrases for them.

The idea is that I never, as Dr. Bruch advised us, serve as a punching bag. Playing rope-a-dope may have helped Ali win fights, but therapy is not a contest with a winner and a loser. Rather it is a learning situation for both, where there is every reason to believe that both parties can "win" as therapist learns from patient, and patient from therapist.

Blaming

This is sustained by patients' conditioned expectation of

criticism. By blaming themselves they hope to obtain mercy; by blaming others, to escape condemnation.

Either mode is paralyzing because it shifts the power to change behavior into the hands of outsiders. Moreover, it reinforces their view of the world as a moral place—that is, a place where every problem is someone's fault.

Here the focus of redirection is to model for them how to be *descriptive rather than judgmental* as they review their pains, treatment, the responsiveness of the "system," and the attitudes of their family and coworkers. Typically I instruct them to be assertive and forthright in their statements: for example, not to apologize by tone of voice or gesture as they report how they feel, think, or believe. *Own your thoughts and feelings!* is the mantra here. Sometimes I nag them to replace the word *should* with the word *need*. That is, not *What should I do?* but rather *What do I need to do?* As they struggle to learn this new language and its message that problem solving is a survival issue, not a moral one, I reinforce its acquisition with careful recognition.

Rambling

In my view this has at least two causes. First it is a manifestation of stress-induced hippocampal organic dysfunction. Emotionally disabled patients forget what point they are trying to make; hence they produce historical information that is discursive, disjointed, and repetitive. The other is a function of past rejections by doctors, family, and friends, leading to the not totally unrealistic expectation that the current dialogue will have the same outcome: rejection. Therefore patients are in a hurry to "get everything in" because they feel they will not get a second chance.

Here, typically after listening for a couple of minutes, I redirect patients to summarize their experiences in short statements. "Boil down what you are trying to tell me," I say, "in six words or so if you can." I explain it is necessary to be brief because otherwise listeners—especially doctors and family and friends—will tune out. Some patients need considerable support and encouragement to learn this style of communication, so it may be necessary to propose such a summary in six words myself, then inquire if it fits. Should it seem to them not quite right, I invite a correction.

If this tactic is properly executed, patients will experience the recognition they need but feared would not be theirs because of past brush-offs by professionals. On occasion it is possible to access such fears with a direct inquiry, such as "Do you ever worry this might be the last time you will have a chance to talk about what is on your mind?"

Finally, sometimes I also recommend treatment with *anti-stressants* (see chapter 9) to "reverse the 'brain scorch' caused by your stress."

Not Listening

Here patients are dominated by a mental cycle of painful worries and concerns related to prior rejections and abandonments. They may seem attentive to inquiries or feedback, but frequently this does not seem to register. Sometimes they are rather unaware of their preoccupation; they apologize and promise to try harder. Others may have more insight, reporting, "My mind doesn't shut down," or something of that sort. A few have little to say, clearly distrustful of engagement.[iv]

Regardless of the cause, and even when dealing with alert and attentive patients, it is important to be concise and focused when making inquiries and providing feedback. I try to limit my responses to a few sentences at a time—I'm not always successful—and then pause to see whether and how my words are assimilated. Things can get lost in translation. This is less likely to occur if I deliver my message in bits and pieces.

Experts in interview techniques advise doctors never to

---

iv. See Mr. Resistive, chapter 10.

conclude a consult with the statement, "Do you have any questions?" This is considered bad form, and may actually come across as a brusque dismissal, they maintain. They seem to think that a well-performed interview leaves no questions. Of course only an expert could reach such a conclusion. There are always questions; that is our nature because we are, to paraphrase the classical definition of mankind, the questioning animal.

Instead, with a genuflection in the direction of correctness, I often manage the ending like this. "I'm going to do something the experts say I should never do. They say I never should ask if there are any questions, so instead I'm going to say 'I'm wondering if you have any questions.'" This usually elicits a laugh and prepares for a smooth closing transition. Or I may say something like, "Well, I'm the one who up to now has been asking questions. Now it is your turn."

Summary

As I stated at the outset, I have devoted these pages to a disability that might seem rather unrelated to Attachment Disability. However, in retrospect I now see that my later understanding and management of attachment issues springs in part from my earlier years of evaluating and treating the disability of chronic pain. While the demographics of each are obviously dissimilar, their dynamics are otherwise similar.

Origin #7: Focus Program, Elk River (Minnesota) School District

In 2002 I accepted a position as child/adolescent consultant at the Central Minnesota Mental Health Center, Elk River office. One of my responsibilities there was new to me: providing outreach services to area primary and secondary schools. Each school would develop a schedule of teachers who wished to discuss their poorly performing students. One by one each would meet with me to discuss an otherwise intelligent youngster who was underperforming academically. We would discuss what the issue might be, and I would suggest a management strategy to deal with it. We then would meet the following month to review and revise. The idea was to give teachers the benefit of my expertise. At least that was the idea.

In fact, I'm not sure if the teachers learned much, but I sure did.

For example, it was my introduction to the primary school maxim *in the first two years kids learn to read; after that, they read to learn.* Reading is the foundation, the essential foundation, the one and only foundation of formal education.

Second, performance issues were most likely to emerge during two transitions, one in the early grades, the other later. The former typically developed as youngsters were introduced to expectations of studying and learning with less direct supervision. And the latter proved to be somewhat similar: changing from the relative order of the middle grades to the turmoil of high school. Again, less direct supervision and greater expectations of independent study.

A third lesson: the vital role of parental support. Underperforming children were not infrequently described as withdrawn or even apathetic, as not at all involved in the class activities. They were there but not there. When I inquired about PTA conferences, phone reports, or notes to the parents, the same seemed true of the parents as well: there but not there. They didn't attend conferences; they didn't acknowledge notes and calls. And the children themselves, even when delicately questioned, tended to be nonresponsive or evasive. Sometimes it was impossible to determine who was in the home.

Only infrequently did these teachers request consultation about acting-out or developmentally disabled youngsters. For the most part such requests came from other community agencies that manage such problems, to which I also provided outreach. One such was the Sherburne County Social Services Department in the persons of two excellent, experienced social workers who tracked problematic children and adolescents, arranging service and treatment as needed. This was also a situation where I was doing most of the learning, in part because of their extensive knowledge of local and state resources, in part because of area customs and mores.

Another agency was the Elk River School District Focus Program, an ALC grades 1 through 12 for students who could not be mainstreamed because of behavioral issues. The program was organized as a school within a school, but was separately administered. Since a number of my office patients were attendees, prospective attendees, or program graduates still in aftercare, it was a given I would regularly liaise with the Focus teachers, Nancy and Sheila, to compare notes.

Each month they presented new or current students, or discussed aftercare once they were mainstreamed. With proper consent we could share our direct observations and insights. As I recall our meetings, Nancy and Sheila apparently assumed that youthful problem behaviors were related to more than just early childhood traumas. Neglect, abuse, and abandonment in later childhood and adolescence had a similar potential. Moreover, Focus teachers and therapists were trained to view the distrust of troubled children and adolescents as a *human response to loss and abandonment,* and they worked with kids to accept and normalize such unhappy experiences.

While we had to bestow the formality of a diagnosis on our proceedings and occasionally discussed psychotropics, most of our discussion centered on parent- and sponsor-child dynamics and behavior management strategies. I do not have any records from these meetings, unfortunately. On the other hand, I clearly recall us reviewing the aftercare tribulations of several (by now) young adults, but whether we framed their continuing issues in terms of lingering attachment-inspired distrust is vague. The same is true of the many child and adolescent Focus students we staffed during the three years I consulted at the clinic: warm memories of productive teamwork, but terminology a blank.

So in November 2014, I called the school to interview Nancy, who, happily, still managed the program. She was pleased to hear from me, and we exchanged reminisces as old friends do at a reunion. Then I described this book and my curiosity about the origins of my conviction about the significance of unrecognized Attachment Disability. And I explained I had the impression that my Focus consulting experience was very instrumental in consolidating my thinking. Therefore, would she consider a few questions about the program's dynamics? Indeed she would.

- Did the staff view attachment concepts as essential to the understanding of their student issues and behaviors?
- Did the "focus" of Focus Program refer to managing the distrust of attachment-disabled children and adolescents?
- Did attachment problems extend into adolescence and beyond to young adulthood?

Her response to all three was unequivocally positive. She added that understanding the fundamental role of distrust in the genesis of Attachment Disability invigorated staffing reviews of children and adolescents at every stage of their participation in the program.

I thanked her, saying it would bring me great pleasure to see this book bring to a wider audience the excellence of the Elk River School District Focus Program initiative.

In retrospect I now see how fortuitous my posting to the Focus Program was. My thirty years' search came to an end. I was now satisfied that the mystery of Dr. Sheridan's "affective interference" was solved. It was his term for Attachment Disability.

Recently I again searched my office records and found that

I first used the adjective "attachment" in 2006. Up until then, I see I used such terms as PTSD or Adjustment Reaction when assessing adolescent disability.

Origin #8: Learning from My Patients

This is a legacy of Dr. Roger MacKinnon, a looming figure throughout the early years of my residency. We rookie psychiatrists needed an overlord to drill us on the basics of history taking, mental status observations, and assessment, a role to which he brought both high standards and a commitment to bringing out the best in us.[v]

Every morning we assembled to present for his and the group's evaluation our emergency room workups of the previous evening. An uncomfortable process if you were up for review, but endurable because for the most part the feedback was fair, honest, and supportive since with one or two exceptions we were all beginners, eager to learn. Now, as you may have already surmised, I certainly was not one of the exceptions. On at least one occasion I was the subject of a stinging critique, fortunately delivered privately, the gist of which was that I had work to do. I emerged from the debacle chagrined, to say the least, but highly motivated to do the "work," which these many years later yet contributes to my career and this book. Dr. MacKinnon, you still loom.

Thus, despite the occasional rigors of being called upon to recite, this morning exercise was highly anticipated and eagerly attended. We appreciated that this was gold, the true north of

---

v. Subsequently in 1971 he published a comprehensive study of the dynamism between personality style and symptom manifestation, *The Psychiatric Interview in Clinical Practice* (republished in 2015, 3rd edition, Buckley PJ and Michaels R, eds. Arlington, VA: American Psychiatric Publishing). I kept this volume on my desk until I retired, and dipped into it occasionally between patients for relaxation.

our clinical compass. Hence at the last meeting of our six-month rotation, as a group we expressed our concerns in the form of a common cry: *Dr. MacKinnon, who will teach us and lead us now?* His reply: *Learn from your patients.* Enigmatic, of course, but so typical of wise teachers. Here's my take.

Of course, some learning from patients is obvious; this is what taking a history and performing a mental status examination are all about. Otherwise how could you perform an assessment? His point was, I think, that not only is it important to provide an assessment (what I call *understanding* in this book) of your findings to your patients, but it is even more important to take note of their response.

A psychiatric or counseling consultation can be likened to a search for the truth in an individual's life, prompted by a request for assistance from the individual or an agent acting on his or her behalf. In this sense you are a detective carrying on an investigation, not of a crime but of a functional disability. As you investigate and compile information, certain items might impress you as significant and you will eventually present them to your client in a (hopefully) orderly and meaningful way. But you do not proclaim in doing so that your presentation is the "truth" of your client's life. Instead you wonder if your assessment provides *clarification*.[vi] And then you solicit a response and listen.

What do you listen for? Three things. Most important, you look for distortions of your message: Does your client seem to believe he or she is being blamed for the functional disability? If so, you re-present the data, perhaps cloaked in different terminology, hoping to minimize the distortion. This may take only a minute or two, but sometimes weeks or months when you are dealing with trauma-related disability because typically such victims were blamed or blame themselves for the trauma. It is ingrained, and for them a (sometimes *the*) significant "truth" of their life.

---

vi. Discussed at much greater length in chapter 11.

You also listen for what part of the message seems to "fit," and if so, how and why. And you listen for the parts that do not seem to fit, again how and why. Using the feedback and the additional relevant data accompanying it, you construct an alternative scenario to present to your client with the hope of providing further clarification, as well as *acceptance* of the trauma or disability, without blame but with an increased ability to *focus* on what can be changed.[vii] In this way, as I sometimes say to my patients, "My job is to help you better understand yourself, to teach you how to be your own detective amid the mystery of your life, and to establish a life path to travel."

But not all learning is auditory. We were also taught to watch what people say and listen to what they do.

For example, Renée:

[CASE STUDY]
Renée: Watching What Is Said,
Listening to What Is Done

Renée is a forty-four-year-old self-referred single physical therapist whom I first saw in 2007. Her major issue is dissatisfaction with her prior psychiatrist, who for several years treated her Bipolar II Disorder and intermittent anxiety with lamotrigine and occasional alprazolam. Interestingly she has no concerns about the quality of her medication management, reporting her functioning as more or less stable, without any intervening hospitalizations. There is a past history of alcohol use since her teens, mutating to unquestionable alcoholism during her work at a government facility, followed by nineteen years of sobriety. Renée has a sponsor and attends AA faithfully. She is studying for an advanced degree in her specialty.

At mental status examination she is cooperative, compliant,

---

vii. See chapters 12 and 13.

bland, smiling, submissive, carefully groomed, without any obvious signs or symptoms of untreated emotional disability. She impresses me as a good historian, as confirmed by my subsequent review of her records, although she pleasantly but firmly demurs from describing the details of her issue with her prior psychiatrist, which I respect. The circumstances leading to her original Bipolar diagnosis remain obscure.

Thereafter our contacts consist of periodic medication checks, at which time Renée typically presents with a bland, fixed smile accompanied by an absence of focal issues or complaints. Yet from time to time she calls to make a semi-urgent appointment, only to arrive somewhat flustered and embarrassed, apologizing for the request for help, her manner suggesting she has overreacted—but to what she is unable to say. Her behavior and interval history are never suggestive of psychomotor retardation or acceleration. As usual, she scoots out of the office, obviously relieved to be gone. After a year or two of this I begin to gently tease her, anointing her as my "mystery of the month," or "today's puzzle patient," and so on. She acknowledges the comment with an uncomfortable smile, makes haste to leave.

Things begin to change in 2012. Renée becomes subject to unpredictable flare-ups of chronic anxiety, at times so intense she is unable to work but otherwise unaccompanied by sustained alterations in her mood. And her studying bogs down. Calls for help become more frequent. Fortunately, brief increases in the alprazolam and brief medical leaves enable her to continue working part time, although at times it is difficult.

Renée's interview behavior also begins to change, becomes more than just a medication check. She remains the full length of the allotted time and sometimes longer, ventilating her distress, weeping yet apologizing all the while for her need for comfort. She begins to report fleeting, very alarming, intrusive flashbacks involving a relative. Eventually her anxiety is so intense she takes extended medical leave.

By 2013 she is coming every three weeks or so. Her intrusive experiences are now coalescing into discrete memory fragments involving several members of her family. She's tortured by the memories. What is she to do with them? About them? What? I suggest the thing to do is to own them. Resist the impulse to bury them, which now is probably impossible anyhow. I say her anxiety is a signal that she can't go back now, that her unmet needs are surfacing. She gulps, says she'll try.

Subsequently Renée's denial slowly crumbles, an excruciating experience as she struggles with the fear of what she might discover versus the fear of revealing herself to others in a search for comfort. She decides she has no choice but to risk the latter and is surprised to discover that her bouts of alcohol craving are less intense.

Her memory recall is more coherent, less fraught with anxiety: for example, her mother's verbal abuse, also her strict admonition that family issues were never to be discussed with outsiders. And now there is a clear memory of repeated molestation by the relative, as well as threats by her mother to have the police come and take her away if she says anything about it. She reveals other betrayals: a former coworker, a former boyfriend, a sponsor, the former psychiatrist who did not protect her confidences. At times she's angry, especially as she recalls another family rule: only mother is allowed to be angry.

Eventually the panic subsides enough for her to return to work to work full time. Then there is a crisis. Exposure to unclad male patients now triggers abuse flashbacks. Renée applies for a transfer to another department, a humiliating request, which is approved in view of her excellent work record and an understanding supervisor.

By August 2013, she is nearing the end of her studies, close to a final examination—now what? I suggest the issue is her difficulty in imagining a life without the restrictions imposed by the lifelong conflicts from which she is just emerging. Because I am no longer consulting at a nearby clinic, we decide to increase the interval between visits, which seems to work out.

Six months later Renée reports some difficulty in finishing her academic work because of anxiety, also because of newly assigned courses. Her plan is to apply for a year's medical extension. Would I support it? Also, she plans to see a female therapist for formal psychotherapy. She has decided she needs a clear and detailed recall of her abuse and the cover-up by her parents, as well as possibly other family secrets. Now there is no question she also sustained intense beatings.

On the plus side, she recently was able to drive past her relative's place for the first time in years, although it was scary. She remains on the alprazolam, but in view of the fact that there is little in her past history to support bipolar tendencies, she has decided to slowly taper the lamotrigine. She reports it is difficult to trust because of so many betrayals, wonders if she ever will.

Just recently, after weeks of mounting agony expressed in a series of desperate letters, she finally writes:

"Well, you listened to my tantrum, so I feel I should tell you the outcome. After arguing with God for over forty-eight hours it came down to either I trust people or from this point on I start going backward. I decided I had no interest in drinking/using drugs, and for whatever reason I don't want to die. I went to my second AA meeting in two days and when it came to my turn to talk I just had to trust the group and let something out or I was going to go backward. I said I grew up being physically sexually and emotionally abused. That was it. I got support. I also found out about a women's group."[4]

The Significance of Renée's Behavior

Initial Interview: The Signal

In my experience this was an unusual transfer-of-care interview. Ordinarily the cause is obvious: perhaps a change in insurance, physician, or locale, a recent discharge, poor compliance, dissatisfaction with results, or indifferent service. But this is different. True, she expresses dissatisfaction, but without the usual litany of complaints: no ventilation, no indignation or frustration that provides the rhythm to the melody of ungratified needs. In fact, there is not even a melody. Despite my demonstrating my customary, welcoming professional attentiveness, she remains bland, smiling, ignoring the opportunity to provide specifics for the change. Where is the emotion, I wonder, the detail? In fact, it soon becomes clear that the continuing lack of feedback is itself a feedback, a red flag, indeed a crimson banner.

Renée's Message

Any professional with even minimal experience interviewing adolescents is familiar with the youngster who remains unresponsive or resistive to prompts, an issue I discuss at length in chapter 10. And the same is true with adults; for example, Mr. Resistive, also discussed in the same chapter, particularly if their participation in the interview is rather unwilling.[viii] But neither applies in this case: Renée is both a mature and willing participant. It seems the message probably is of the category *there are things I am not ready/able to discuss.*

It pays to heed a warning of this sort—by this time, after forty years of polishing my interpersonal footwork, even the good Dr. MacKinnon would acknowledge I had graduated from the "project" stage—so I table further inquiry for later investigation and finish the interview according to the usual format: reviewing medications, discussing management and follow-up, and so on.

---

viii. Mr. Resistive was a young man also reluctant to reveal himself, in this instance because of his issues with authority. Youngsters whose silence is protective of family members will frequently signal with looks and glances at the vulnerable adult their concerns about speaking up.

Renée's Management

As discussed in chapter 2 with case Helen, ordinarily my "med-check" routine incorporates two activities, one wearing my "doctor" hat, the other my "therapy" hat. In the guise of "doctor" I perform all the usual stuff of follow-up med checks: initial complaint, interval medical and psychiatric history, medication compliance, medication side effects, and medication benefits. Then, depending on the time, I might actually announce I'm "putting on my counseling hat, which means open agenda, we can talk about anything." Many patients find an unstructured interview of this sort rather uncomfortable, apologizing after a moment or two that they have nothing to say. I might then provide some structure, perhaps explaining that just because there is silence, that does not mean learning is not taking place, or suggesting an update of a prior topic, and so on. This usually serves to reduce the discomfort about taking more responsibility for the proceedings, in the process reinforcing the potential for learning that assertiveness and taking the initiative are not always dangerous.

    This tactic also serves to change the dynamic of the interview. Rather than engaging in an ofttimes desperate search to present what will be pleasing to me, patients now receive encouragement to focus on their needs. Sometimes I clarify the change with a comment, such as "Now we are going to work on what might make you happy other than trying to keep Dr. Curran happy." Of course this is an extremely burdensome expectation for some individuals with attachment issues, one residual of which is a preoccupation with serving others.

    This does not happen with Renée. She typically flees the interview as soon as the "usual stuff" is transacted, not giving me the opportunity to assume my therapist guise. The same is true even with her semi-urgent calls for an appointment; ordinarily a patient is anxious to ventilate an issue of some urgency. Not so of Renée. It is as if the call for help never happened. Eventually I judge sufficient trust has been established to gently and indirectly comment on her behavior by anointing her an enigma. From a psychodynamic perspective, this is an example of what Dr. MacKinnon called "speaking to the unconscious." There is no doubt that her ambivalence signals a powerful conflict about help—help is dangerous—but to directly address the conflict risks aggravating the conflict before she is ready to deal with it. After all, as she much later reveals, the last time she sought help she was threatened by her mother with abandonment, perhaps even imprisonment. From an attachment perspective, on the other hand, it is clear that I am addressing the weeping, wounded child hiding within the adult, that I recognize the hurt, that it is okay to remain concealed until things feel safer.

Renée's Surging Anxiety

After five years, this routine becomes punctuated by bouts of surging, occasionally disabling anxiety. I view anxiety as *a signal of change, whether immediate or pending, whether real or symbolic*, a definition I will discuss at length in the next chapter. Hence for Renée the question is, What change does she foresee? "Foresee" is a misleading term in this context because it implies a conscious process, not applicable here because Renée lacks insight: she is a mystery not only to me but to herself as well. It would perhaps be more accurate to say that it is a burgeoning awareness of danger that she cannot suppress, the full significance of which she cannot comprehend. Moreover, it cannot be relieved by a hasty med-check contact. Something more is needed; thus did our meetings begin to include therapy because of her necessity for comfort. Help has become less dangerous than no help.[ix]

---

ix. A familiar human dilemma, this. Do we sit by the campfire alone in the darkness, trusting just our own resources, or do we ally with a companion, trusting he or she will not fall

The question now becomes, What is the looming yet intangible danger? Thus reformulated the answer is obvious: flashbacks. Something in her life is triggering previously powerfully suppressed trauma memories: her denial defenses are crumbling.

We "use" denial defenses to manage need conflicts, to prioritize and order survival needs based on which are more important versus less. On occasion this is a totally rational and deliberate calculation: for example, my balancing the language I use in this book to engage attention without offending. But most of the time our reasoning has long ago been formatted and relegated to a routine assessment of our survival issues that runs in the background. Life would be impossible if we had to approach every survival occasion de novo without an automatic appraisal capability to deflect, minimize, or otherwise ignore needs. This is what denial is all about. But if it is too rigid, denial can lead to catastrophe when circumstances change. And the one thing we can count on in life is that circumstances will change. So our survival program needs a subprogram that alerts us when circumstances become non-ordinary, unique, exceptional.[x] Its name is *anxiety*; its function is *survival*.

Not all flashbacks necessarily provoke anxiety. In fact it is likely that over the years Renée experienced some off and on. Perhaps in the past she managed them with alcohol, or otherwise was able to ignore or suppress then. But she renounced alcohol years ago and now her ability to suppress is collapsing; we have no idea why. Perhaps later in her therapy with the help of her counselor she will come to a more complete understanding of what changed. But for now it is clear that, whatever the cause, things are different. Flashbacks are beginning to dominate her life: more precisely fear of flashbacks because they evoke

---

asleep while on watch? Neither way totally banishes anxiety, of course.

x. Excessive denial can destroy a society and presents some threats to ours. See volume 2.

a return to helplessness that was part of her original trauma experience.

In my experience with trauma victims and survivors, it is precisely a sense of powerlessness and abandonment that is *the* significant horror. Whether the trauma is physical or sexual abuse, or a military or civilian catastrophe, or witnessed or sustained, it is the sense of utter impotence that cripples. Moreover the experience may be recalled as endless despite the original, objective time sequence. It goes on without end. This is what catastrophe survivors have in mind when they repeat the familiar saying "It was like my entire life flashed before my eyes." They were unable to intervene either on their own behalf or on behalf of others. A living death.

In short, Renée's flashbacks represent a return to the terrors of her childhood, which she had finally escaped by becoming self-sufficient.[xi] Now she must be on guard that a flashback would be precipitated without warning, rendering her flustered, tongue-tied, briefly paralyzed, and unable to function. Much as the classroom became dangerous for Dyllen, the workplace has become dangerous for her.

Living with Anxiety

Originally Renée had signaled there were things not to be discussed, a message I honored for a number of years, apart from prodding her off and on regarding her reticence. Now things are different. She cannot help but mention the unmentionable, threatening as this is. Not speaking is becoming unendurable, but speaking is also troubling because as she hears her words give life and structure to her formerly vague inner world, she can no longer hide her suffering and misery from herself. What

---

xi. Her choice of a life career in health care is not unusual for an abuse survivor. Other attractive career choices for abuse survivors include nursing, parole officer, teaching, social work, and service agencies.

is she to do? Now what? How to regain control?

I suggest that her task is to practice acceptance of what cannot be changed—for now.[xii] It is important for her to learn that the anticipatory anxiety is now part of her life. She can't go back. To attempt to return to her former state of denial and pretending would be like trying to perform a mental lobotomy on herself. It wouldn't work, and the failure to do so risks precipitating a profound drop in her self-esteem as "weak-minded." Moreover, the burgeoning traumatic memories are a sign of unmet needs. Following the memories wherever they might lead creates the possibility of tapping into the energies associated with the needs, with the potential for personal and professional growth. I interpret her suffering as a sign that it is time to do something different: identify life situations where she is in fact not the helpless kid of her childhood. Now she is an adult with an adult's power and freedom to experiment; in other words, she can focus on what can be changed.[xiii] And eventually she does begin to experiment, visiting the locale of her abuse, for example, choosing to begin a more formal, structured counselling arrangement, electing to begin a lamotrigine taper and, in an ultimate expression of choice, her "coming out."

Renée's Future

While she is now prepared to fully address That Which Must Not Be Discussed, on the other hand she would prefer to deal with a woman rather than a man, a common preference in such situations, I might add. It will be interesting to see if her therapy leads to an exploration of the circumstances leading to the

---

xii. See chapter 12 for a more extended discussion of this therapeutic principle.

xiii. See chapters 12 and 13.

original Bipolar diagnosis. In my experience decompensations precipitated by an overwhelming traumatic experience are frequently misdiagnosed as a Mood Disorder. If this proves to be the case, the lamotrigine taper may work out well.

Origins: Summary

Any personal recollection is by its very nature subjective. But that is true of history as well: what is written depends not only on the historian's selection of facts, but also the significance he or she attaches to them. With regard to the origins of my concept of Attachment Disability, and by way of recapitulation, what seems most relevant to me is:

- The fundamental role of anxiety in promoting or undermining trust and attachment (discussed in chapter 8)
- The token economy confirms Winnicott's notion of acting-out as a call on society for need relief; management more effective if it is disability focused
- "Affective interference"—the missing link in student underperformance and dropping out—is an attachment issue
- Truly effective management may require active intervention
- The impact of loss and experience of death during adolescence
- The similarity between adult chronic pain disability and adolescent attachment disability
- Attachment issues extend beyond early childhood into adolescence and young adulthood
- What I learn from my patients

Part 4

Attachment Disability, Anxiety, and Depression

8

Attachment Disability and Anxiety

We can understand anxiety as the response to the prospect of separation, whether immediate or pending, whether real or symbolic.

Anxiety, with its impact on trusting, is one cornerstone of this book. It has the power to both stimulate and suppress, to create and crush, to unite and separate. And anxiety feeds distrust.

Webster's definition of anxiety is "a painful uneasiness of mind over an impending or anticipated ill." This is a pretty handy definition. I find that such is what patients generally have in mind when they use the word, although not all of them are able to connect the experience with any specific event. It seems to be "free-floating" for some. It such cases it is not uncommon for anxiety to be mistaken for "depression" when some patients describe their anxiety as a "black cloud coming over me." In fact anxiety and "depression" generally coexist, a linkage I will discuss shortly.

Regardless of the language or behavior cloaking it, anxiety

can always be *understood*. This has the advantage of drawing us together because we all experience anxiety. While we cannot truly say to the other that we know *how* they feel, on the other hand we can truly say we understand *what* they feel. The idea here is to focus on the "what" of anxiety rather than the "why" or the "how" of it. *What* is happening is much more important than *why* or *how* it is happening.

A Definition of Anxiety

The "what" of anxiety is this: *anxiety is always the prospect of separation.*

This dictum was conveyed to me by Dr. Lawrence Kolb, the director of the New York Psychiatric Institute (PI) during my residency training there in the 1960s, under circumstances memorable precisely because they were so mundane.[1]

PI is located in a fifteen-story art deco tower crammed into the west end of the Columbia University medical campus, perched on a bluff overlooking the Hudson River. The tower dates from the 1920s, charming but cramped with antiquated mechanicals. At the time, its elevators reflected its age: pokey, inadequate, confined. One morning I was on my way to the library on a higher floor when the elevator paused and the doors opened to admit Dr. Kolb, evidently on his way to his office above.

There were just the two of us trapped in this groaning, slowly ascending contraption, so not to engage in some sort of polite discourse would have been very ill mannered. Besides, we knew each other well from his prolonged supervision of me the year before. We began to chat about the different ways to conceptualize anxiety. The elevator finally reached his destination, its doors opening. He stepped out. As he turned away he tossed off a final remark, something like, "Of course, it's all due to separation."

The elevator doors closed and he was gone from my sight, but his words were grit in the mind's eye. Despite my respect for him, I didn't buy it. I remembering thinking, *How can he be so dogmatic?* But you don't readily forget an unambiguous, authoritative declaration of this sort. It turns out I was not alone in not signing on to the concept. A very recent epidemiological survey determined that not only is separation anxiety a worldwide phenomenon, but a high percentage is of adult onset. Yet it has been ignored by American psychiatrists. "Our nosology may have avoided ... what so many of our patients find humiliating, childish, and undermining of their sense of autonomy and competence. We all have collectively looked away and cannot afford to continue to do so."[2]

I pondered the idea for a while, then filed it away, a kind of psychiatric curiosity amid the orthodoxies of that era.

Then I encountered Rebecca.

[CASE STUDY]
Rebecca: "Treatment-Resistive Depression"

I'm sitting with Rebecca, a woman I first saw in 1968 at Minneapolis General Hospital when I treated her for phobias and "depression." When I entered private practice, she continued to see me. After she improved, her husband left her and their three children for another woman. For years thereafter her symptoms waxed and waned. At times she was quite paralyzed by these problems, but at other times she was able to work and function normally; for example, ride the bus. Brief trials of a host of psychotropic medications were without any lasting benefit.

A very significant change occurred when her father died in 1975 and her sister moved in. Immediate conflicts developed between the sister and Rebecca's son, Marc, and Rebecca was not insightful or shrewd enough to avoid being sucked into their battles. She became very "depressed," guilty and self-blaming regarding her inability to keep the two of them happy, a chronic problem that will never be fully resolved until her children move out. In the meantime I prescribed yet another Antidepressant, she reported relief, and then in a few months she reappeared, frustrated and apologetic, complaining of a return of her "depression," panic, and anxiety. And we repeated the same cycle. Eventually I settled on a combination of an Antidepressant and a minor Tranquillizer, resulting in only incomplete symptom relief.

Now it's 1982 and I'm gloomy and distracted, mentally reviewing my rather meager therapeutic effectiveness while Rebecca is again describing feeling "depressed," as usual because of the situation with her sister and her son. There is no flash of lighting to unhorse me or heavenly voice, yet it dawns on me that what she actually is reporting is her worries about the lad. Will he to end up like his father as her sister prophesies? What would people think then? Everyone would say it is her fault!

I correct her, prompt her to use the term "worry" to refer to her anguish, not "depression." I also point out that her son is now a teenager, that she has very little control over him or her sister, and that her major responsibility is to inform him as needed what she thinks is best for him regardless of what her sister thinks. What happens after that is his responsibility.

This clarification proves to be huge. Much of her "depression" is actually her frustration with her sister, a housebound nagging recluse who routinely second-guesses Rebecca's parenting, a replay of her childhood. Furious but unable to assert herself for fear of losing control and alienating her sister, Rebecca has to suppress and stuff her anger, thus remaining "depressed." Moreover, she has become contaminated by her sister's phobic avoidance, hence has withdrawn from maintaining or establishing relationships. She has lost her husband and she is losing her son. She therefore cannot risk jeopardizing her only remaining attachment, as painful as it is.

Later I shift the focus of her counseling by suggesting she continue to report her problems to me as she always did, but with two more rules: no apologizing for her problems, and no using the word "should." Subsequently her fears of anxiety and panic begin to recede as these phenomena now seem understandable and meaningful in the context of her life experiences. She begins to accept that it is impossible to make everyone happy. We also examine her hidden belief that her anger is lethal if revealed openly, a residual of her being raised by an emotionally abusive mother.

Thereafter the picture becomes one of progressive, albeit uneven, improvement. At one point her sister even calls me to complain that Rebecca is becoming more withdrawn and not "happy." Actually what is taking place is Rebecca's pretending less and stuffing less whenever she is troubled, and being more honest about her own conflicts and frustrations ... and anger. With me she becomes more logical and direct, and more accepting that medications have little to offer her beyond the relief they are already providing, and that further prescription changes are unlikely to be of much use. The change is dramatic: less medication seeking, less focus on parenting, more discussion of how to manage her sister, less frowning and frustration, even laughing and kidding herself about the unrealism of her fears.

In June 1986 she reports that her last child has graduated and that her two other children are now permanently out of the house. In fact, she has just traveled by plane—her first plane trip ever—to visit her daughter in Texas. Moreover, she has obtained her driver's permit and is looking for work. For the first time ever, weeks and then months go by without her reporting any anxiety or panic.

My last contact with her is in October 1987, to complete a pre-employment physician's statement on her behalf.

What did Rebecca teach me?

The Need for Clarification

Many adolescents and adults are untutored when it comes to describing their suffering. They lack a vocabulary to describe their inner world and therefore resort to more global words such as "unmotivated" or "procrastinating" or "upset" or "miserable" or "unhappy" or, as in this case, "depressed." While it is important to record what they have to say, you must move beyond the general to the specifics, to the phenomena that give rise to the global complaint. This can be particularly arduous with adolescents because they are so close to their trauma, so to speak. That is, the resulting anxieties suffocate not only introspection but subsequent attachment restoration as well. Kids collapse into a state of paralysis and disability, which is what brings them to my doorstep. As I will discuss at greater length in chapter 11, management of Attachment Disability begins with clarification of anxieties about trust.

Where does "depression" fit into the picture? In this book I prefer to restrict its use to designating a *negative cognitive assessment*—self-blaming, in other words, which I signify by italics: *depression*. In Rebecca's case her *depression* was provoked by an anxiety-induced paralysis of functioning. She was convinced that if anyone in her life was unhappy, most notably her sister, it was her "fault." She then began to project her negative regard onto all her relationships, expecting everyone to be critical of her like her sister was. This further contaminated her ability to trust anyone, causing her to withdraw into herself, avoiding social contacts. And when she did venture out of the house, she panicked, expecting either criticism or rejection or both. She became homebound, able to manage only household chores and her self-care: in essence, disabled. She showed up at my office frustrated, distracted, guilty—and complaining of "depression."[i]

In chapter 9 I will again discuss the importance of *not accepting such a self-characterization without an investigation of its referents*. That is, upon hearing the word, you must mentally swap your therapist's hat for your detective's fedora and plan a search for the behaviors, emotions, and thoughts that the term encompasses for the individual. This may prove to be an exhausting and lengthy task, especially with non-insightful individuals, but such a clarification is a vital first step in the understanding and management of attachment issues. My delay in doing so prolonged Rebecca's Attachment Disability for years.[ii]

---

i. Researchers refer to this phenomenon as "cognitive bias." They surmise that the primary effect of Antidepressants is not mood enhancement but mitigation of a state of amygdala hyperactivity that predisposes to a negative assessment of life events; for example, facial expression or vocal emphasis. MRI studies reveal that normalization of amygdala activity after the first week of Antidepressant treatment leads to a later report of mood improvement. For a brief summary of this recent development, see the report by Bruce Jancin, "Target: Cognitive Bias-PReDicT seeks earlier depression results." *Clinical Psychiatry News*. October 27, 2016. See also the chapter in volume 2, "Are Antidepressants Effective?" in which I similarly conclude that the therapeutic effect of Antidepressant treatment is first anxiety relief—the clinical manifestation of reduced amygdala hypervigilance—and then less "depression."

ii. True, feedback between disability and self-critical appraisal of the disability—*depression*—has the potential to transmute a cognitive assessment into a life-threatening Endogenous phenomenon, what I term in the next chapter the "Phenomenon of Endogenicity" in order not to give credence to the notion that the term "Depression" has any reliable content. Its use is archaic. This I will also discuss at length in the next chapter. Fortunately, this complication is relatively uncommon in children and adults.

The Profound Significance of Rebecca's Abuse

Nowadays everyone, professionals and nonprofessionals alike, is aware of the devastation of child abuse. Multiple media accounts are a daily occurrence. But the role of abuse in the genesis of adult psychological disability was not only ignored by psychiatry forty years ago, but it was not even understood. Fortunately things have changed … somewhat. Although inquiries about abuse are now a routine part of all medical and psychological evaluations, too often the emphasis is on current relationships; for example, between spouses or partners or lovers. But, as I have discussed above, the residuals of childhood and adolescent abuse, whether witnessed or sustained, can manifest later in the form of serious and persisting adult disability, one aspect of which is the paradox of the abused clinging to the abuser. At times the intensity of this attachment overwhelms even ingrained self-preservation instincts.[3]

Another complication is misdiagnosis, in Rebecca's case my accepting her complaint of "depression" as a textbook case of Depression. I am sure she appreciated my interest and energy, most likely the reason for her faithful compliance over the years. But she needed more.

Ultimately it became clear the emotional abuse she had sustained during her childhood and adolescence had paralyzed her, sucking the vitality out of her, rendering her colorless and subservient and clinging. Perhaps this is why her husband left her once she improved, figuring now she could manage without him. But when her older, domineering sister moved in, forecasting doom regardless of circumstance and tolerating no voice other than her own, Rebecca sustained a relapse. Once again she was trapped.

Anger Paralyzes

Two things happen to youngsters raised with an angry parent: they emulate anger or they suppress it—sometimes both. Emulation serves to promote distance and maintain safe boundaries, while serving as a disguised call on the environment for help. Suppression is actually more disabling because, as it begins to percolate into awareness, it prompts fears of retaliation and obliteration should anyone—anyone!—suspect its presence. Hence Rebecca's home boundedness and hidden social anxiety.

Some anxiety is quite apparent. Consider my years managing Charles.

[CASE STUDY]
Charles: Cancer Cures a Phobia

He storms into my office indignant about the way he was treated the night before in the emergency room of the hospital across the street from my office building. He had gone there concerned about a "sore" on his tongue and was brushed off. So I suggest I take a look at it. It turns out to be more than a sore. On the left margin of his tongue is a nasty looking, inflamed, deeply ulcerated lesion. Although I am more than ten years away from my surgical internship, I have no doubt I'm looking at a carcinoma.

I had inherited him years before when I signed on at MGH, where he had been an outpatient for several years and had succeeded in exhausting everyone's patience. My first afternoon the director of the outpatient department, Dr. Tony Pollock, called me to his office to instruct me on my duties, or so I thought.

In fact it turned out his plan was hand over to me, the newbie staffer, the care of Charles. If you have any experience in the corporate or medical world, you will recognize this as a familiar ritual, the baptism by fire. By this time a veteran of more than three years of state-hospital bureaucratic combat, I immediately recognized the gambit and the expected counter. So I kept my mouth shut, nodded, and looked agreeable as Tony provided me with a case summary.

This consisted of him ventilating at length about why Charles was such a royal pain in the behind, particularly his habit of calling Tony at his home, sometimes several times a night. Nothing could satisfy him: not extra appointments, not threats to terminate him. And for certain, no medication had helped. Nothing fazed him. He would still call Tony or hassle the emergency room staff, demanding to be seen. Since the hospital was a public space, he could not be denied entrance, plus the exasperated ER staff was so tired of dealing with him that they would just wave him on through. Many a morning he would be perched outside Tony's office. Therefore it was understandable that when I hove into view, Tony, an experienced and ordinarily empathic figure, nonetheless concluded his tirade with a certain relish by delivering Charles into my hands.[iii] Not surprisingly, Tony never asked for a follow-up. Charles was all mine.

Over the ensuring years, I obtained his history by bits and pieces. In 1970, for example, after I resigned from MGH and joined a private practice, he followed me there and I discovered he had an old chart from the 1940s when he had been evaluated by one of my senior partners. He had been referred for examination because at an induction physical he stated he thought he was pregnant. He was diagnosed as Schizophrenic and classified

---

iii. My dear sister-in-law, who for years served as a hospital ombudsperson, would have said that he had simply "run out of nice."

4-F.ⁱᵛ Apparently he was never hospitalized. Later he went into the insurance business and enjoyed a successful career until he became totally disabled by a cancer phobia, which brought him to MGH for treatment. I never did establish what precipitated his disability, nor did he reveal much about his background. However, I now recognize that his very stormy ambivalence toward medical figures was a manifestation of significant trust issues nonetheless. Was it due to prior exposure to an angry parent?

At examination it was obvious Schizophrenia was not the problem. Charles proved to be a very intelligent, very charming, very handsome,ᵛ very extroverted, and very gay man in his middle fifties. He had a lifetime partner, "Wilson," who supported him. He did not cruise but otherwise was well known in the gay community both locally and nationwide. For example, he maintained that whenever Liberace was in town, he would throw a party for him. He loved to titillate me with tidbits about such functions and the many eminent doctors, lawyers, judges, and so on, who attended. But always the gentleman, he never named names.

On the other hand, Charles was clearly very needy, very demanding, very rejection sensitive, and very, very cancer phobic, with an especially painful dimension: he was very frightened of doctors, afraid that one day they would confirm his worst nightmare. He haunted emergency rooms and doctors' offices while avoiding a clear statement of his concerns: a classic approach/avoidance paralysis. He was unable to venture more than a few miles away from the hospital and had not traveled for years. No wonder he was seen as Schizophrenic. Indeed, on one occasion, gripped by an unusually intense dread, he made a threatening call to the White House, knowing the Secret

---

iv. In those days Schizophrenia was overdiagnosed. Now it is Mood Disorder.

v. He bore a striking resemblance to the English actor Charles Gray.

Service would detain him and he would be forced to submit to a physical while in custody.

Although he was reluctant to explore the dimensions of his fears, it soon became obvious that the idea of cancer prompted fears of death, which he visualized as being trapped in a coffin, alone and helpless.[vi] In other words, for him cancer symbolized separation. I eventually realized that his midnight calls served to not only relieve his sense of isolation and powerlessness, but to reassure himself that I was still alive. What helped in such dark moments was not what I had to say, but simply the action of calling and hearing a voice, proof that he was not alone and helpless and abandoned, and that his ceaseless demands had not caused me to give up on him or make me sick.

In response, by trial and error I developed a protocol, the gist of which was to abbreviate our nocturnal dialogue yet instruct him that I would make room to see him the next day. He did not always take advantage of this offer, but typically when he did the emergency had evaporated and we would pass most of the time with him entertaining me with insider gossip, political scandals, and intrigues, things of that sort. Slowly, very slowly, the frequency of his nocturnal calls diminished.

On the other hand, he continued to hang out in emergency rooms, but less now at MGH, more at the ER across the street. His reception there proved less than genial, at times rude, even hostile. Now, as the above history suggests, Charles was not a timid soul in all respects, certainly not one to accept a brush-off meekly, so he got into the habit of marching over to the medical staff office and camping outside it until it opened the next morning, then berating the secretary, Peggy, about the way he was managed.

Now, I must admit that by this time I was neither Peggy's nor the administration's favorite because of my rather dyspeptic view, shall I say, regarding the benevolence of medical

---

vi. Note an early verification here of Dr. Kolb's hypothesis, but I guess I still needed more evidence.

administrators. I should have been more discreet with my observation that hospitals and doctors were like politicians and newspapers: natural enemies that yet needed each other and that would therefore strive to manipulate the other. I would warn my peers that unless physicians were careful not to sell out, the way things were going the administrators would soon dominate medical care, and that at crunch time, we doctors would be crunched in the name of "the good of the patients."

So it was surprising that one day Peggy was on the phone beseeching me to "do something" about Charles's most recent protestations. Exercising surprising (for me) political adeptness, I refrained from reminding her of the obvious: if the hospital did not want to be troubled by the likes of Charles, all it needed was to turn off that sign that said, EMERGENCY ENTRANCE. In other words, once you open your doors to all comers, some are going to be difficult to manage. Instead I simply told her to send him over, not only then but any time he showed up on her doorstep with a beef. "Just wave him on through like the staff did at General. He's used to that." Which she did.

He soon got into the habit of coming directly to me with his complaints, which in fact was my plan anyhow. Calls from Peggy ceased. And the frequency of both his midnight calls and impromptu visits declined. He seemed to be more at home with his health worries.

Then one day he storms in about another ER rebuff, with concerns about what turns out to be a serious health issue. What to do?

> *Dr. C., deciding directness is the best approach:* "I can see why you are worried. That does look like trouble. It could be cancer."
> *Charles: Silent.*
> *Dr. C:* "In fact you should have an expert take a look at it right away."
> *Charles, with surprising calm:* "Okay."

> Dr. C., scribbling a note on his prescription pad: "Down the hall is the office of a surgeon with an excellent reputation. Dr. U. He's an older man, a bit gruff but very qualified. Take this to his receptionist and tell her you'll wait until he can see you."
> Charles: Nods, accepts the note, leaves.

He does not return to give me a report, then or thereafter. No midnight calls either.

Two months later I see he has an appointment. He shows up on time with half of his neck and tongue missing. Obviously the ulcer was a carcinoma with positive nodes, surgically treated via a left hemi-glossectomy/radical hemi-neck dissection. Hardly able to articulate and barely to rotate his head, thinner, looking like a concentration camp survivor, he's smiling and vivacious as before, regaling me as usual with his interim adventures, medical and otherwise, but without bitterness about physicians and/or health concerns.

In the months thereafter he makes an amazing recovery. He regains lost weight, neck strength, and normal articulation except for a very slight lisp. Moreover, there is no evidence of a cancer recurrence. He no longer calls at night. And the interval between visits increases; sometimes I do not see him for months. At one point he mentions that he and Wilson just returned home from a lengthy tour of the Black Hills and Mount Rushmore, a place he has always wanted to visit. It's obvious he is no longer housebound. In fact, later they plan to fly to Arizona for a winter vacation.

After a while I realize it's been a year or two since I last heard from him. Obviously he has dropped out. Thereafter I think of him now and then; it's hard to totally forget such a flamboyant figure.

A few years ago, after more than twenty years since our last contact, I get a notion to see if he is still alive, so I do an Internet search. I stumble upon a perfunctory mid-90s obituary notice, same name, no address, no funeral home contact, no cause of death, no survivors, but the 1920s birthdate fits. It's likely he's dead. I'm a bit melancholy; it would have been nice to dream that Charles is still out there, touring with his life partner, entertaining, gossiping, cancer and phobia free.

Discussion

What to say about this remarkable man, his remarkable recovery, and, most of all, his remarkable management by Dr. U? I will begin with the man.

Charles the Man

Unfortunately I do not have his office file, shredded per protocol years ago. As garrulous and loquacious as he was, even if my notes were available for review now, I do not think I would glean from them much more information than I have summarized. He was very circumspect, I now realize, careful to conceal — what? Certainly not his identity; he practically advertised his gayness, this at a time when coming out was neither fashionable nor admired. Indeed, as I reflect on my experience of him, it now seems he used his identity as camouflage to distract me, to escape pointed inquiry. Nonetheless the very nature of his complaints provides some clues.

Most understandable is his bitterness and distrust of hospitals. I recognize that in the 1940s most doctors would have difficulty comprehending a young man expressing a belief he was pregnant. Moreover, this was not an era noted for enlightened treatment of Schizophrenia. Recommended methods included fever therapy, coma therapy, and transorbital lobotomy, not to mention commitment to an institution.[vii] If Charles had been

---

vii. Psychiatrist Jeffrey A. Lieberman provides a summary of these unhappy decades in his informal history of psychiatry's

exposed to any, he never said. And whether any treatment played a role in his subsequent successful career in insurance is also unclear. Some twenty-five years later when I first met him, he was still labeled Schizophrenic but without any of the primary or secondary signs characteristic of that illness. Perhaps his enduring distrust of and anger with things medical represented a residual of his treatment experiences. If so, he never said.

Less understandable are the origins of his cancer fears. But once present, his cancer apprehensions ignited a secondary apprehension. Many, many people experience and live with fears of cancer. Only a very, very small percentage become disabled by them, incapacitated by a fear of fear, so to speak. Typically the incapacitation is partial: say, not allowing them to travel out of town, or move more than ten or twenty miles away from their family doctor or—in this day of peripatetic physicians and insurance plans—favorite clinic. Charles was unique, a sort of Ancient Mariner, becalmed on a sea of cancer dread and physician distrust.

All professionals have encountered phobic avoidance although many times it is not recognized as such. Sometimes it is rather subtle: a patient not appearing for an appointment arranged by a doctor's or dentist's office or, as I learned during my outreach work at the Central Minnesota Mental Health Center, a parent missing a PTA conference. Sometimes less subtle and therefore more noticeable and potentially more irritating is the patient who calls for an appointment and then does not appear. I remember one man so tortured that after such a series of misses I suggested we dispense with making appointments, inviting him to just show up when he felt the need, promising I would fit him in, if only briefly. He did call a few times to say he was going to come—same result. I finally

---

struggles to understand and cure mental illness, *Shrinks: The Untold Story of Psychiatry* (New York: Little, Brown and Company, 2015, 153–66).

offered to arrange for him to seek comfort in our Urgent Care department by sitting in the waiting area without having to register. What could be more informal? He agreed, but he never appeared.

Of course, some patients eventually do appear, typically with an excuse for the prior skip: their ride didn't show, there was a last-minute emergency at work or a sudden illness at home, things of that sort, which I would accept without comment if the no-show was not part of a pattern. But if a pattern of such behavior did seem to be present, at some point I would gently inquire if something about seeing a physician was threatening. Some patients would continue to deny or minimize such a problem. Some would be more frank and reveal a fear of being listened to. Others the opposite; that is, not being listened to. With the former, the concern is that by listening the doctor will confirm their fear that they need treatment: say, medications or even "being locked up." With the latter, the concern is that their issues will not be taken seriously, that they will sustain another rebuff, the story of their life. Charles manifested both, simultaneously and intensely.

Contemplation of death is not always fearful. In chapter 11 I will discuss Hans Castorp, the protagonist of Thomas Mann's *The Magic Mountain*, bewitched by "an inborn attraction to death," who, realizing that death gives meaning to life, descends from the mountain to participate in the turmoil of life in the flatlands below. Moreover, some already immersed in the turmoil, most famously Hamlet, and certainly scores of my "depressed" patients, consider thoughts of death a consolation, a symbol of peace and relief from suffering. In the midst of hopelessness about life, they find hope in the prospect of death, an escape from suffering and helplessness. They reassure themselves they are not totally powerless: *I can always kill myself,* they think. Paradoxically, such an attitude gives them the courage to continue on with life.

On the other hand, perhaps once a year or less, a patient will seek or be referred for consultation precisely because of death fears. I always inquire if the fear of is one damnation. The great majority deny such concerns, expressing a belief in a Merciful Almighty. Rather, their concern is separation. A few like Charles worry they will end up alone, unable to communicate, a kind of cold, eternal purgatory. For most, however, the separation takes the form of concerns about loved ones left behind. Who will look after them, take care of them?

Charles's Recovery

The diagnosis of a tongue carcinoma forced Charles to confront his two nightmares: doctors and cancer. As I described, I was surprised by his equanimity about and his forthright acceptance of the referral. I surmise that he may have previously concluded that his problem was more serious than an ordinary canker sore, which would account for his fury and rage about the brush-off. Perhaps this explains his subsequent undemonstrative trek down the hall for his consult with Dr. U.

What happened thereafter remains a mystery. I should note here, however, that the Behavior Therapy literature dealing with phobic avoidance describes a therapeutic maneuver known as *flooding.* For example, in theory, one way to get over, say, a fear of heights would be to skydive one or twice. In practice, however, few therapists would ever recommend such an extreme measure, although I suppose some tortured souls have self-prescribed the technique. The more standard approach for phobic avoidance of things medical, however, would be to recommend an exposure/response-prevention (E/RP) protocol,[viii] perhaps combined with hypnosis. I have recommended this for at least three patients traumatized by otherwise life-saving sustained hospital treatment regimens. Two were survivors of extensive burns, which required a series of very painful debridements to remove devitalized tissues and refresh

---

viii. Discussed in chapter 13.

dressings. The other had sustained a weeks'-long intubation to preserve respiratory function while recovering from a tenacious pulmonary infection. All three experienced nightmares and flashbacks while expressing enduring apprehension at the prospect of hospitalization. Hopefully a combination of both E/RP and hypnosis would help them learn progressive relaxation to manage their anxieties and reframe the notion of the hospital as the locale of healing rather than suffering.

But Charles, without the advantage of either, plunged right in and was cured not only of his tumor, but of his fears as well. I attribute this to his management by Dr. U.

Charles's Remarkable Management

In retrospect, after not having reflected on my experiences with Charles for decades, and only prompted to do so now by my realization of how his life dramatizes the dynamics of anxiety, I am puzzled by my choice of Dr. U. It could not have been the proximity of his office. I was located across from the hospital in a four-story medical office building, the locale of a variety of medical specialists, including a host of surgeons. And we had not established a social or consulting or referral relationship as I had with many of the physicians on the medical staff. We had never entertained each other, never hung out at staff functions or parties or picnics. In fact I can't recall ever talking to him in the staff lounge or sitting at the same table at lunch with him or hearing him participate in chatter about travel, sports, hunting, economics, politics—all the usual things doctors gab about with time on their hands. Now and then late in the afternoon I would spot him in the lounge engrossed in the newspaper, apparently finished with rounds, on his way home or to the office. If he noticed me it was only with a nod, not necessarily one of recognition. He was a contemporary of our group's senior partner; perhaps that was the connection.

Also, as I now think about it, he would have been approximately the same age as Charles.

Nonetheless, whatever my calculations, my choice proved to be an inspired one judging from the results. I imagine Dr. U., after a brief but careful examination, announcing something like, "It is cancer. You have to go into the hospital at once to have half of your tongue removed, also all the neck tissues on that side, except for the skin and muscles, to get all the lymph nodes out." And I imagine Charles again nodding in agreement. He knew this was no drill, that he had to leap into the abyss or die. So he jumped and lived.

Well, it would be fitting if I had a feel-good anecdote to wrap up this tale of my brief collaboration with the remarkable Dr. U.—the two of us, say, if only one afternoon in the staff lounge exchanging a glance or a nod or a fist bump, a symbolic victory lap. But nothing of the sort transpired. All of us passed in the night and went on to live productive lives, and how could one not be content with that?

But there is a denouement nonetheless, a byproduct of my experiences with Charles. I learned how to manage midnight phone calls. Once in solo practice, I now had the freedom to leave my home phone number on my office phone, later my cell phone number as well once that capability became available. The need for this service was obvious once my experiences with Rebecca and Charles and others had convinced me that Dr. Kolb's pronouncement of years before was unquestionably valid: all anxiety was indeed related to separation. Providing a lifeline in the form of around-the-clock phone contact would mitigate feelings of isolation and promote anxiety relief, especially if the caller faced a problem for which there seemed no solution.

I evolved a three-step protocol. After listening for a minute or two I would ask if it was an emergency. If so, I would advise the patient to go to the nearest ER for an evaluation, and give the examiner my phone number for a phone consultation regarding their findings. If it was not an emergency, they could make an appointment to see me the next day.

The next step was to interpret the motivation for the call by, as Dr. MacKinnon would say, "speaking to the unconscious." I would reassure callers I was alive and well. What was I addressing here? Many patients fear that their concerns are so burdensome, even toxic, that they will drive their therapist nuts, or to drink, or to suicidal despair, even to leave the profession because of burnout. Typically a call of this sort is most likely the evening after an earlier intense therapy session, particularly with patients whose trust has been damaged by abuse or rejection. For such individuals to finally begin to ventilate emotion feels lethal, liable to provoke retaliation or abandonment or both. Hearing me respond to such lurking concerns with a seeming non sequitur, that *I'm okay,* is profoundly therapeutic.

The final step was to provide reassurance that no matter the seeming intransigence of their problem, not having an immediate solution was not their fault, that problems came with the territory of life. Yet the territory of life was also unpredictable, that things would look different later, perhaps even tomorrow. No need to succumb to hopelessness.

Eventually with new patients, after explaining my availability via phone, I took to rehearsing the protocol in advance so they would know what to expect should they call. As I grew older and more susceptible to restless sleep, I would add a footnote to the effect that they had to give me a minute or so to get over my crankiness about being awakened. It was the rare patient who called. Most left messages.

Dr. Kolb's Dictum Modified

In view of the epiphany I experienced during my encounters with Rebecca, Charles, and others, some of which I am including in this book, I will pass on here with a slight modification Dr. Kolb's pronouncement, not as a rigid law but as a rule of thumb to assist in understanding and managing student underperformance and dropping out as well as adult emotional disability. The idea here is to get into the habit of looking beyond the behavior—whether entangled or underperforming or avoidant or resistive or "depressed"—to determine if it rises from a background of separation.

> We can understand anxiety as the response to the prospect of separation, whether immediate or pending, whether real or symbolic.

One might say this amounts to an insignificant difference, simply substituting "separation" for the dictionary's impending or anticipated "ill." But the apparent simplicity of the reformulation is deceptive because the perspective it reveals is vast. Change always incorporates some kind of separation and loss. Think about it. Think not of the obvious changes that bedevil life—birth, death, marriage, relocation, school, promotion, retirement, layoff—but the very minor fluctuations we all experience in the day's flow of events: traffic jams, the headlines, our partner's behavior, the coworker who butts in, the coworker who doesn't acknowledge a greeting, and so one. Each blip, or the absence of an expected blip, ignites a passing appraisal of its significance, the gist of which is *Does this affect the security of my relationships?*[4] Of course, most such appraisals do not rise to the level of consciousness, unless the blips multiply and evolve into a major disruption of life's flow. Then they might ignite what I call a *What if?* thought ("awfulizing" is how a friend puts it, or "Igor talk," Dr. Anderson would say).

The consequences of what-ifness thinking depend on the context of the appraisal; for example, our loss and separation history, the trauma embedded in our neurons, the degree of support in our environment, and how much blame—Whose fault is it?—rules our life. We might judge the blips as no threat to our security status. Or certain blips might motivate us to an enhanced state of performance. In short, some anxieties possess survival value.

On the other hand, we might find certain blips signal ominous portent: the prospect of separation, perhaps even loss and feelings of abandonment. The latter has the potential to trigger a body/brain combat mode, preparing us to contest the loss of security, or replace what might be lost, or both. So we are transformed into a pumped-up state, an activated state, a state of stress, the duration of which can range from a few seconds to a lifetime. The longer the duration, the more likely the disability. Conversely, successfully overcoming the challenges evoked by change can enhance one's self-acceptance and self-confidence.

Adolescents or young adults coping with abandonment and distrust of closeness precipitated by life changes face persisting disability if their attachment issues are not recognized and managed.

For example:

[CASE STUDY]
Julie: The Dangers of Recovery

A young adult, Julie had been married for only eight months when her husband collapsed and died while playing hockey. She experienced profound grief accompanied by severe weight loss, became unable to function, and remained so for eighteen months thereafter despite continuous and exhaustive psychiatric treatment including three hospitalizations (one via commitment following an overdose), one course of electrotherapy, and trials of six different Antidepressants. Moreover, if treatment seemed to be helping, she became noncompliant.

Eventually she consulted with a therapist, who succeeded in gaining her trust and who referred her to me to restart one of the Antidepressants that had worked in the past.

When I inquired of what I suspected, she did admit she

blamed herself for ever having married. "If I had not fallen in love and married I would not be hurting," is how she explained it. Thus her habit of aborting successful treatment: it protected her from the risks of the relationships that health and recovery would inevitably bring into her life. But this "solution" carried a huge cost. She was unable to function because of persistent but unwitting anxiety that the next person she trusted would also drop dead ... and again the loss and grief would be her fault, because once again she had foolishly given her trust to another.

This vignette, brief as it is, illustrates a number of fundamental attachment issues.

Unmanaged Attachment Issues Linger

While her Depression was profound and even life threatening on occasion, the attachment conflicts driving it were never addressed. Suicidal behavior or ruminations of any sort always—always!—signal an emotional or physical pain, occasionally both, the relief of which the sufferer has come to believe is hopeless. *So-called Depression disables, but it is hopelessness that kills.*

Thus Julie remained vulnerable to relapse and retreat into disability.

Not all relapse is due to noncompliance, as was the situation here. Not infrequently it is caused by a change from a brand medication to a generic substitute or by a switch between generic equivalents, or by a change to a different generic from the same class of medications. Or relapse is precipitated by a new stress; for example, a rejection or promotion or offer of promotion (as was the case of Dyllen), or a new romantic interest (as illustrated by Amanda in chapter 4). Or by an apparently autonomous upsurge of anxiety; for example, as happened to author William Styron, which I will discuss in the next chapter.

Here, however, relapse was clearly related to her discontinuing otherwise successful treatment since "improvement" symbolized once again risking attachment with its inevitable possibility of subsequent abandonments. To change to a state of health was *dangerous,* to be disabled was *safe.* In short, while her several treatment experiences relieved the obvious disabilities, they did not address her underlying and persisting hopelessness: she would never be free of the possibility of loss and abandonment.

Adolescents are susceptible to the same dynamic. But it is the rare youngster who can articulate this issue as clearly as Julie. Typically it is only after years of reflection that we develop some understanding of how our life's path is determined by our unwitting navigation of youthful miseries. Until then we stumble blindfolded through the minefield of life.

The Mystery of Life

Julie's fears of connectedness are not so difficult for us to comprehend since we all suffer the stresses of change and have experienced the loss of the beloved. We know how we feel and have felt; therefore little imagination is necessary to understand the devastation of her loss and reluctance to move forward. On the other hand, it is not at all clear how her current therapist was successful in gaining her trust. This is the Catch-22 of therapy: if you are good at trusting, you wouldn't be sitting in a therapist's office to begin with.

A Vignette

Toward the end of my psychiatric training, several of us were wrapping up a psychotherapy seminar with one of our professors, an eminent psychoanalyst. He had struggled with us for a year to polish therapy techniques, the gist of which was learning when to say something and when to say nothing. Once a month we would gather at his mid-Manhattan office and take turns presenting an update on our therapeutic (mis)adventures, offering critiques of our own and each other's performance. When things got murky and one of us started to founder, the professor provided clarification and suggestions. By year's end the proceedings were informal and relaxing. We all had bonded and we all knew we were going to graduate; it was, in fact, rather relaxing to pile into a car and go for a ride downtown to his office while taking a break from our official responsibilities as senior residents. Indeed, our final meetings were more like a conversation among equals, with him sharing his views on the wider world of psychiatry and psychoanalysis.

During one such audible rumination, he tossed off a comment: "Of course, when it comes to therapy, technique is about twenty percent. The rest is trust, and that is up to you." I remember thinking, *What the #$%&! I wish someone had told me this at the beginning. I would have had a better idea of what I was trying to do.*

He was right, of course, but the deeper significance of his words escaped me then. The disability of Attachment Disability is precisely a wounded ability to trust. Relationships are dangerous because they create the risk of abandonment, or exploitation, or betrayal, which amount to the same thing. Therapeutic relationships present the same hazard. Effective therapeutic technique consists of a constant vigilance and assessment of the injured party's trust tolerance and adjusting the trust boundaries accordingly. Out of this 20 percent of expertise, we hope the other 80 percent of chemistry will flourish. I presume that Julie's therapist was effective because from the very first he or she was focused on the delicate task of trust building. Julie was very fortunate.

To be sure, her physicians, after a good deal of trial-and-error prescribing — not unusual in my experience when it comes to Antidepressants — happened upon a regimen that was both tolerable and effective. Her fight/flight mode was mitigated, her overt disability relieved, she was pronounced improved, and she was discharged. But her attachment concerns were not relieved. True, she had a clearer picture of the problem, but her insight came unaccompanied by a remediation strategy. Hence her "solution" of noncompliance: safer to be sick.

Acceptance of Grief

It is vital to understand prolonged grief not as a "depression" but as a natural component of the human spirit. Otherwise we professionals can become trapped into a misguided alliance with attachment-disabled adolescents and young adults who come before us complaining they cannot "get over" grieving. Rather, it is important to investigate the possibility of a hidden anxiety about subsequent loss. If present and not addressed, it remains underground, leaving in its wake a lost, unhappy, perhaps bitter and angry soul. Moreover, the sufferer risks becoming avoidant, withdrawing from making an emotional commitment when the opportunity for subsequent relationships arises.

In short, there has been a double loss, not only of the beloved but also of the social support that ordinarily would be available to sufferers if they were not so wary of accepting it. Therefore when an adolescent or adult reports they are unable to "get over," say, the death of a friend or parent or grandparent, it is critical that this be understood as a double death, so to speak. That is, there is not only the tangible loss of the valued figure, but the intangible loss of a potentially supportive network, and with it the possibility of adaptive learning.

Grief requires acceptance, not treatment. The loss of the beloved is never and cannot be rectified. For Julie to heal does not mean "getting over" her loss, but finding the courage to go forward in life with the understanding it could happen again. If her awareness of risk were to be submerged, she would remain susceptible to a more-or-less mysterious "collapse" whenever the prospect of relationship intimacy sails into view.

A somewhat analogous situation occurs during recovery

from addiction. Addicted individuals who achieve sobriety are to be congratulated because they have discarded a maladaptive behavior. On the other hand, they need awareness that while they have overcome a "bad solution" to a life problem, there remains the task of finding a "good solution" to the problem. This is why recovery consists of both sobriety and support. Without the support of AA, or aftercare, or relapse prevention to promote awareness and adaptive learning, addicts remain at greater risk of falling back into their addiction.[ix]

Similarly, while psychotropic medications have the potential to relieve so-called Depression they cannot remove the underlying vulnerability to recurrent episodes. Medication is necessary but not definitive. The underlying life problem needs to be addressed as well. This is supported by a survey of the comparative effectiveness of Depression treatments by Dr. Steve Balt. These show that medication helps, or therapy helps, but the combination is more helpful than either alone. After a careful review of a host of studies, Dr. Balt concludes they support the conventional notion that all Antidepressants are basically equal in effectiveness. He also remarks, "The quality of the therapeutic alliance … is sometimes a better predictor of patient outcome than which drugs are prescribed."[5]

If upon examination much of so-called Depression consists of unexamined and poorly understood anxiety, which is my position in this book, does the term have any meaning at all? I will address this question in the following chapter.

---

ix. I will present a more exhaustive discussion of addiction in volume 2. See chapter 12 below for the need of addicts in recovery to learn acceptance.

9

Attachment Disability and Depression

*Depression is a spectrum phenomenon rather than
a collection of discrete illness syndromes.*

Trauma promotes distrust, dissociation, anxiety, and maladaptive learning. How survivors manage depends on their pre-trauma adaptive skill set, which is likely to be less extensive with adolescents and children, rendering them more vulnerable than adults to attachment anxieties.

For example, some traumatized individuals may have previously been trained in meditation practices; they may resort to such techniques in order to "float" with their anxieties without becoming disabled by them. However, it is important to recall that they became adept after first learning to manage the body processes over which they had some direct, conscious control—such as muscle tension, and respiration depth and frequency—through rhythmic exercise, chanting, or prayer. In other words, successful emotion management of this sort requires prior successful body management.

Others are protected by the activation of automatic protective wired-in nervous system defenses that wall off the threat of overwhelming activation. The activation goes underground, so to speak, lurking in the background, dissociated, more or less separated from consciousness. This comes at the price of a constricted life, however, burdened by the lingering threat of unexpected symptom outbursts such as nightmares, flashbacks, anger tantrums, and so on. Moreover, even the activation of joy and happiness is experienced as potentially dangerous and therefore must be suppressed. True, the dissociation enables victims to survive, but life at its best is rendered dull, flat, boring, endless, and monotonous: in short, fertile ground in which to nourish hopelessness.

Still others resort to substances, marijuana in the case of Dyllen and alcohol in the case of William Styron, whom I will discuss later in this chapter.

But some remain unable to float or dissociate or medicate away the anxiety that is embedded in their distrust. Therefore they have little choice beyond struggling to regulate and manage it via exercising "will power," not realizing that to harness anxiety they must first focus on harnessing the body. Failure is inevitable, but they continue to strive, often in response to encouragement from well-meaning family or friends—and too often, incompetent therapists—who advise, "Don't dwell on your worries" or "Think about something else." Of course the result is another failure. It takes a very stout mind to not succumb to what is the usual outcome of repetitive failures: lowered self-esteem, heightened self-blame, pernicious self-criticism. Failed "will power" practitioners who experience this *self-deprecatory triad* frequently characterize it as "depression."

But it is important to be very clear here. The anxiety of distrust is an *emotional* process. In contrast, the deprecatory triad is a *cognitive* phenomenon, an error of judgment generated by a failure to control the uncontrollable, in this case the emotion of anxiety.[i] Unfortunately this cognitive self-assessment is too

---

i. Obviously trauma fallout is not the only life circumstance

often uncritically accepted by psychiatrists and therapists as Depression, which may result in a second error of judgment: treatment with Antidepressants. This places survivors at risk of being shuffled down a blind alley leading to their being designated as "treatment resistant." In fact, they are actually *medication resistant* since, in my experience, a posture of self-deprecation is unlikely to respond to psychotropics.

Therefore, any discussion of attachment disability is incomplete without some consideration of the notion of "Depression."

A Definition of "Depression"

This is a term that escapes terse characterization, which is reflected in *Webster* where, in contrast to anxiety, the definition of depression is broader: "... dejection, as of mind ... lowering of vitality or functional activity ... negative attitude ... abnormal state of inactivity and unpleasant emotion ..." Interestingly, as unwieldy as it is, the definition accurately reflects the bimodality of "depression," a bimodality that incorporates the domains of the psychological and the physical.

In fact, everyday use of the term is even broader that *Webster*. Attachment-disabled youngsters and adults also make use of it as they refer to stress and anxiety phenomena such as minute-to-minute changes in affect, worry, looming apprehension, and so on. Indeed, surveys suggest that 48 to 78 percent of depressive illness is accompanied by an anxiety disorder.[1] But not infrequently patients cram all issues of whatever sort into the portmanteau of "depression." This is what derailed my

---

that generates attempts to control the uncontrollable. Consider, for example, how we try to manage the behavior of our children or coworkers or supervisors, or how we attempt to shape our career and life choices. If we are not realistic about our limits, any change, whether foreseen or unforeseen, risks igniting the deprecatory triad with its potential misinterpretation as "depression."

treatment of Rebecca for years: my uncritical acceptance of her use of the word "depression" to denote her suffering.

A Proposed Clarification

Yet it really is impossible to carry on a discussion with youngsters or young adults or their sponsors—or author a book, for that matter—without using the term. Hence, to repeat the convention I proposed in the introduction, when I enclose the term in quotes—"depression"—I refer to its popular use in everyday conversation. But when I use the term capitalized without quotation marks—Depression—I have in mind its more technical meaning within the professions. Finally, to denote the specific meaning I have in mind for the purposes of this book only, italicized—*depression*. That is,

- Popular use—some kind of uncomfortable feeling or behavior, signified by quotes: "depression."
- Technical use—as defined in standard psychiatric textbooks, signified by uppercase: Depression.
- My use—persistent self-criticism, a psychological phenomenon, signified by italics: *depression*.

The Benefits of Clarification

Accordingly, I encourage adolescents, their parents, and adult patients to clarify, if possible, their use of the word "depression" in reporting problems. I explain that the idea is for them to focus on the underlying phenomena, the behaviors and feelings lumped into the term. For example, a not uncommon description of "depression" is "a black cloud coming over me." Typically, a careful analysis of the circumstances reveals that the "black cloud" is actually the sudden onset of free-floating anxiety. In some cases I will advise patents that "that the word 'depression' is forbidden in our conversation, so we have to converse without using it."[ii] Sometimes I forget my own rule, which is usually good for a laugh.

To be sure, clarification of this sort is not accomplished in one or two visits. The idea is to establish this as a goal of management: the development of a different mental language, so to speak, which requires patience and time. As I will discuss further along and at greater length in chapter 11, the first of the three steps of disability recovery—*clarify* the disability—addresses in part the problem of ambiguity.

Another reason for clarification, beyond its utter necessity for effective attachment disability management, is to make some sense of the debate in the literature about the utility of Antidepressants in children and adolescents. Some authors report there is little evidence to support their use in the treatment of youthful Depression. For example, Jureidini et al analyzed randomized controlled trials of newer Antidepressants, typically Selective Serotonin Reuptake Inhibitors (SSRI), published during the interval 1989–2004.[2] They concluded that Antidepressant efficacy was exaggerated, demonstrating little additional benefit versus control groups. Moreover, there was a tendency to minimize adverse effects. They concluded such Antidepressants could not be recommended as a treatment option for childhood Depression. More recent surveys reach the same conclusion.[3]

Yet other researchers confidently conclude there is considerable evidence that Antidepressants are of definite benefit in childhood and adolescent disability. But the catch is that they limit their analysis to selected anxiety disorders, excluding Depression.[4]

So the question is, Do Antidepressants help or not? Perhaps

---

ii. In the volume 2 chapter, "Are Antidepressants Effective?" I earnestly implore all of psychiatry to abandon the word, arguing it is without meaningful content, somewhat similar to the phlogiston concept employed by alchemists to "explain" combustion.

a part of the answer rests in considering the role of trauma in the genesis of Depression. In 2003 Dr. Charles Nemeroff, studying treatment of adults with Major Depression, discovered that those with a history of childhood trauma responded better to psychotherapy alone (48 percent remission) than treatment with Antidepressants alone (33 percent). For almost half of the study patients, the trauma was physical abuse, for about one-third, parental loss.[5]

A more recent study of Major Depression Disorder (MDD) in three- to five-year-old preschoolers provides additional evidence of the influence of trauma on subsequent mental health.[6] Taking their cue from a well-established correlation between such early onset Depression and guilt, these researchers note that while the early development of guilt requires more study, a host of reports points to the influence of genetic and environmental factors such as "… experiences of adversity, stress, and trauma." Via MRI evaluations, they then compared the size of the Depressed youngsters' insula—that part of the brain that processes self-conscious emotions, especially guilt—to the brains of normal preschoolers. They discovered the brains of Depressed children demonstrated a significant size reduction versus non-Depressed peers.

Of course it is possible that the structural changes were the consequence of a preexisting genetic factor, thereby promoting an increased susceptibility to guilty ruminations evoked by the stress of adversity and trauma. On the other hand, the latter may be primary. Regardless of the direction of the dynamism, the takeaway here is the role of trauma in either case.

Nonetheless, the question remains: Do Antidepressants help or not?[iii] Even taking such studies into account, there will always remain a significant proportion of youngsters with trauma-related Depression who do not respond to therapy alone

---

iii. I will discuss the theoretical aspects of this issue at greater length in volume 2, but the practical answer is you never know until you try one.

and therefore may require a trial of Antidepressants.

I face this question when adults, sponsors, and an occasional adolescent request a formal, let's say "authoritative," definition of the concept, especially if an Antidepressant may become part of the management plan. These are valid and legitimate requests for information, and they require a thoughtful and considered response. This is not an easy task because the meaning of the word depends on who is using it. Is it the public? Or the author of a textbook of psychiatry? Or the author of this book? In my view, each use is valid within its context. With the above distinctions in mind, I will return to the above question shortly. But first an explanation of why I confine *depression* to the cognitive domain only.

Depression Revisited

A Little Background

For many years the tradition within psychiatry was to view Depression as two separate and distinct types, with little in common: *Reactive Depression* versus *Endogenous Depression*.

Reactive Depression, as its name implies, was seen as a reaction to a life circumstance, typically the *prospect of change* and its consequences, as discussed in the preceding chapter. Sometimes the change is openly acknowledged as such, but just as often the precipitating agent is unrecognized, minimized, denied. In either case it is the paralysis and disability induced by the accompanying stress reaction that brings patients to the office.

In contrast, Endogenous Depression seems to come on without an obvious precipitant, gradually but progressively, threatening a crushing disability, even death, if not checked. The concept of Endogenous Depression has a venerable history, roughly corresponding to what the Greeks called *melancholia*, thought to be caused by an excess of black bile, one of the four humors. That is, they identified a type of sadness that was not only unremitting but seemed to have no external cause, and therefore had to come from within. An Endogenous Depression bears the some connotation and, in addition, is accompanied by apathy, disturbances of sleep and appetite, neglect of personal appearance, confused thinking, ruminations, withdrawal, and extreme risk of suicide. Fortunately, Endogenous Depression is relatively uncommon, in my experience, perhaps outnumbered by Reactive Depression ten or more to one.

Throughout the 1950s and 1960s researchers labored diligently to establish the presence of two clinically distinct Depressive populations in which the symptoms of one conformed to the Reactive prototype, the other to the Endogenous prototype. As is the case with most clinical research, the results provoked controversy. No sooner would one group claim to have established a clear and reliable demarcation of syndromes than another would reanalyze the findings and claim that the data actually supported the opposite conclusion.[iv]

Perhaps in part because clinical support was lacking, this simple classification was modified in the 1970s when the American Psychiatric Association published its third revision of psychiatric diagnosis categories, *DSM-III*. The expectation was that diagnosis and treatment of mental illness would be enhanced if each illness manifestation was carefully defined by a specific set of symptom, complaint, presentation, and exclusion criteria. Thus Depression evolved from two categories to a half

---

iv. A similar controversy of that era was the effort to define a blood pressure cutoff point for hypertension, a debate sustained for years in *The Lancet*, the official journal of the British Medical Association. Eventually a definition was established by consensus. Today's cancer research is similarly blessed/afflicted, as is most clinical research on chronic disease. Much of the ambiguity arises from gathering control and illness populations according to defined selection criteria, a difficult task indeed.

dozen or so, setting the stage for decades of intense research seeking to uncover laboratory tests specific to each.

The search goes on, and while it has yielded a number of intriguing and promising findings, reliable and reproducible lab tests are not yet available. In the meantime categorizing Depression by subtype does not seem to predict Antidepressant response.[7] So psychiatrists in practice still rely on patient history and findings at examination to diagnose. In short, the idea of Depression-as-collection-of-categories has not paid off for the profession.

It is in the midst of this ideological fatigue that conceiving Depression as a *spectrum phenomenon* presents, to my way of thinking, a refreshing alternative.

Spectrum thinking is a recent development in the professional literature: the idea of illness presenting as a *continuous phenomenon* rather than a collection of discrete illness syndromes. This seems especially applicable to those illnesses, for example fibromyalgia, where diagnosis is based largely on history and physical examination rather than laboratory findings. Thus fibromyalgia is viewed not as a discrete disease but as a disability of unclear origin on a continuum between rheumatoid disease at one end and sustained postural-repetitive motion trauma at the other.

In psychiatry, diagnosis also remains based for the most part on history and findings at examination. This situation joined to the spectrum concept suggests that so-called Depression might be viewed as a continuity of signs and symptoms rather a series of isolated entities unrelated to each other. In other words, spectrum thinking, when applied to psychiatry, pictures Depressive differences as a matter of degree rather than kind. Moreover, the spectrum concept does not automatically rule out the concurrent presence of anxiety symptoms.

Interestingly, spectrum thinking as applied to Depressive phenomena revives Reactive/Endogenous thinking, but with a vital modification. Rather than being seen as mutually exclusive, the two categories are now understood as polar but nondiscrete exemplars on a continuum. Consequently, every so-called Depressive condition has the potential to manifest both Reactive *and* Endogenous phenomena. I have found spectrum language quite handy when discussing "depression." It is concise and relatively nontechnical, and does not exclude the role of stress and anxiety in the genesis of "depressive" phenomena.

One Pole of the Spectrum: The Phenomenon of Reactivity

I interpret one spectrum pole as embodying *Reactivity*; that is, a patient responding to a change of some sort—perhaps just a "blip" as I discussed earlier—either present or impending, either tangible or symbolic, that signals separation and loss. This activates the fight/flight stress response, also discussed above, to mobilize energy to overcome or replace the loss. If the stress response becomes sustained, which can happen even if the loss is rectified, the energy mobilization backfires and the patient begins to experience *disability* rather than enhanced *ability*.

Stress symptoms increase, and if the incremental energy mobilization does not rectify the disability, patients become at risk of blaming themselves for the reduced capacity to perform. Should the self-blaming and negative thinking become fixed and not respond to changes that signal restoration of the loss and separation, this constitutes a state of *depression*.

In short, the Reactive pole has two components: the stress response itself and the cognitive significance attached to it by the patient. To clarify the two I recommend using the term *"stression"* to signify the stress response while reserving the term *depression* to denote the self-critical thinking induced by the *stression*. Further, I recommend that Antidepressants be viewed as *"antistressants"* in view of their widely recognized anxiety- and stress-reducing properties.

To oversimplify, *stression* rests more in the physiological domain, *depression* in the psychological. In practice, of course, the two domains are entangled and interactive, so these distinctions must be viewed with caution. They reflect a reality but are not the reality itself.

The self-blame and negative thinking frequently become much more disabling than the stress symptoms themselves. The psychological domain eventually overwhelms the physiological as sufferers project self-blaming and negative self-talk onto other figures in their world, infecting previously stable relationships. They begin to withdraw in order to protect themselves from rejections that they now figure are inevitable: *Who would want to keep company with such a miserable wretch as I?* The increased psychological isolation precipitates an even greater vulnerability to stress and a greater risk of a self-critical assessment. Eventually a disability develops about the very fact of being disabled. Ultimately this is what cripples, with Rebecca, for example, and with Dyllen. In his case it was not the panic itself that ignited his underperformance and eventual dropping out, but his fears that others would detect his fears.

Antistressants have the potential to mitigate stress and anxiety, but correcting the cognitive fallout precipitated by the stress is another matter.

Which provides an answer to the above question. In my experience, Antidepressants are very helpful with *stression* but not especially helpful with *depression*.

The Other Pole of the Spectrum: The Phenomenon of Endogenicity

The other pole, as I interpret it, embodies *Endogenicity*. Here the precipitating change is muffled or even—apparently—absent. The fight/flight response runs amuck, the physiological overwhelming the psychological to the point of paralysis. Apathy, withdrawal, low motivation, confusion, preoccupation, and neglect of self-care predominate. The patient is barely able to communicate. The task of describing and communicating the whirlwind of stress and anxiety within is impossible. Only later, upon recovery, might the whole story emerge, as it did with Julie and in her case, only after months of arduous treatment.

The mainstay of treatment is medication—notably Antipsychotics rather than Antidepressants—or perhaps even electrotherapy. Day treatment or hospitalization may be necessary. Dr. Balt remarks that Antidepressants are even less effective in Bipolar Depression, which is somewhat equivalent to my notion of Endogenicity.[8] Therapy here is more supportive. Its corrective potential should be reserved for later when there has been some recovery of psychological adeptness.

Recently, reviving the notion of Endogenicity has received some support. In 2010 a group of eminent professionals proposed a return to the idea of *Melancholia* by adding it to a pending *DSM* revision.[9] They cited the long and distinct history of a unique type of Depression without an obvious precipitant, characterized by blunted affect, psychomotor slowing, cognitive impairment, sleep and appetite changes, and profound hopelessness. In addition they noted specific biological features that served to distinguish it from all other categories, such as characteristic changes in the sleep cycle and excessive production of circulating steroids. But the category of Melancholia was not added to the revision. However, I strongly recommend that professionals and sponsors not be deterred by this lack of official endorsement from making use of the concept, which is the equivalent of the *Phenomenon of Endogenicity*.

Fortunately, most adolescent so-called Depression tends toward the Reactive pole of the spectrum. Unfortunately, the phenomena these youngsters manifest—dark essays (or drawings, journal entries, letters, and such), declining grades, resistiveness, irritability, withdrawal, suicidal thinking or gestures—are commonly misunderstood as an indication for treatment with an Antidepressant. In truth they reflect an underlying hopelessness about ever being free of some kind of pain—typically emotional—that is perceived as unending without the possibility of escape. Death offers the prospect of relief, peace, the absence of suffering. These children and adolescents do not actually wish to be dead, just to be free. Antidepressants cannot hope to excavate the buried hopelessness; hence the reports by Jureidini and colleagues. Counseling is imperative in such situations, which he advocates.[10]

Now, if in the process of clarification, anxieties emerge—I prefer the word "worry"; what kid does not "worry" about his or her parents, sibs, or friends, especially if the parent is separated or disabled, or the friend or sib is suffering—then the use of an *antistressant* might be indicated. Certainly it needs to be discussed. And should one be prescribed, it is vital that Dr. Schiele's notion of a target symptom or behavior be specified as the therapeutic goal. So I might inform youngsters and their sponsors, "I'm hoping the medication will cut your 'what if' thoughts, so when you return I'm going to ask how that is going. If your worries are less, you might not feel so hopeless about stuff."

The Spectrum Concept of Reactivity/ Endogenicity Compared to the Categorical Concept of Depression

By no means, of course, does my interpretation of so-called Depression represent mainstream psychiatric thinking. I simply offer it here as a platform for clarifying the discussion of treatment modalities with adolescents and their parents. It is rather unlikely that spectrum thinking will replace the categorical approach embodied in *DSM*. This is somewhat unfortunate because, as noted above, it is unusual for Depressive phenomena to appear unaccompanied by anxiety phenomena. The spectrum concept has the benefit of being nonexclusive when it comes to anxiety. That is, stress and anxiety are recognized as a possible symptom component across the spectrum, Reactivity pole to Endogenicity pole.

Indeed, this notion is supported by a recent analysis developed by Dr. Kenneth Kindler, perhaps our most distinguished psychiatric researcher. He selected nineteen standard textbooks of psychiatry or psychological medicine, all published circa 1960. Then he examined each one to identify how Emil Kraepelin's 1899 classic description of "affective illness"—what we now term Major Depressive Disorder—is variously characterized, identifying and tabulating what each author considered cardinal signs and symptoms of the illness. One of his findings is that "various aspects of anxiety, including panic attacks and obsessive fears, were noted by fourteen authors, but anxiety is not included in the DSM criteria for Major Depressive Disorder."[11]

In short, separation and loss, while obvious in most instances of Reactive disability, play a powerful if hidden role in Endogenous disability as well.

Here are two examples, one literary, the other clinical.

[CASE STUDY]
William Styron: Endogenicity

Novelist and Pulitzer Prize winner William Styron's memoir *Darkness Visible* is a compelling description of the paralysis and suffering accompanying his plunge into the darkness of an Endogenous Depression.[12]

In 1985 he suddenly develops a revulsion for alcohol, his "true friend" of some forty years when it came to soothing feelings of anxiety and dread, "a shield against anxiety." He begins to experience a daily midafternoon "gloom crowding in at me, a sense of dread and alienation and, above all, stifling anxiety." Slowly but progressively, he becomes gripped by the cardinal signs of melancholy: joylessness, an overwhelming feeling of worthlessness, forgetfulness, sleeplessness, and loss of appetite, occasionally accompanied by bouts of "dreadful, pouncing seizures of anxiety." After two months of barely endurable mental pain, he finds himself no longer with "faith in deliverance."

He begins to plan his suicide. This would require destroying a hidden journal he had never meant to be seen. He tells us how he methodically and ceremoniously wraps, tapes, and boxes the notebook, stuffing it deep into the garbage to be incinerated, a symbolic "annihilation of self." Later he sets about composing a suicide note, a task he, a gifted writer, finds fatuous and embarrassingly banal. He tears it up.

That night, contemplating his impending demise and unable to sleep, he passes the time watching a movie featuring a scene set in a music conservatory with an unseen voice, "a sudden soaring passage from the Brahms *Alto Rhapsody.*" The sound pierces his numbed heart "like a dagger." He is flooded with all the joys his home has witnessed: laughing children, festivities, commotion, endearing pets. This is more than he can abandon, he realizes, nor can he inflict on those connected with these memories "what I had set out so deliberately to do." He awakens his wife, arranges to be hospitalized, and begins to heal.

At one point he describes his belated recognition at age sixty of the lifelong profound effects of the loss of his mother at age thirteen. In passing he tells us that he came to suspect "that devastating loss in childhood figured as a probable genesis ... I felt loss at every hand." Only later, upon recovery, does he provide any detail.

Recovered, he reveals a fuller understanding of his melancholic affliction. He recalls his father's lifelong struggle with Depression and the death of his mother. He reviews the idea that suicide is the culmination of a lifelong incomplete mourning and finds it applicable in his case.

> If it is also true that in the nethermost depths of one's suicidal behavior one is still unconsciously dealing with immense loss while trying to surmount all the effects of its devastation, then my own avoidance of death may have been belated homage to my mother. I do know that in those last hours before I rescued myself, when I listened to the passage from the *Alto Rhapsody*—which I'd hear her sing—she had been very much on my mind.[13]

In retrospect, he reports, he now understands that Depression hovered at the margins of his life throughout the years. In his books three major characters commit suicide. Rereading his work, he is "stunned" by how precisely he had delineated the turmoil of mood his doomed heroines experienced. Hence Depression, when it finally came upon him, "was no stranger … it had been tapping at my door for decades."[v]

The Significance of Styron's Experiences

Lifelong Impact of Childhood Loss

In a book intended to explicate childhood and adolescent attachment issues, it may seem irrelevant to review the adult Styron's struggles with a potentially fatal Endogenous Depression. But the child is parent to the adult. Only after recovery was the adult Styron able to perceive the weeping, lost child within. His sparse yet poetic account of his passage from life to near death to life offers much to contemplate about the vicissitudes of attachment and loss. This book is my hope that by recognizing early the significance of behavior that shouts loss and abandonment in

---

v. Some years later Styron experienced a return of symptoms and received a series of electroconvulsive treatments. One has to wonder if he had been visited by another loss, real or symbolic.

youngsters who lack the insight and language to express it, we can help them avoid lifelong suffering such as his.

Hopelessness Kills

Styron's touching memoir also provides insight regarding the lethal potential of Endogenous Depression.

Examined carefully, these excerpts reveal that it was not the Depression itself that drove him to methodically plan his suicide but his hopeless belief that it would never end. That is, the lethal potential of his melancholic state rested not in the melancholy itself, but in his conviction that he would never experience relief. In the presence of pain, whether mental or physical, it is hopelessness about "deliverance" that kills, not Depression. When adolescents ruminate about death, incorporating thoughts of suicide in their tweets or essays or journals, their wish is to escape, not die. Death equals peace. Which is why media accounts of suicide not infrequently include observations by shocked friends and acquaintances that the departed one "actually seemed to be recovering" The "recovery," in fact, is the peace of mind sufferers experience when they have finally decided to end it all. Now they no longer feel trapped—they at last have found a way out.

That hopelessness kills is actually part of our culture. Recall the four-verse, sixteen-line poem that many of us memorized in eighth-grade English, Edwin Arlington Robinson's "Richard Cory." The first three verses are a setup in which Robinson provides us what psychiatrists call a *collateral history*. He presents Cory as rich, elegant, and handsome, the envy of his townspeople: "he fluttered pulses." Everyone wished to be in his place. Obviously no hint of melancholy here. No apathy, no neglect of self-care, no withdrawal. Yet the punch lines of the fourth verse:

> So on we worked, and waited for the light,
> And went without the meat, and cursed the bread;
> And Richard Cory, one calm summer night,
> Went home and put a bullet through his head.

I was once asked by an attorney to investigate the circumstances of a grandmother's apparent suicide. He had been hired by her estate to contest a denial of life insurance benefits, the insurer invoking a suicide clause in her contract. That she had taken her own life was not in dispute. She had ridden her bike to a rail crossing, was seen waiting for several minutes, and then stepped in front of a freight train. But the bike contained books she had just checked out from the local library. At home there was no note. Moreover, in the kitchen there were a recipe and ingredients for the evening meal. Was it really suicide? asked the attorney. Would I perform a psychological autopsy?

He provided me with her medical records, which revealed that many years earlier she had been briefly treated in the local hospital for anxiety and Depression. Reading between the lines, I sensed she was a bit of a perfectionist. Thereafter she occasionally experienced panic attacks, well managed by her family doctor with low doses of an Anti-anxiety medication. His records indicated she had been symptom and medication free for several years prior to her death, confirmed through interviews with family members. They were stunned. They described her as optimistic, outgoing, and fully engaged in family and community life. She had just seen two of her grandchildren off to summer camp.

What had happened?

I suggested that on her way home from the library she had experienced the return of panic, perhaps generated by separation from her grandchildren. I speculated this plunged her into an intense state of despair and hopelessness. That painful, dreadful out-of-control feeling state, which she had though she had licked forever, had returned. She would *never* be free. But she was not totally helpless; she could kill herself and escape the pain. So she turned aside on her way home and rode to the crossing, now calm and serene.

To illustrate that suicide did not represent a wish to die but, rather, an escape from pain, in my report I discussed the 9/11 jumpers, whose behavior was the subject of much speculation in the media just then: Was it suicide or not? I suggested that jumpers, facing the inevitability of an agonizing death by incineration, chose immediate relief. Their behavior did not reflect a wish to die, but a wish to escape. Similarly with my proxy client. Thus her death was not suicide.[vi]

Although here the distinction between Depression and hopelessness did not sway the court, life is not a courtroom when it comes to assessing adolescents. There are certain situations, especially with *attachment-entangled* youngsters, where there is no notable, objective paralysis or disturbance in functioning despite a profound but hidden negative self-assessment. This is the setting in which suicide can take place "out of the blue," without any external evidence of a prior Depression. Which is why so much teen suicide comes as a surprise — classic signs of Depression are frequently missing. An apparently happy and smiling school attendee one day, dead by overdose or hanging or reckless driving the next. If there is a note, typically it is little more than a terse plea for forgiveness, that the pain is too much to bear.

Thus indications of hopelessness are *the critical element* when I am evaluating youngsters — and adults, of course — whose speech or schoolwork or journals or Facebook postings contain references to death and others being "better off" without them. Recently a new clinical disorder, Acute Suicidal Affective

---

vi. As I prepared my report, I had to admit to myself that, despite the brilliance of my logic, from a legal point of view she did unquestionably die by her own hand; therefore her death was suicide, regardless of intent. Apparently, the court agreed with the insurer's argument, dismissing the family's argument, although that decision was later reversed.

Disturbance (ASAD), has been proposed to account for suicides not attributable to the usual causes such as impulsivity, disordered mood, or substance use.[14] According to the originator of the concept, Dr. Thomas Joiner, ASAD is characterized by a sudden increase in suicidal intent, hopelessness about relief of suffering, and extreme agitation. In his experience its most common precursors are personality and anxiety issues; it is also age independent.

A Cardinal Sign of Hopelessness Is Inattentiveness

Styron provides a striking description of how inattentiveness can signal suicidal preoccupation. He describes how his pervasive sense of worthlessness intruded into a celebration to honor his acceptance of a notable literary prize. Totally preoccupied, he somehow managed to struggle through the award ceremony, then contrived an excuse to skip the subsequent luncheon, which was at first misinterpreted by his hostess as rudeness rather than a sign of his developing illness.

Inattentiveness of this sort has a distracted and unfocused quality. The patient opposite you seems to be listening to two voices, yours and an inner one. The hypervigilance of resistiveness or the pressure to ventilate every issue before you tune out—as if there never will be another opportunity to "get it all in"—is not present. The patient is not concerned about loss and abandonment because that inner voice is saying that is no longer the issue. The issue now is life or death.

Hence the gaze is inward or, if directed at you, seems to peer through you as if searching a distant landscape. Responses to questions or comments seem just a bit off, absentminded. Thus, in the midst of the usual pointed inquiries about depressive signs and symptoms, I throw in open-ended questions such as *Does it ever seem things will never get better? Does it ever feel that nothing you do is good enough? Do you ever feel that everything is your fault?* In chapter 12 I will address the circumstances in children's lives that create the need for such inquiries. But for now I simply wish to emphasize that hopelessness signaled by inattentiveness is the central dynamism impelling suicidal behavior. And the primary focus of management, whatever the modality, must be directed toward protecting adolescents from surrendering to the belief that their pains will never remit.

Such distractedness is easier to detect in young adults and grown-ups. Adolescents are more practiced at covering up, mainly because they don't want you to worry about them. So they pretend, minimize, and deny. They don't need another soul whose happiness depends on them, another figure to prop up. It is vital that the concerned sponsor, teacher, or counselor come across as a reasonably secure adult who doesn't avoid asking the tough questions when it comes to evaluating death thoughts and preoccupations, yet doesn't panic should such concerns float to the surface.

Loss of a "True Friend"

It is not unusual that after years of heavy use, individuals abruptly stop drinking. Typically some external event is the precipitant. A mate threatens to leave, or health deteriorates, or there is a decline in performance at work. Styron's case is unusual: alcohol suddenly becomes repulsive. What is not atypical, on the other hand, is that now he no longer has the defense of alcohol to keep his lifelong anxiety and dread at bay. Recall that in the midst of his suffering from what is most certainly the phenomenon of Endogenicity, Styron frequently refers to a component of anxiety and panic. He assumes that a sudden intolerance to alcohol, for forty years a "shield against anxiety," leaves him vulnerable to his "demons." (Similarly, Dyllen experienced a return of anxiety when he stopped smoking marijuana.) Lifelong abandonment anxieties previously managed by the alcohol now began to flood Styron's life, gradually paralyzing him, setting the stage for his descent into "darkness visible."

The Energizing Potential of Loss

Eventually, Styron tells us, he recovers completely, which he attributes to the pacifying effect of the hospital and the devotion of family and friends. He ends his memoir with a brief discussion of the causes of his Depression and, by extension, all such potentially lethal "madness." In his case he accepts that genetics undoubtedly was a factor—his father was hospitalized for a condition that greatly resembled his, he now realizes. More important, he believes, is the death of his mother when he was thirteen, which precipitated a lifelong state of unrecognized "incomplete mourning." Such energies possess both destructive and creative potential. No doubt they are the source of much world art and literature through which "the theme of depression has run like a durable thread of woe."

Styron's predicament is hardly unique. Many a disabling mood swing, whether Depressive or Manic, is precipitated by the unexpected return of attachment issues. But sometimes the presence of a precipitant is obscured by the turmoil it unleashes. For example:

[CASE STUDY]
Rose: From Convent to Convict

She is a forty-eight-year-old married, unemployed, childless woman whom I have been following since 1999 because of Rapid Cycling Mood Disorder. Now she returns describing a sudden return of "depressive" symptoms and suicidal feelings despite excellent medication compliance. She is disheveled, dejected, gloomy, discouraged, defeated, obviously exhausted from lack of sleep, and under-spontaneous, patiently waiting while I again review her copious records.

I note that twenty years previously, while a novice in a religious order, she developed panic attacks, became dependent on the novice director, and was subsequently briefly hospitalized because of suicidal thinking. After her discharge she was asked to leave the order. There was no follow-up treatment until 1999 when she started counseling for an Obsessive-Compulsive Disorder. Shortly thereafter her therapist referred her for medication management. This was not especially helpful until I added a Mood Stabilizer.

In the meantime she demonstrated a series of decompensations and hospitalizations provoked by a variety of stresses: the Christmas holidays, a broken engagement, the therapist's vacation, the overdose of a friend from her therapy group. In the midst of this turmoil, her therapist discharged her after she ran thirty-six miles to the therapist's home and then later brought a knife to her office with the intent of mutilating herself. She was served a restraining order, which she violated. She was arrested, charged with terrorist threats, but pleaded down to a gross misdemeanor.

Subsequently she violated probation on two occasions for making contact with the former therapist and was once sentenced to a weekend in the workhouse. Thereafter she continued to pine for her therapist, but she settled down, resisting the impulse to see her, possibly because she (Rose) had married a loving and supportive fellow. The cycles continued but were not as intense.

She was let go from her job as a lay church secretary, in part because her productivity had decreased due to burnout, in part because of budgetary constraints. After two attempts to become qualified in the health care field did not pan out, she found work as a food shelf coordinator. She did well at first but, as the onset of the 2008 depression flooded the food shelf with greater numbers of needy clients, she found her work increasingly burdensome. She began to experience flashbacks of her brother's prior physical abuse of her, possibly precipitated by the deaths of four relatives within eight months.

She then was witness to the delirious ramblings of her mother, who was recovering from anesthesia after surgery. This provoked a recall of her mother's verbal abusiveness. Rose lost sleep, became manic, eventually had a "breakdown" at work. In 2009 she was let go because of "behavior problems." She had no luck finding work.

In the meantime both parents began to demonstrate cognitive and physical declines, which touched off squabbling among her sibs over the family's meager assets. She began to report feeling like she had lost her family, that she was dead, that she no longer had a mother.

Eventually her unemployment benefits were exhausted. Later she caught on as a part-time substitute receptionist/coach at a neighborhood exercise studio where she had been a regular for years. Eventually she was awarded a full free membership. The payoff was financially meager but psychologically enormous. She felt uplifted, also later by her mother telling her she loved her, later still from being awarded Social Security disability benefits in June 2012.

Things seemed to turn around. Slowly, painfully, she extricated herself from her siblings' concerns, focusing more on the decline of her mother and the impending sale of her childhood home: "My childhood is disappearing piece by piece … my home base." Thereafter she occasionally experienced suicidal feeling. Nonetheless her thinking was more linear as she recognized and processed her grief. "I feel like an orphan … trapped … can't go to see my mother … my mother kept me stable but nothing to make me feel good."

Now she is back in the office, obviously severely Depressed.

Dr. C: "What's happening?"
Rose: Reports no obvious trigger. In fact, except for the

financial strains, things actually are going better: no parental crises, her husband has two job opportunities, she's exercising, going to church. Yet recently she's been dreaming of how she was fired from her last two jobs: "Angry … I feel so much pain."

Dr. C, asking the obvious: "How is the exercise studio going?"

Rose: "That is something I'm angry about … now I'm sitting on the sidelines." *It turns out there was a merger with another studio and to save money the owner let her go without notice. Shortly thereafter, the dreaming began.*

Dr. C: "Could that be the trigger?"

Rose: "It sure fits."

Dr. C: "Here's some homework. I want you to return next week to determine if it still fits, and in the meantime make a list of rejections you've experienced in your life."

Rose: Agrees. Leaves.

Rose: *Returns a week later rested, composed, less drained, insightful.* "I did my homework …A lot more rejections that acceptances … I survived … current rejection is piled on by the past." *Also,* "I have fatigue and lack of energy … Some anxiety, but I'm not desperate."

Dr. C.: *Slapping himself on the forehead,* "Duh—now I finally understand that goofy stuff with that therapist years ago. Obviously an entangled attachment issue!"

Rose: *dryly,* "Well, sometimes you are kind of slow."

Dr. C.: "You know I should put this in my book."

Rose: *Delighted agreement:* "You could call it 'From convent to convict.'"

Subsequently she continues to experience mood fluctuations, but never disabling ones. At a later visit she remarks she had been thinking about my notion of her "fear of success," that it still didn't seem to fit. Then, "I never accepted responsibility for pain, always felt it was someone else's fault." Subsequently she is rehired at the studio, and now is leading both an ACOA and an Al-Anon group.

At a subsequent visit:

> *Rose: Brisk, upbeat, focused.* "Just want to let you know I'm in a good mood ... some anxiety, jittery ... my mood depends on the day, but more good than bad ... do they come from codependency issues? ... hard to tell ... I'm trying to work on my issues."
> *Dr. C:* "It is always related to abandonment."
> *Rose: Identifies some abandonment feelings when husband leaves for work in the morning. Then reports her mother, who has been more lucid recently, is planning to move to an assisted living facility nearby.*
> *Dr. C:* "Will this be a solution or a problem?"
> *Rose:* "It depends ... I could make it into a problem ... I will have to set some boundaries."

Apparent Lack of a Precipitant

In summary, the two of us have struggled for almost fourteen years to relieve her turmoil and distress. Clearly she is afflicted by a severe and intermittently disabling Mood Disorder only partially responsive to Mood Stabilizers because of Rapid Cycling features. And clearly some of her mood swings and disorganizations are reactive. On the other hand, we were never able to establish that there was a pattern or rhythm or predictability to her decompensations. Depressions came and went willy-nilly, as did bursts of euphoria and ambition without preamble, only to be heralded by a call for assistance when she crashed. Typically she would appear in the office obviously quite distressed but without any insight or awareness of a precipitant. We would labor to uncover a plausible cause, perhaps adjust her medications a bit, never with much certainty regarding an underlying dynamism, if any. Not an unfamiliar scenario, as any psychiatrist knows.

Belated Recognition of Entanglement

When I first met Rose, her infatuation with her therapist was a puzzle to everyone: to the judge—after the third or fourth time she was hauled into court on a probation violation, he just told her to go home and stay out of his courtroom—to Rose herself, to me. At that point in my career I had not yet grasped that not only could attachment issues persist well into adulthood, but they could also manifest as an entangled relationship rather than as acting-out or avoidance behavior. Her desperate clinging was not only an attempt to heal the many rejections she had sustained, but to repair the suffering in others to which she was exquisitely sensitive. This led to rebuffs, years ago by her novice director, later by her therapist. Fortunately she is learning to channel this energy more appropriately through coaching at the exercise studio and through leading AA and Al-Anon groups.

Ultimately we achieved some clarity, as the above vignette demonstrates. She deserves most of the credit—or rather, her unconscious does. It was as if she had assembled all but one of the parts of the puzzle in the right order, waiting for me to insert the missing piece. As if she needed permission to use the concept of "rejection." But the point here is not her acuity or my dullness. Rather the point is that even the most severe Depressions have a reactive component and that prevention of subsequent episodes requires both medication management and addressing underlying abandonment vulnerabilities. This does not mean that Rose now may anticipate a life free of mood swings. But with a greater understanding of her rejection sensitivity, she may learn to anticipate triggers and protect herself in circumstances that otherwise might precipitate a profound decompensation.

Indeed, just recently she returns, five days after her father's death while hospitalized. This is not unexpectedly in view of his long history of declining mental and physical health, yet a shock because he again seemed to be rallying. She is distraught, guilty, confused by a sense of loss despite his lifelong alcoholism and neglect of her, and furious with both the hospital … and with me because I was not more supportive earlier when she first called: "You blew me off!" In truth, I had done so. After listening for a few minutes, I had ended the call, saying that we could discuss things at her next appointment. Now here she was, feeling utterly rejected, both by her father and me.

I do not deny her angry accusation. I say she is correct, that I did give her the brush-off, an acknowledgement that soothes her somewhat.

It turns out that the sibling squabbling had extended to funeral arrangements, with threats of having private security officers available at the proceedings to exclude some from attending. Tired of attempts by both sides to suck her into the struggle, Rose finally sent an angry email to one sib demanding to be left alone. She established a boundary, for which I compliment her.

I also repeat a prior suggestion: perhaps now that she is more aware of her entanglement proclivities, it is time to retry counseling. "You need to expand your support system," I say. And I note she has avoided hospitalization, which, given her past history, would have been the likely consequence to a crisis of this intensity.

Subsequently she continues to struggle with boundaries, as well as the reality of my eventual retirement. She accepts a referral to one of the clinic's therapists, recognizing her need for additional professional support.

Rose: Review, Summary, and Illustration

Above I described how effective management of chronic disability, whether attachment or pain related, is founded on three principles: *clarification, acceptance, focus.*

The ease of this characterization of management principles belies the toughness of their implementation, akin to traveling a maze in the dark, as certainly was the situation here with Rose. As an introduction to the later chapters, therefore, I will highlight the dynamism of each in her case:

- *Clarification:* our belated recognition of her lifelong Attachment Disabilities
- *Acceptance:* her conclusion that her pains were not others' responsibility
- *Focus:* her realization that she needed to work on boundaries

Our work together as we navigated from dark to light offers an excellent illustration of the utility of these principles as guideposts in the recognition, management and remediation of Attachment Disability.

Part 5

Managing Attachment Disability

The idea of therapy is to help you better understand yourself, to teach you how to be your own detective amid the mystery of your life, and to establish a life path for you to travel.

10

Management: Strategy and Tactics

Management is simple: avoid making things worse.

Trauma injures trust, perpetuates dissociation, and suffocates adaptive learning. The goal of the preceding chapters was to develop an understanding of these consequences. Here I will discuss their management, the goal of which is not making things worse. If we avoid reinforcing maladaptive behaviors, more adaptive behaviors will spontaneously flourish, driven by the activating energies of unmet needs. The adaptive will crowd out and displace the maladaptive.

This sounds simple in concept but is not easily executed. It means we ourselves need to acquire certain adaptive skills to effectively manage traumatized children, adolescents, and adults.

I divide these skills into two categories: strategic and tactical. The former are more general. They involve three dynamisms potentially applicable to any encounter with trauma survivors: 1) recognizing their power to resist, 2) dealing with their inattentiveness, and 3) timing feedback. Tactical skills come into play in more specific situations; for example, security arrangements or working with family members, sponsors, or involved professionals.

Then in chapters 11 through 13 I will apply the three principles of management—*clarification, acceptance,* and *focus*—using case presentations that incorporate a mixture of strategic and tactical considerations. It is important to recognize that the application of these three management principles is not linear, but rather jumbled. Therefore the spirit of these three chapters is more tentative and suggestive than formulaic, but always directed toward not making things worse.

Management Strategy

Young people are dynamic; things are always changing for them. At any given moment, half of the average high school enrollment feels gloomy and defeated; tomorrow, it will be the other half. Teachers, sponsors, and professionals need to take advantage of the mercurial temperament of youngsters and young adults by avoiding making things worse. If they succeed in this, the odds favor eventual improvement. Effective management of this sort is enhanced by constant awareness of three critical constraints: *resistiveness, attentiveness, timing.*

The First Constraint: The Power to Resist

[CASE STUDY]
Dr. Searles Meets "Mr. Resistive"

Occasionally Dr. Kolb would import professors from other training programs to lecture on their research or clinical interests.

One such was Dr. Harold Searles, an eminent psychoanalyst on the staff of the famous Maryland private mental hospital Chestnut Lodge. His books and articles were recommended reading because of his insights derived from years of intense therapy with Schizophrenic patients. He was also recommended because of his unique notion that countertransference—feelings evoked in the therapist by the patient—could be an effective therapeutic tool when shared with the patient. Thus when we heard that Dr. Searles was to visit to demonstrate his interview technique, we were delighted.

In medicine the time-honored protocol for a demonstration by a visiting fireman calls for the most senior resident to select an in- or outpatient volunteer to be examined. An unofficial corollary mandates a game of stump-the-expert by selecting a candidate notorious for difficulty of diagnosis or treatment. Psychiatry is no different. Eventually our chief residents settled on a young male whom I'll call Mr. Resistive.

My recall of the venue is hazy. It seems to have been rather intimate, no doubt to conform to the nature of the proceedings, probably a ward dayroom since this was long before the advent of closed-circuit TV. The place was crowded with residents, faulty, nurses, and attendants. This was like the reigning Masters Tournament champion giving a swing demonstration, so anyone with a professional interest had to be present. The place hummed with anticipation.

Dr. Kolb: Introduces Dr. Searles.
Dr. Searles: Introductory remarks.
Assembled multitude (AM): Comfortably attentive.
Mr. Resistive: Enters, takes a seat.
Dr. S: Draws up a chair perhaps five feet opposite, no intervening props. Sits, greets.
Mr. R: Silent, impassive.
Dr. S: Briefly explains the exercise.
Mr. R: Silent, impassive.

AM: Posture stiffer.
Dr. S: Asks what his problems are "these days."
Mr. R: Silent, impassive.
AM: Posture tense.
Dr. S: Silent, impassive.
Mr. R: Silent, impassive.
AM: Restless.
Dr. S: Silent, impassive.
Mr. R: Silent, impassive.
AM: Audibly restless.
Dr. S: Silent, impassive. Then, thoughtfully reports, "This is one of times I wonder why I ever became a psychiatrist."
Mr. R, AM: Explosive laughter.
Thereafter: Interview proceeds swimmingly.

What happened here? We were witnessing a power struggle: Who would be the dominant party? A response, verbal or otherwise, to Dr. Searles's apparently innocuous question would place him in charge of the proceedings. Refusing to acknowledge his very presence made Mr. R. the winner. Our growing discomfort reflected the intensity of this interpersonal arm wrestling. After a few minutes—which seemed like hours to us—Dr. Searles recognized that the odds of prevailing were not in his favor since he was the party expected to perform. On the other hand, Mr. R. had already met expectations by simply showing up and demonstrating his signature behavior: passive resistance. And most likely he was enjoying showing off this particular skill that, no doubt, Dr. Searles came to appreciate as he listened to his own countertransference. *This guy can sit here all day and relish the chance to make a big cheese like me suffer. I can't win. Why did I ever answer that call from Dr. Kolb? Why did I ever get up this morning?* Thus his gracious and humorous surrender. Rather than challenging Mr. R's power, Dr. Searles recognized it.

This demonstrates a most important principle: the power of the other to resist engagement. Human transactions do not occur by chance. Rather, they are driven—activated—by unmet needs. Transactions thus involve the exchange of needed goods and services, hopefully by agreement, which is the basis of social organization. Peaceful exchanges proceed via a reciprocal exchange of power. But each always has the power to resist, if only passively as did Mr. Resistive, as long as there is a power imbalance.

More specifically, youngsters beset by attachment issues are prone to resist because of their distrust of power and authority. Bitter experience has taught them that transactions risk entanglement, betrayal, abuse, or abandonment, typically combining elements of each. It is safer to resist.

In short, we as parents or teachers or counselors must guard against being seduced by the power of our position. No matter the honors or responsibilities, formal or informal, that accrue to us via society's favor or laws, those nominally subordinate to us always retain the power to resist—for example, tune out, skip class, or become truant. Thus we must approach all interactions without an expectation of automatic obedience.[i]

The Second Constraint: Attentiveness

To return to my training years, in our bull sessions as residents we not infrequently addressed the issue of how to deal with attractive patients. How do you resist the seductiveness of intelligence or beauty? How do you avoid being snared by the

---

i. Automatic obedience in youngsters always stirs my suspicions. When I find kids enthusiastically agreeing with my formulations or recommendations, I always inquire if they "really agree" or are "just being nice." They typically assure me that, of course, it is the former, which makes me even more dubious, but I leave it at that. Time will tell.

very traits that no doubt played a part in bringing the patient to your office for help? I can't recall any of us coming up with a definitive answer. Nor did our professors. Yes, they would agree, that can be a problem, but it is something you need to discuss with your analyst to understand better what your conflicts are. Not having an analyst, I never did find out what conflict had to do with the attraction of one human being to another, although it was clear that attraction could generate conflict; hence our question.

Well, once in practice I discovered I was, indeed, very susceptible to seduction … by attentiveness. I was a sucker for the patient who in the course of an interview might say something like, "Dr. Curran, I was thinking about what you said before." My pulse would accelerate, my pupils dilate, my thinking transfixed by loving surrender: *Oh, what a beautiful, perceptive being it is that worships before me.* Whether the patient agreed or disagreed with my observations was irrelevant. The listening, that was what was significant, for it offered the possibility of developing a treatment contract. Now we could proceed to explore the data upon which the patient's opinion is based. Where did we agree and why? Where did we disagree and why? Now we were both poised to learn.

On the other hand, if the party, no matter how good looking or smart, chattered on regardless of the astuteness of my prior observations, I found myself feeling like Dr. Searles must have felt: *Why was I born?* No doubt something of the sort was going on during my years struggling with Rebecca and her complaint of "depression." I can't recall, as it was so long ago, but it is more than likely. I was younger and more stubborn then and I wasn't going to give up. Determination is certainly admirable, but I should have been more sensitive to my feelings of being ignored. I should have been wondering, *What is going on here*? Perhaps Dr. Kolb's voice from on high might have visited me sooner if I had been doing a better job of listening to my countertransference.

In short, feeling ignored has the potential to undermine a therapeutic relationship. If you surrender to your client's inattentiveness with a corresponding lack of attention, no learning—which is the goal of disability management—will take place. You must remain vigilant and be prepared to interrupt and restructure and refocus the proceedings.[ii] For now it is important to note that when a client floods you with words and irrelevancies, ignoring responses to questions and so on, the behavior most often represents underlying abandonment issues. Such clients feel overwhelmed by a need to get "everything in" before you disappear from their life, which is their experience.

This style of inattentiveness is different from that of the hopeless patient, discussed previously in chapter 9 and next in chapter 11. The hopeless patient does not flood you with words but rather waits to be prompted, is distracted, lacks the overproductive intensity of the patient fighting to get it all in. On the other hand, if my attempts to refocus and restructure do not succeed in gaining my patient's attention, I consider the possibility that more than abandonment disability is present: for example, hypomanic activation, intoxication by street or prescription drugs or other substances, post-concussive residuals, developmental issues, pending psychotic decompensation—things of that sort.

The Third Constraint: Timing

To return to my residency years once again, recall my sense of frustration when our supervisor offhandedly remarked that while cultivation of trust was the basic ingredient of psychotherapy, it was something he could not teach us. He could only teach us the art of psychotherapy—essentially when to say something and when to say nothing. What I have come to appreciate is that, in the world of disability management, trust

---

ii. I will discuss these techniques at greater length below.

and art are reciprocally connected: each builds upon the other and each has the potential to undermine the other. A mistimed comment can be just as intrusive as a failure to comment. And an intuitive remark or companionable silence can generate notable anxiety relief.

With Amy, for example, it soon became apparent that providing her with an opportunity to tell her story, my customary interview technique, was backfiring. She was becoming even more defensive while collapsing into what seemed immature helplessness. My expectant attitude of respectful silence proved unnerving; why, I wasn't sure. So I took her off the hot seat by turning to her mother and then adopting a role familiar to her: the teacher in front of the class giving a lecture. As she relaxed and became more engaged, it became clear that entanglement was a vital issue for her, one that even contaminated her ability to engage with me, a stranger whom she had just met. Eventually the timing seemed ripe for an interpretation, which I introduced by drawing her attention to the notable change in her behavior over the course of the interview, which she couldn't deny. That's when I said something rather than nothing … and generated some trust.

Of course, one well-timed intervention of this sort is not going to heal entrenched distrust, but it is a beginning.

Here, on the other hand, is an example of a poorly timed intervention.

[Case Study]
Owen: The Unworkable Child

He is fourteen years old, seen with his mother, who works in health care. She reports he needs follow-up because his previous psychiatrist had terminated care: "She said she could not work with him." With his mother, he had been sent to an emergency room, where he was seen, placed on a psychotropic, and then referred on to my office.

In the waiting room he is very overactive, standing on chairs, straightening pictures, things of that sort. At first he refuses to complete a symptom inventory, but when both my receptionist and his mother say this is okay, he promptly changes his mind and fills it in. His handwriting is the scrawling work of a second- or third-grader, and the effort is hasty and sweeping. He simply circles the negative column for all categories ... except for one mood item: "Thinks she/he is the smartest, best person in the world." Here the response is positive, with the marginal comment "I am."

But despite what appears to be a touch of grandiosity in the midst of massive denial, other comments suggest higher-level introspective functioning and conflict. Next to his global denial of all anxiety items is the comment, "I don't know, kinda." At the bottom, "almost 14 ... I'm just a teenager ... I don't know what this means ... my mom doesn't get me ... I have to do these things, not my option." As for his strengths, he describes these as "good" in school, "good happy" socially, but "don't do anything" at home (frowning face).

His mother's rating of his behavior is a different story. She endorses a host of items in the attention, oppositional, and mood categories, plus three in the conduct category. Only when it comes to the anxiety/worry items does she agree with her son, checking none but also adding a marginal comment: "Anxiety with life." She dates all the lad's problems to the toddler years. She cites his strengths as art, also as "more accepting to foreign or disabled people." But at home, "We struggle, not much positive."

The registration sheet indicates Owen also takes two other psychotropics and has been seeing a counselor for two years.

Dr. C, addressing Owen: "Well, what brings you here?"
Owen, clean but poorly groomed, bulky build, resistive, poor eye contact: "I don't know."
Dr. C: Judicious, expectant attitude.
Owen: Tries to change the subject.
Mother: "Dr. V. says she can't work with him. Says she doesn't usually work with adolescents."
Owen: Giggling, immature, provocative, defiant, mocking.
Dr. C: Beginning to understand Dr. V's sentiments.
Mother: "He does not want to take the medicine."
Dr. C, thinking of Dr. V.'s reported difficulties: "I doubt if he takes it anyhow."
Owen, smirking: "How did you know?"
Dr. C. "Well, that's not going to be a problem for me."
Owen, full eye contact, delighted: "I like this doctor!"
Mother, icy: "I don't think it is good for him to hear that message."
Dr. C, scrambling to buttress his posture, cites his four decades'–plus experience with adolescents, how to address the fear behind the resistiveness and noncompliance: you have to take it off the table as an issue. If Owen has been willful since he was a toddler, telling him now to follow orders would be fruitless, and so on.
Mother: Maintains a tight-lipped silent glare despite my impressive display of expertise.
Dr. C, finally accepting he's blown it, suggests that perhaps he's not what she's looking for in a psychiatrist, that maybe she might obtain another referral from Dr. V; waives his fee.
Mother leaves, Owen in her wake.

Clearly I played my hole card too soon. I should have finessed the issue of compliance. I should have turned to Owen, perhaps feigning surprise, with a bland inquiry: Could mother's allegation about not wanting to take medications possibly be true? This tactic softens resistiveness. Whether there is a response or not, the repetitive seeking of a response conveys a subtext: you can't make me give up or get mad by ignoring me. This is where having the sponsor in the room, as I will discuss further on, is critical. Engaging the sponsor via, say, taking a history, provides pertinent data and offers an opportunity to slowly engage the resistive party. With Owen, the idea would be to slowly undermine the desperate noncompliant posture that colored his view of grown-ups and authority. To comply would be to lose his identity.

I might justify overplaying my hand by saying that the inventory data plus Owen's behavior made it clear to me from the start that a major issue here was developmental. This implied that effective management would depend primarily on Owen participating in a skills-training agenda. Or, to put the matter differently, medication was not the answer—at least not now. That could come later; now he needed engagement. Therefore it was not dangerous to downplay the medication issue, as I did, because other matters were more important.

But medication was the most important matter for Mother because it symbolized her hope that power emanating from a doctor could make her child behave at last. In short, my job was to be a cop.

Now, doctor-as-cop is an expectation not unfamiliar to any physician who deals with adolescents, young adults, and their sponsors. It is important to neither buy into nor rebuff such an expectation, but to gently explore its dimensions. In today's other-directed[iii] society, sponsors and parents typically experience a good deal of anxiety should their kids not be well

---

iii. The concept of the "other-directed" society, discussed in volume 2, comes from *The Lonely Crowd* by sociologist David Riesman and associates. In fact the book is mistitled: it should be *The Anxious Crowd*.

mannered or studious. It is when discussions have not helped that they turn to an outsider, hoping that lectures from an authority figure will make a difference, and sometimes it does. For parents who struggle with their children's developmental issues, the anxiety-provoking potential of poor manners generally ranks high. Getting them to fit in at all, that's the issue, and it had been the issue with Owen since he was a toddler. But Mother, obviously intelligent and motivated, also had an issue. She had not learned from experience. She had not figured out that one more exercise of authority, whether hers or others', was not going to be the answer.

I recognized this and, based on my four decades' experiences with medication noncompliance, knew that if compliance remained the primary goal of treatment the inevitable outcome would remain persisting noncompliance. So, aiming to disqualify myself as an enforcer of medication compliance, I put my cards on the table, hoping that I could take compliance off the table. But I was trumped by Mother's exercise of her authority; she removed Owen from treatment.

The question remains: Could I have obtained Mother's cooperation by first addressing the compliance issue directly with her, rather than indirectly via Owen? Should I have stated there were some issues more important than medication? Should I have noted that medication was a symbol of power for both Mother and Owen—as it is for many youngsters and their parents—and that therefore the basic issue here was a power struggle? That we needed to focus on the two of them learning how to get along? I doubt it—the two were so entrenched. Nonetheless, I could have been more patient.

Management: Tactics

Interview Participation of Parents and Sponsors

I have found that the management of attachment disability is best addressed by including parents and sponsors in interviews whenever possible. Some of the advantages of this arrangement are:

Collateral Information and Feedback

To repeat, an adequate workup rests on three legs: patient and collateral history, mental status examination and testing, and psychodynamic formulation. The cases I chronicle here occurred long before the era of the pre-interview questionnaire and symptom inventory that now are routine for all medical and psychiatric initial evaluations. I recall as a medical student a good deal of the responsibility for collecting collateral data fell upon us lowly creatures once we began our third-year clinical work. It was a tradition to assign such scut work to us, given our status without any "real" therapeutic responsibilities and therefore with the time to perform such investigational duties. So we passed a lot of time on the telephone tracking down obscure records of prior medical treatments, or we hung around the ward during evening visiting hours to buttonhole relatives and friends of patients for information about events preceding hospitalization. Once in a while we might stumble upon a nugget of dramatic portent, but for the most part I found it tedious and uninformative, although most informants were gracious and forthcoming.

Not so with adolescents. Given their propensity for denial and resistiveness—think of Dyllen here, or Mr. Resistive—and since most of us do not have the interview skills of a Dr. Searles to elicit data, one-on-one interactions are likely to flounder. So when youngsters show up in my office I always invite their escorts to sit in. Most escorts, though not all, are quite happy to do so. Occasionally parents or sponsors will resist my invitation to sit in, and then are eager to escape, hoping to dump their child in my lap, a striking if silent collateral statement.

This arrangement includes an escape clause. I waive the requirement if adolescents are able to make it to my office on their own, without someone riding shotgun, so to speak. Taking on this responsibility is a tangible sign of an adolescent's emancipation, one consequence of which is that our discussions become confidential unless there is clear and current evidence of danger to self or others. But confidentiality does not extend to parents or sponsors who might call to apprise me of developments; I make it clear I will discuss such matters with their youngster. When a call or letter comes to me prefaced with a directive not to reveal its source, I immediately disclaim agreement. Otherwise I risk acting as a parental surrogate, which undermines the uniqueness of my therapeutic role. Finally, if the issue is emergent, I recommend the youngster be brought to an emergency room for examination with instructions to the examining doctors to contact me with their findings.

Just as important, if not more so, is the nonverbal child-sponsor interaction, which speaks directly to the quality of the attachment bond. Does the interaction fluctuate, alternating between resistiveness and affection? Is it conspiratorial? When a sponsor describes provocative behaviors — "It seems like he does it deliberately to bug me" — does the youngster smile in guilty affirmation? When an angry child finally admits to the fear of loss behind the anger, does the parent accept or reject the child's expression of love and concern? The context of a joint interview offers a richness of insight otherwise difficult to retrieve; to again paraphrase our professors, listen to what people do and watch what they say.

Similarly, framing my formulations in terms of underlying and unrecognized loss and attachment issues is more illuminating if I present it to parents and youngsters together.

[CASE STUDY]
Ryan: The Danger of Growing Up

I see in consultation a twelve-year-old lad with a long-standing history of violent and aggressive behaviors that have resisted seven years of consultation and therapy, including months in a day-treatment program. As I listen to his despairing mother, the youngster, obviously intelligent, remains distant, unattached, and uninvolved, pretty much ignoring my prompts to clarify or amend his mother's report. Finally I suggest to the mother that while her son likely has developmental and attachment issues—both concepts she understands—there is another problem: "I think he's afraid that if he gets better and grows up something awful will happen to you."

Shocked at first, she exclaims that she nearly died eighteen months earlier from an allergic reaction. He then makes his only remark, muttering, "I don't want to talk about it," pulls his hoodie over his head, and slumps back into his chair.

Clarification! I recommend a psychotropic for his anger outbursts and suggest they return in two weeks to review his records for further clarification.

Of course, clarification of this sort is no guarantee that management will be successful, but in its absence, any management strategy is doomed to fail. And without a joint interview we would never have achieved such dramatic clarification.

Security

As I described in chapter 7, when I joined a small private practice in 1970, one of the services our group offered was the medical-legal evaluation of individuals claiming psychiatric disability. In such situations the client was not the individual but the referring party, typically an insurance company, occasionally a government agency, to whom I was to submit a report after the examination. Some insurance companies were quite persnickety about not allowing family members to be present at the interview, other companies not so. Eventually I discovered that having a chaperone present, so to speak, produced a better interview because the interviewee, feeling safer with a familiar face in the room, was more forthcoming. So at every opportunity I welcomed family and friends into my office.

The same is true of adolescents. One will, on balance, hear and see more if a parent, sponsor, friend, or sib is in the room. Occasionally a youngster will arrive in my office accompanied only by a buddy, obviously to provide moral support for what is an intimidating encounter under any circumstances. I always invite the friend to join in the proceedings. Perhaps things might have worked out differently for Dyllen if the school counselor had invited him to bring a trusted friend along. He might have been less defensive.

It is true that occasionally this arrangement means there are some things I will not hear about. Just recently I saw a youngster who previously felt constrained not to report sexual abuse while hospitalized because her abuser was present during her interview. (Obviously, the truth eventually emerged.) This is why I use the qualifier "on balance" because I must take into account the things I won't hear or see should I conduct a solo interview.[iv]

In medical school we were trained to always weigh the downside potential of any treatment decision, including the decision not to treat. The same holds true for managing adolescent attachment issues. There are risks and benefits associated with any interview technique. Nonetheless I strongly recommend seeing adolescents in the presence of a third party. Indeed, I will generally refuse to see an unemancipated youngster without one.

There is another security interest to consider here as well:

---

iv. For example, Samantha (chapter 11), who took advantage of the emancipation option to see me without her mother being present, which impeded clarification.

mine. Interviewing an adolescent or child alone increases the risk of the youngster feeling trapped or overwhelmed, especially if one is too friendly. Kids with attachment issues distrust closeness and offers of friendship, which, in their experience, are the prelude to exploitation or risks of renewed loss. Such fears fuel anger, provocation, and attack. Bystanders dampen the fire because there is safety in numbers.

I will shortly discuss Mr. POP, a very angry fellow, enraged and frightened because he was forced into treatment. Staffing him followed our usual protocol: he was seated closest to the exit and we across from him with a table in between, ensuring he felt protected and free to escape the room. Thereafter I was careful to avoid one-on-one contacts, interacting with him only in public, and in passing at that. Because we always had his — and similar patients — security concerns in mind, we never had violent physical encounters at staff-patient conferences. Years later when I was a consultant at a residential treatment center for youthful sexual offenders, I always conducted interviews in the presence of our nurse, with the same seating arrangement, primarily for security reasons.

Co-option Prevention

Many youngsters who arrive on my doorstep are accompanied by a history of troubles with authority. Teachers, parents, and sponsors hope that one of the benefits of management will be the development of an attitude more receptive to their authority. Sometimes the message is naked: *make them behave!* Here, if I am not careful, I risk being used as a club in a fruitless attempt to beat the recalcitrant one into submission. At other times the manipulation will be more subtle, usually taking the form of my words being misquoted. This is most likely to occur when parents or sponsors request a private conference before or after I meet with their youngsters. It is amazing how what I think is an identical communication to both parties in private suffers in translation, not infrequently ending up with both forming an alliance against me because trust has been undermined, each thinking I am taking the side of the other. True, I am most interested in what parents or authorities have to say, but I always preface my listening with the reminder that I will not hold the information confidential. Sometimes I have to explain that otherwise it is useless, especially if there is an element of danger.

In short, my expertise as an authority is less likely to be undermined and co-opted, whether intentional or not, if I invite all parties to every meeting. For example, as parents and youngsters enumerate problems or issues, both parties can amplify, correct, or deny for the record. But there is only one record—admittedly ambiguous—rather than two. Better the ambiguity of two voices in the same room than the illusion of clarity provided by each voice alone. Clarification—the first step of disability management—includes facilitating a consensus of voices rather than judging the merits of each.

Co-therapist Recruitment

It is rare that a youngster or young adult who has been referred to me for consultation arrives without a current or proposed counseling relationship. In fact, a fair number of my referrals come from therapists or counselors themselves. Thus my time with a youngster is limited compared to theirs, at best a half hour every two weeks versus an hour, sometimes two, per week. And their time in turn is constricted compared to the hours youngsters pass each day in the company of parents and sponsors.

Now, it is a safe bet that prior learning methods—lecturing, admonition, suspension, grounding—administered by parents and sponsors have been tried and failed. If these techniques had worked, the adults would not appear in my waiting room with their youngsters. So the kids who come to me will require:

1) repetitive presentations of 2) different styles of attitude and behavior that compose the three principles of attachment disability management. But I suffer a profound time-on-task disadvantage when it comes to defining and demonstrating the steps. I need co-therapists.

The presence of sponsors and parents in the room is a potential resource. By observing how I restructure dialogue and fashion responses to their youngsters' behavior—whether withdrawn, resistive, provocative, or angry—I am modeling a repertoire that they can take home and continue long after the hour is over. That is, they can observe and practice my stagecraft. I will discuss the idea of "stagecraft" at greater length later, but here let me provide a few brief examples:

An Unending Litany of Complaints

Here youngsters hide behind a wall of words. They have learned, when parents attempt to focus on one complaint, to switch to another, and then another, until their parents either tune out or are tempted to attack with their own complaints. When adolescents try this gambit with me, I listen for a while and then interrupt and ask them to "boil things down to six words or less." Some can; most are stumped. So I might say, "You feel they are not fair" or "They are too strict" or "They don't care" or "They don't take care of their health." If used consistently, this serves to focus issues.

Heated Rhetoric

Here again, the younger's goal is to stay safe, but now by provoking an angry, rejecting reaction. In response to a blaming, angry tirade of this sort, I might say, "Let's see if you can tell me (or them) what the problem is without raising your voice." The idea is to transmute an argument into a discussion, hopefully setting the stage for a mutual understanding of how to proceed.

Resistiveness

I do not have the skills of a Dr. Searles, so I need help when it comes to resistive youngsters. Typically such youngsters respond minimally if at all to open-ended, unstructured inquiries. For example my routine opening question usually is "Well, what brings you here today?" or "How are things going?" With these kids, at best I might get a grunt or a dismissive "Fine" if there is a reaction at all. Cold rejection here. Rather than withdrawing into a tired, ruminative recycling of all my past rejections, for help I turn to the parents or sponsors in attendance. This gambit serves both my personal and professional needs. It also advances management.

I am a human being. If I choose to participate in an interaction, I will need feedback and recognition. We all do. We cannot long tolerate the presence of another who, for whatever reason, ignores us. If this persists, we will either withdraw or go out of control. So to feed my social nature, I engage the other parties at hand, whom I have invited into the room foreseeing I might need protection from rebuffs. Thus I nod briskly to the silent one after being stiffed—as if I had just been gifted with a singular insight—then turn to the parents with the same question. They typically are more than happy to converse with me; my soul is enriched.

And professionally, of course, I need information. Not that the dimensions of the problem are not apparent—the behavior signals fear of attachment, fear of engaging. But I need to fill in the blanks. So I conscientiously record their information and review whatever records or reports they may provide.

Now, in the midst of all this busyness, from time to time I will turn to the (ostensibly) uninvolved one—who is usually quite attentive beneath a cloak of feigned indifference—and brightly check out a snippet of data. "Is that so?" I might ask, or "Is that what happened?" My intent here is not really verification or otherwise, but to undo the previous rebuff by pretending it never happened. My message is not *I am going to make you talk!* Rather it is something like *You can't make me disappear or go out of control by ignoring me.* After a few seconds I return to the dialogue I have briefly interrupted.

This is how I melt resistiveness. I plan on it taking a number of visits; resistiveness does not spring forth or vanish overnight. Of course, when the resistive barrier begins to weaken and my inquiries elicit more than stony silence, it is most important not to overreact despite my thirst for recognition.

Stagecraft

My introduction to stagecraft, although I did not recognize it as such at the time, took place the first afternoon of my first day as a psychiatric resident in 1962. I have no recollection of that first morning: probably I was too preoccupied with conforming to the usual mustering-in routine that initiates a new career.

The afternoon was a different matter. We were assigned to work in the outpatient department, where we were greeted by our preceptor—a slender, brusque, unsmiling, master-sergeant type that company commanders rely on to run the outfit—who, without flourishes, began to lecture us on rule number one: never be too friendly with a paranoid patient. He then modeled an officious minor bureaucrat: narrowed eyes, impatient pencil tapping, suspicious expression, all reminiscent of a pre–World War II, grade-B Hollywood foreign intrigue thriller. His point: anger is the only emotion a paranoid understands. Any display of, say, friendliness or sympathy will simply elicit suspicion and anger. In short, he was recommending we mirror our patient's emotional state to establish a boundary and maintain distance across which we could establish a cautious connection. Recall that this was precisely one of the effects of the token economy (chapter 5). It clearly defined the contingences of staff-patient interaction, therefore reducing the probability of boundary violations.

Stagecraft Is Pervasive in Society

Some parents may object to "stagecraft" tactics as "dishonest" or "manipulative." When I suggest they may need to learn to "outmanipulate" their rebellious and defiant child, they are horrified: "She's too manipulative already!" Some don't return. Such parents are still gripped by the archaic notion their kids are supposed to do what they are told despite years of evidence to the contrary. (See the mother of Owen, above.)

Recall my earlier remarks that children are learning machines. The issue is never *are they learning?* Rather, it's *what are they learning?* Which means that from breath one, that child has you, its parent, in its sights. You are under constant surveillance. Your every move or lack thereof goes into its memory bank, as does the effectiveness, or lack thereof, of its behaviors to obtain need gratification. Long before its first words, your child has you figured. And will work you. Manipulate you. Expertly. It behooves you to develop some manipulative tactics of your own. So to ameliorate your discomforts about acquiring such skills, here let me put in a good word about "manipulation."

Manipulation is the heart of politics. Think of Spielberg's movie *Lincoln* and its portrayal of the president as an accomplished wordsmith using language to unite both his government and the nation to support the Emancipation Proclamation. Society in general could not exist without such manipulation. Society encourages negotiation; it promotes the use of words to obtain a peaceful, nonviolent exchange of goods and services. Dale Carnegie's *How to Win Friends and Influence People* still sells eight decades after its publication in the 1930s. But now we refer to manipulation as persuasion and salesmanship.

Of course, artful manipulation can also be disruptive. When we were second-year residents, one of our professors enjoyed spicing up a presentation by leaning back, staring absently into the distance, then (darkly) wondering whether the resident was being "manipulated" by the patient. This usually enlivened and refreshed the proceedings. It took me years to realize the comment itself was manipulative. I put this insight to work on one occasion during a medical-legal deposition when the attorney for the insurance company asked, "Dr. Curran, could the patent be manipulative?"

"Could be," I said, "I get manipulated all the time. In fact, for all I know you could be manipulating me right now." The attorney solemnly assured me he wasn't.

Counter manipulation of this sort also has its uses outside of case presentations and courtrooms to avoid aggravating the social disability of severe mental illness. Let me illustrate.

[CASE STUDY]
Mr. POP Is "Outmentalized"

Some twenty years after leaving Anoka State Hospital, I am once again back in the state hospital system, this time consulting at the Saint Peter (MN) Regional Treatment Center. I am assigned to an unlocked admissions unit. (I do not have available the case records from my experiences there. But let me offer a reconstruction of the shtick I evolved to defuse antagonism, also as an example of not pathologizing anger.)

It's late afternoon now and we are all tired. We've been staffing new admissions for three hours; only one to go now, a young man under commitment, pissed off and hostile, ready to argue and debate. He stalks into the room, strides to the table, and glares at us, shouting. We look at each other and by unspoken consent decide to let him ventilate. We offer him a place at the table; he sits.

> *Mr. Pissed-Off Patient:* "Who says I have to enter the hospital? Who has the right to make me stay? Everyone is against me! You are against me!!"
>
> *Dr. Curran (Taking a cue from the others, I switch from my concerned professional stance into my officious irritated routine, beckoning him closer—I've learned to counter shouting with gestures—waving the commitment papers):* "You won't believe this," *I hiss impatiently, as if dealing with a slightly dull student,* "but some people actually think you are mentally ill. Look! It says P-A-R-A-N-O-I-D S-C-H-I-Z-O-P-H-R-E-N-I-A. They think you are crazy!"
>
> *Mr. POP (ignoring me):* "I'm not crazy. You are the crazy ones. You are corrupt. You are just in this for the money!"
>
> *Dr. C (again waving the papers, continuing my petty bureaucratic shtick:)*[v] "You don't understand. Look! This is from the probate court—they are committing you to St. Peter Regional Treatment Center. They actually think there is some kind of a problem. I know what a wild idea it is, but they think you need some kind of treatment."
>
> *Mr. POP (starting to tire; he's had a long day too):* "Everyone is against me. No one cares!"
>
> *Dr. C (switching to a different bit, the indifferent caretaker):* "Look, it's not my problem whether people are against you or whether they care. My problem is getting this interview finished because I want to go home. And at the end of the week collect my check."

---

v. Another lesson here, this one from my patients: keep repeating yourself. That's what made Ronald Reagan the "Great Communicator."

Mr. POP (threatened by my change in manner): "You are just trying to trick me!"

Dr. C: "True."

Mr. POP (further threatened by my agreeing with him): "I'm out of here!" *(Gets up to leave.)*

Dr. C (not letting him have the last word): "Hey, things would work out better for me if you never cooperate because it means permanent employment for me." *(Now I'm at the doorway shouting after him.)* "And if you want to elope, that's okay too. The door down the hall is unlocked by day—be my guest, just don't stop at the state border, just keep on going, and if you are detained don't tell them you are on the run from Minnesota. And for goodness sake don't mention my name!"

A week later we have a follow-up interview.

Dr. C (suspiciously): "What's this? The staff says you're taking your medications, controlling your behavior, not talking about your strange ideas, cooperating with the hospital rules and regulations. Trying to con us into giving the court a good report, huh? What's this cooperation bit?"

Mr. POP (disgusted): "Knock it off—you're just playing a game. What kind of a doctor are you, some kind of a quack? I'm just doing it so I can get out of here. I'm not cooperating, I'm in charge, not you." *(Walks out.)*

A few weeks later we meet in the hall.

Dr. C (rhetorically): "What—you're still here? What are you hanging around this place for?"

> Mr. POP (ignores me, brushes by me, mumbling something about not having a place to go, no money).

Later I hear from a staffer that he's complaining about me: "Dr. Curran is outmentalizing me." Obviously, he's been thinking things over.

His stay remains uneventful. We discharge him in five weeks. He never returns. We never have a follow-up report.

Mr. POP's Presentation

Although Mr. POP presented with a diagnosis of Paranoid Schizophrenia, it is immediately clear to us, experienced observers of the newly committed, that he does not demonstrate the disorganization of behavior and thought that normally is part of a psychosis. It seems he has responded to his current Antipsychotics. True, he is angry, defiant, and provocative, yet he seems ready for a debate and his denial defenses are intact. Moreover, he responds to social cues. It appears we are dealing with his disability, not with the disease.

Mr. POP's Expectations

It soon becomes clear that beneath the bluster he feels lonely and rejected—no one cares, people are against him—yet he would feel quite threatened by any sign of caring. He expects more rejection, verbal combat, perhaps even a fight if he can get us worked up enough. In this respect he is rather similar to Jackie, whose provocativeness also precipitated her commitment. This is quite familiar to us since it is a common reaction by the newly admitted, whether committed or voluntary, regardless of diagnosis. Whether by design or habit, such patients maneuver to establish a boundary, a bulwark to keep us at a distance in order to feel safe. It also allows patients to enjoy the support offered by the hospital—food, shelter, entertainment, activities—without recognizing dependency needs: that is, without feeling like a kid. In short, in Mr. POP's case, it is very suggestive that attachment issues are part of his disability.

Mr. POP and Stagecraft

In deciding upon the stagecraft for Mr. POP, the idea is to respect his boundaries while providing him the opportunity to develop less disruptive, more socially congruent techniques to maintain distance. In other words, we hope to promote his capacity to exercise choice and learn from experience. So we don't treat him as a prisoner or behave like his superiors or captors—which is his expectation. Instead I greet him as if he was just one more pain in the hind end. Playing the role of an impatient, irritable, officious, petty bureaucrat that I was taught years before, I allow him to read his record and note that he will have the freedom to refuse medications, even elope: whatever; more money for me. The team, used to this gambit, plays along.

Later I play another hole card, a second switcheroo: I add to my guise the persona of the suspicious cop, accusing him of trying to con me by following the rules. The staff play "good cop," supporting his grumbling and beefing about an authority that did not match his punitive and tyrannical expectations. He complains of being "outmentalized," his term for *cognitive dissonance*. His only recourse is to escape by working the system and getting out of Dodge.

It would have been a mistake to openly recognize his compliance, and for two reasons. It would suggest an intimacy, admittedly rather tenuous, that would threaten his need for distance. And it would imply that his compliance would now be the expected norm. As I will briefly discuss later in this chapter, when a patient finally does something right, it is important to recognize the achievement, of course, but with what I call a "backward" compliment: one that endorses the performance without an implication of subsequent consistency.

Mr. POP's Experience

Apart from his blustering and presumptive psychosis, it's clear that Mr. Pop is not unintelligent. His description of his experience—he's being "outmentalized"—is revealing because it implies he recognizes he is himself manipulative in the way he manages authority. Of course, this is a dangerous game because it invites physical retaliation. Possibly he is aware of that as well, and indeed may have in the past provoked an assault or two because of his rants. Perhaps he even figures he needs to make some changes and at some level welcomes the opportunity to be "mentalized," thus making only a token fuss now and then to maintain his self-respect.

I would like to stress here that our goal was not to revise his emotional functioning, only his social functioning in the hope of providing him with a broader behavioral repertoire from among which to choose in social situations. The idea was to promote adaptive flexibility, not enhanced empathy or trust.

Mr. POP's Future

What to make of the fact that we never hear of or from him again? No return to us, no requests for his records from other hospitals, no inquiries from the court for a recommendation regarding his commitment status, no letters from social service agencies, no complaints from the community to the medical director as had happened years before to me at Anoka State Hospital (chapter 4). Nothing at all. This is most unusual considering his youth, sex, diagnosis, and degree of disability. Young males of this sort weave in and out of treatment facilities for years, in my experience, only settling into a more stable, less socially visible lifestyle as they learn from experience, or "burn out," or cobble up a support system, or most likely some combination thereof. Is his "mentalization" permanent?

I have thought about him for years, wondering how he is

doing. I have imagined him, now in his late forties, medication in hand, thinking something like *Do I really want to keep taking this stuff? It's a drag having to go to the clinic, get a script, go to the drug store ... and it is making me fat ... Why not stop it? ... But better not, I might end up back in that hospital ... last time that happened it drove me sane!*

Caution and Clarification

In presenting this vignette it is not my intention to imply that patients who are committed because of hallucinations and delusions are not psychotic. Nor am I implying that institutions—or society—are the cause of their psychosis. Rather, as I learned during my years at Anoka, what is true of all medicine is true of psychiatric medicine as well: you must distinguish between the illness and the disability associated with it.

Individuals vulnerable to psychotic decompensation can learn to recognize the early signs of trouble—usually a change in the sleep pattern—and take steps to abort it: for example, resuming or increasing medications, seeking consultation, reducing stress, or decreasing substance use. But they have to be given the opportunity to learn; that is, the opportunity to make choices and experience consequences. And I will repeat here, because it is such a vital but pernicious dynamism in persistent mental and emotional disability, that I sometimes tell certain patients, "You have a problem worse than your mental problems—not learning from experience." Hopefully the way we managed Mr. POP helped him learn something about his predicament and how to live with it.

In short, stagecraft is teaching by another name. Recall again the manipulative dynamic embedded in the token economy we devised years earlier at Anoka State Hospital. Patients could acquire tokens—ordinary washers available at any hardware store—either by working the program or, once they earned a few privileges, by taking a bus into town and surreptitiously buying a supply for a dollar or two. Whether or not "cheating" of this sort ever took place is unclear—rumors of this sort never came to us via the patient grapevine. However, we did discuss the possibility, concluding that it was very adaptive behavior.

In group therapy, one constant instruction to our patients was that they had to learn how to work the system—especially the greater one outside the walls—and learn manners, rather than fighting against the system or with each other. We concluded that if a patent should "bust out" of the hospital by fancy finagling, this demonstrated the sort of foresight and impulse control that would merit discharge anyhow. Moreover, it seemed that an unofficial honor system developed in which patients maintained surveillance on each other, an unexpected dividend of the social cohesion fostered by the manipulative powers of a cheap metal washer.

Familiar Adolescent Manipulations Calling for Stagecraft

Count yourself lucky as sponsor, therapist, or teacher if your adolescent or student tries one of these on you. For these gambits mean the youngster has not given up on you, still aspires to a relationship, and still hopes to remain attached, although on terms that keep you one down and at a certain distance. In one way or another all these manipulations are anxiety driven; that is, driven by youngsters' concerns to secure relationships, especially with peers, in which they feel relatively safe. And since, as I will discuss in volume 2 of this series, in an other-directed society sponsors are gripped by peer-group anxieties of their own, it is difficult to manage the discomforts such tactics elicit unless you are prepared.

"You (They) Are Not Fair"

Youngsters thrive in a predictable, ordered environment: in other words, an environment of rules. As adults we have learned—perhaps bitterly—that following the rules does not always pay off. And, as Dr. Mary reminded my sister-in-law, in fact in life there are no rules.[vi] Or they don't pay off. In my practice a frequent referral is the forty-year-old father who, after a lifetime of following the rules as instructed, finds himself not happy or fulfilled as he had been promised, which is the reality of the so-called "midlife crisis."

If you have not already reconciled yourself to the unfairness of life—and an astute youngster will intuit this about you early on—you will be especially vulnerable to this manipulative ploy. So when you hear this from youngsters, there are two reactions you need to resist: apologizing/giving in, or attacking/belittling. Both cater to youngsters' developmental immaturity by treating them as too young to tentatively face the unfairness of life, or too ignorant to have figured things out.

Statesmanlike leadership is called for, the kind that recognizes the reality of unfairness and accepts it without blame, yet supports the validity of striving for lawful rights. With older adolescents a response might be the question, "Well, what would be fair?" Or, more baldly, "I see what is in this for you, but what am I going to get out of this?" In other words, where is the exchange? Interestingly, for some adolescents such a reply is de facto evidence of your unfairness because you are treating them like an adult. That is, you are expecting them to behave like a grown-up and accept responsibility for their behavior, while they wish to remain a kid and have you accept responsibility. Which is what the unfairness indictment is all about: you are unfair because you expect them to grow up. This is a great learning opportunity for all. Rise to it.

---

vi. See chapter 6.

"Everyone Else Is Doing It"

A little background here. We Curran kids grew up on Saint Paul's West Side, an enclave perched on hundred-foot-plus bluffs above the Mississippi River, separated by its broad gorge from the rest of the city across the way. A rickety, half-mile long bridge dating from the horse-and-buggy era connected the two sides: the legendary—and notorious—High Bridge. Legendary because all West Side kids of that era swam under it, biked over it, and walked the bluff trails beneath it. To climb its girders and venture forth over the river below was the test of manhood. Notorious because we country club caddies would whisper among ourselves about how ol' man so-and-so on his way home from a night at the club drove off the bridge—and he survived! Thus did the High Bridge loom large in our imagination and life.[vii]

Now to the unfairness complaint. I think at one time or another, Mom must have heard each of us whining how other kids could do stuff we couldn't—say, go to the game or hang out late. In other words, "Everybody else" could do it. Not even bothering to look up from her housework or hear us out, she would snap back, "Well, if 'everybody' jumped off the High Bridge, would you too?" We would walk away crushed, or at least I did, feeling, *Aww, Mom ... that's so unfair.*

In volume 2 I review the conjecture that our era is witnessing the consequence of a cultural shift in ruling emotion. According to sociologist David Riesman, human culture was formerly controlled by tradition-based shame or rule-based guilt. But now, in our consumption-driven culture, both parents and

---

vii. It's long gone now, replaced years ago by a presumably safer structure but with a grimmer reputation as St. Paul's "Suicide Bridge." Susan Du, "The long wait for prevention barriers on St. Paul's Suicide Bridge." *City Pages*: May 3, 2016. I discuss the recent increasing frequency of youthful suicide in volume 2.

children are ruled by anxiety. Clearly this was not true of Mom. She was a creature of rules.

The interesting thing, as I look back on it, is that the rules were implicit, rarely enunciated. She was guided by two beacons: the Rosary Society and Mrs. Schmidt.[viii] The Schmidts, of more comfortable means, lived a few blocks away in a more genteel neighborhood. There were ten or eleven kids, a number of whom eventually entered various Catholic orders. As the mother of an Irish family in a German parish, according to my older sister, Anne, Mom was very conscious of the Schmidt way of doing things, and we were inculcated accordingly. She never said, "Well, if one of the Schmidts jumped off …" or the like. She didn't have to say it because we got the idea. So, if Mrs. Schmidt did spring cleaning, so did we dust, break out the furniture polish, take up the carpets. If Mrs. Schmidt brought baked goods to the Rosary Society … and on it went. I can see now that Mrs. Schmidt was the embodiment of what later was enunciated by John Mortimer's doughty but long-suffering character *Rumpole of the Bailey* as the SWMBO (She Who Must Be Obeyed) rule.

I often muse, while listening to parents' struggles with their adolescents, *Where are the Mrs. Schmidts to provide leadership?* SWMBO is deceased, replaced by CTMBO (Crowd That Must Be Obeyed). Modern motherhood, you will need to be creative here.

"You Can't Make Me"

The truth of the matter with this one is that as a parent, you can't. Your ability to command the compliance of your youngster begins to erode at birth, a deterioration that accelerates once the child is walking. As the energy and determination of your child swell, yours diminishes. Here you are outmatched. So thoughtfully you turn to a combination of leadership, stagecraft,

---

viii. During our upbringing Anne was more privy to Mom's concerns than I.

good humor, and tolerance to achieve compliance ... hopefully.

Sooner or later, however, into all parents' lives rain will fall in the form of the ominous words *"You can't make me!"* And you can't. You are not going to turn your home into an armed redoubt from which escape is impossible. Not if you are sane. And you are not going to organize a posse to snatch the recalcitrant one from the grip of peers of dubious character and reputation. Not if you wish to retain any credibility. So what do you do?

You might begin to enumerate the consequences of transgression. This I do not recommend because sooner or later you will be tested, and then you will have to follow up or risk loss of credibility. If you must take this approach, it's better to say something like, "Well, I can't stop you, because it's clear you are going to do what you have to do ... but then we will see what I am going to do." Never put your cards on the table; in a situation like this your hand will always be weak. You need to bluff, hoping it will pay off.

Better yet, however, is to acknowledge that the defiant one indeed speaks the truth, is bigger, stronger, perhaps even wiser. Then you can add, thoughtfully, something like, "You know, no matter what you say or do, you cannot change my mind about what is best for you." Now, to be honest, none of us ever heard this from Mother Curran because we all already knew that nothing was going to change her mind. Her truth was fixed, immutable, revealed. I can imagine, however, if one of us dared to threaten to jump, she would have sniffed, "Go ahead." What a killjoy!

An illustration.

[CASE STUDY]
Maddie: Defiance Concealing an Entangled Heart

Maddie is an adolescent girl seen with her foster father because of anxiety, cutting, experimenting with drugs, and declining schoolwork.

The immediate issue is the tragic death of a schoolmate in a diving accident. One weekend the boy and some buddies were goofing around at a state park, diving off a cliff into a river. Apparently he hit a concealed rock, was knocked unconscious, and drowned before anyone realized what had occurred. Everyone was shocked by the event, of course, but hers was more profound for she lapsed into a numbed, persisting withdrawal, now perhaps accentuated by the Antidepressant she is taking: "feeling blank and neutral in my head."

There is a background of family stress for which she has been seeing a therapist, some eighteen months now. One problem is financial; her foster father is unemployed because of health issues. And a younger foster sister is severely disabled because of lupus.

At examination in the company of her foster father, she presents as a preoccupied young lady who looks older than her stated age and who sports a vividly colored mop of hair—the tint of which would subsequently change from visit to visit—suggesting a resistive and rebellious spirit. Instead she proves to be a cooperative, compliant, tense, restless, haunted, and discouraged child, at times close to tears. "I worry about the weirdest things ... the what ifs ... always worry ..." She needs little encouragement to reveal how this recent catastrophe has further upended her life.

I find her a very sad girl with many worries about her foster family and friends. I recommend she discontinue the Antidepressant and suggest she return in two weeks, at which time she seems improved. Several weeks later, however, she reports that contact with a relative of the lad killed in the accident "brought back memories ... my mind, always going ... don't want to sleep ... I think about things that happened long ago." She avoids discussing things with her therapist: "If I talk to her, it freaks her out, wants to fix things." I recommend a trial of another Antidepressant, which perhaps is more helpful than the first; she later states she is less concerned about being a burden.

During the course of these visits I am struck by two things. One is the tolerance, insight, and patience of her foster father. The two of them are comfortable with their mutual affection. (I later learn he is determined not to repeat the mistakes he made years earlier with a son by another relationship.)

The second is her entanglement in her peers' affairs. For example, she feels "weighed down" by some of her boyfriend's problems. Later she brings him home and her foster parents take him in.[ix]

One afternoon I receive an emergency call from her foster father. It seems she and the fellow they had been harboring had concocted a scheme to run away. Dad disagreed but otherwise did not intervene—did he do the right thing? I fully support his obviously painful decision. Afterward I wonder if she had precipitated the crisis, hoping to extract herself from the suffocating presence of her needy boyfriend.

She returns with her foster father one month later, at which time they provide me with a blow-by-blow, hilarious account of their showdown, which I will attempt to reproduce here.

> *Foster father, upon hearing her threat to take off:* "I don't agree, but I'm not going to try to stop you."
> *Maddie, incredulous:* "What?"

---

ix. Not uncommon, in my experience. Despite limited means, families of troubled adolescents sometimes simply take in and informally "adopt" a stray, estranged youngster. More celery and oatmeal are added to the meatloaf and another place is set at the table.

FF: "Go ahead, go."
Maddie: "You are not going to stop me?"
FF: "No!"
Maddie leaves, returns twenty minutes later with police in tow.
Police: "We had a call there is an abuse situation here."
FF clarifies.
Police: "Oh."
Maddie: "Take me to a foster home."
Police: "No, you are going to detention." Depart with her in custody.
FF then makes his call to me. I reassure him he did the right thing, that as a parent myself I understand how painful it must have been, but she is now in safe hands.

Maddie and foster father, one month later, smiling.
Maddie: Chagrined, rueful as she relates her weekend in detention, like a boot camp with bad food, and not much of it at that. Now she's back home. The boyfriend is out of the picture, back with his old girlfriend.
FF: Says they are now in family counseling. "She's able to open up ... gives her a springboard ... she's made great progress, her behavior, her attitude."
Dr. C: Wonders if the whole affair was to manipulate herself out of the grasp of her boyfriend.
Maddie agrees: "He was an emotional leech ... I can't figure out why I'm not more upset [now that he's gone] ... we helped each other."
FF: Reports that her behavior helped him recognize the pain he caused his own father.
Both: Joshing and kidding.
Maddie: More serious. It turns out that things began to fall apart more than two years before when her

> *trust was betrayed while trying to help a girlfriend with her problems. Afterward she felt so dumb and ashamed she couldn't reveal it until recently.*
>
> FF: *On a brighter note, reports just recently his twenty-four-year-old unemployed homeless nephew appeared at the door one day, pregnant wife in tow, seeking shelter. Now they are part of the family.*
>
> Maddie: *Excited, glowing; now she has a new foster brother and a new foster sister whose baby is due the next day.*
>
> Maddie, thoughtfully: *"You know he [the foster brother] took me aside and told me that six years from now none of this stuff about friends will be important, that I will have forgotten all about it … funny, that's what everyone else had been telling me."*

Six months later she continues to do well at home and at school, still thrilled by her new family. Still later I read she has graduated with honors and has been awarded a partial scholarship.

Discussion

It would have been intrusive, given the drama and intensity of their healing and reconciliation, for me to have inquired what prompted Maddie to finally speak of the unspeakable. And perhaps it is not necessary to know what finally dissolved her shame. Perhaps taking in her leech of a boyfriend was her way of atoning for the misery she had caused. Indeed it is likely that Maddie herself would not be able to explain what happened, only that she suddenly felt free to reveal what was formerly forbidden. I suspect, however, that her foster father's firmness—and perhaps the "tough love" of the cops and the detention center—convinced her that not everyone would be freaked out by the truth, as was her therapist previously. No less than all of us, youngsters need firm leadership.

But what about the future? Under most circumstances, years of Attachment Entanglement create a lingering, powerful impulse to protect and console others perceived as vulnerable and needy, an impulse that is at times difficult to resist. Ordinarily, it takes months, even years to recover from Attachment Entanglement, to acquire a grip on your own needs and feelings firm enough that is unlikely to slip away in the face of the suffering of others. I would expect, therefore, that Maddie's path will be rocky, that her enchantment with her new family will sour a bit, that the old boyfriend might reappear with enticing distress signals aloft and fluttering, that she and her foster father might butt heads again in the midst of her mission—no doubt a function of being raised with a disabled sibling—to rescue the wounded and crippled. In short, it will take a while for her to learn to live with the largeness of her heart.

However, I am sure her foster father will not waver, and this is a powerful argument in favor of a positive outcome over the long run. Moreover, her academic performance is another positive note. Finally, a third and very influential factor here is that despite her years of tortured secrecy, Maddie never once demonstrated suicidal behavior.

Let me clarify. By suicidal behavior I have in mind tangible behavior—for example, overdose or hanging or carbon monoxide poisoning—that involves a foreseeable lethal consequence, as opposed to suicidal talk or ruminations. No doubt at times Maddie was preoccupied with the latter but there is no history of the former. In my experience suicide intent or attempts always involve an unmentionable shameful secret, such as sexual abuse, identity issues, betrayal, fear of disability, incest—things of that sort. Eventually the pain becomes too much to bear because it seems to loom on without end. Life appears a prospect without hope. Then suicide becomes a "solution" because it offers an end to suffering. Recall Styron's plan to kill himself. In short, whenever a client, and especially a youngster, presents with a history of suicidal behavior or intent—as opposed to rumination or talk—think hidden secret. Or presume hidden secret until proven otherwise.

But Maddie, despite harboring her shame for years, never did engage in suicidal behavior. True, she acted out here and there, but as I discussed at length earlier above, acting-out is a positive sign, a disguised plea for help on the part of an unhappy and distrustful youngster who yet has not totally given up on adults. Ultimately Maddie is a believer in the goodness of humanity, she has hope, and this will steady her as she navigates life's path.

Recognizing Achievement

I began this chapter by noting that the emphasis of this book is *management* of attachment disorders rather than their *treatment*. The idea is that if you as a sponsor or teacher focus on not making things worse, good things are likely to happen. Attachment-impaired youngsters, despite their trust issues, are just as dynamic as their less troubled peers. If you are patient, eventually the most hapless of adolescents will do something right.

Therefore, when a youngster finally makes a long hoped for adaptive maneuver, my habitual practice is to run a shtick I have perfected over the years:

Adolescent: Describes achievement.
Dr. C: Incredulous: "What?"
Adolescent: Repeats self.
Dr. C, amazed, boisterous, bellowing: "I can't believe it! *For once* you did it right."
Adolescent: Shy smile.

The critical piece here, of course, is the *"For once."* This recognizes the achievement without any subtext implying continuing performance. To do otherwise risks triggering success fears. The message must be *you did good* without the implication *I expect the same from now on.* And never so state. We who help must remember we are dealing with impulse-ridden beings who, even if they firmly desire to tread the straight and narrow, cannot guarantee with any certainty their future emotions and behavior. In chapter 11 I will present the case of Samantha, an entangled teenager whose recovery I may have sabotaged by forgetting to exercise such caution just as she started to demonstrate assertiveness with her peers.

11

The First Management Principle: Clarification

The goal of clarification is to differentiate attachment disability from the blaming it can precipitate.

Above I presented the case of Rebecca, whose chronic "depression" persisted despite my years of treating her with a series of Antidepressants. It was not until I realized that she was actually describing chronic anxiety that we began to make any progress. Until then *clarification* was the missing ingredient. Here I will discuss this in greater detail.

The Management of Attachment Disability Begins with Clarifying the Problem

The goal here is to *differentiate attachment disability from the blaming it can precipitate.* The idea is to distinguish between a damaged ability to form trusting relationships and its cognitive consequences—fears of future trauma. In other words, there are both *disability* and *a disability about the disability*. For example, Dyllen's performance anxiety was not the cause of his progressive academic difficulties and eventual dropping out. The cause was his apprehensions about how his peers might react were he to reveal his concerns openly. Hence his avoidant behavior. Note: Dyllen did demonstrate learning here, but his learning was maladaptive—more and more social isolation—not adaptive.

Clarification involves two (not necessarily sequential) processes: softening *denial* and promoting *insight*. The former is rather familiar. That is, we all have had the experience of finally admitting to ourselves the presence of some facts or truths in our lives that previously we overlooked, ignored, or minimized.

And the same is true on a larger scale. For example, by the end of the nineteenth century, the devastating effects of rapid-fire automatic weapons on massed attacks by African tribesmen had been widely studied and reported by military observers. Yet because of their conditioning, World War I generals persisted in ordering bayonet assaults against entrenched machine gun positions, sending hundreds of thousands of infantrymen over the top to their deaths. It took two years of carnage and stalemate to finally stimulate rethinking of military tactics, and the concept of an armored mobile assault capability evolved … the tank.[1] In volume 2 I will discuss Jared Diamond's thesis that societies collapse and disappear because they "choose" to do so despite evidence of their pending doom.[2] But I argue it is not "choice" at work in such circumstances but conditioning. Like the generals, societies too may be unable to change.

But adolescent denial is less powerfully conditioned or deeply entrenched because it has had less time to evolve through repetition. It is important to remember that conditioned denial, like most conditioning, tends to be subcortical for the most part, operating apart from conscious awareness. Thus directly confronting denial is not only ineffective but risks enhancing and reinforcing it: *confrontation strengthens denial*. An indirect approach is called for, one that gradually and kindly reveals the behavioral contradictions and inconsistencies of the adolescent's life in which denial protects from pain, but at the price of disability. Avoiding direct confrontation deprives the conditioned denial of support and therefore makes it easier to extinguish. Something like this happened with Mr. POP. We avoided a direct debate about whether he was mentally ill or not, simply revealing what the court thought, presenting ourselves as weary, minor bureaucrats following orders, our only interest collecting our paychecks.

Softening Denial

One consequence of our highly evolved cognitive skills is the ability to *deny loss and ignore the threat of subsequent loss*. But the capacity to experience mental/emotional discomfort is also an essential component of our survival kit. In fact, the ability to experience, assess, and respond to threat is hardly a hallmark of our species alone.

We humans have developed the capacity to overlook danger, with both adaptive and maladaptive consequences.

Life would be unsustainable if we could not evaluate stimuli and filter out "white noise." We would be paralyzed by too much data. We rely on an ability to focus our attention on the important tasks at hand. For the most part this is a nonconscious—as opposed to unconscious—process. On occasion, with conscious effort the filtering becomes so extreme that threat awareness is totally suppressed: for example, when parents rush into a burning house to rescue their children.

However, such adaptive use of extreme threat denial is quite unusual under the ordinary circumstances of day-to-day life. Much more frequent are its maladaptive consequences, such as denial of bullying.

In their perceptive analysis of the causes and management of school bullying and violence, Tremlow and Sacco devote an entire section to what they term "the denial mind-set."[3] They find that it is denial of threat awareness that renders youngsters vulnerable to exploitation by bullies. They discuss the "allure of denial." To maintain awareness of danger made sense in the long-ago world of our ancestors where violence from man or beast was the routine. But in our modern world, the cost-reward benefit of unceasing vigilance is skewed toward anxiety without relief, except by mentally "closing your eyes." Tremlow and Sacco describe a host of strategies that vulnerable kids employ to blind themselves to danger: a "Pollyanna" view of the world as basically good, risk seeking, avoidance, dissociation, identification with the aggressor, and so on. In their view such strategies may lead to collapse, the "giving up/given up on syndrome." They also argue that when the many figures in the victim's world—peers, teachers, principals—practice the same denial techniques, a school evolves a culture of bullying. Hence their conclusion that "bullying is a process, not a person": bullying is a social dynamic fostered by denial. If it takes a village to raise a child, Tremlow and Sacco would also say it takes a school to bully a child.

Now, youngsters rarely end up in my office with outright complaints of being bullied. Their sponsors may identify it as an issue but it often lurks in the backgrounds of youngsters who are not doing well in school. Typically it accelerates attachment issues of kids already rendered vulnerable to demeaning behaviors because of a background of loss or exploitation. Bulking up their innate denial capabilities has helped them carry on despite their suffering. But in consequence, they now tend to minimize the bullying as well. So they pretend. Moreover, many feel it is somehow their fault because perpetrators blame their victims. It is too shameful to admit.

When youngsters deny a problem—"I don't care ... It doesn't hurt ... So what?"—this simply perpetuates the problem and sets the stage for progressive disability. Excessive denial, in this sense, is worse than mental or emotional illness because—here

Clarification

I'm practicing the principle of *repetition* that I learned from my patients—it leads to failure to learn from experience. They are doomed to endless suffering.

Eventually the maladaptive pretending or denying starts to erode performance in school, on the job, or at home. At this point, hopefully, youngsters (and adults), willing or otherwise, appear at my office for help. Sometimes this recognition by self or others that help is necessary undermines denial and jump-starts the clarification process. Clients may be more or less forthright. With prompting, they will describe the multiple dimensions of attachment and loss issues: trouble concentrating, anxiety, "depression," anger, acting-out, substance use, and so on. Perhaps they will even address bullying if it is present. Such frankness and the surrender of denial it represents promote clarification and enhance disability management. However, frankness of this sort is uncommon. More likely is one of the following denial styles, or a mixture thereof.

Entrenched Denial

Sometimes, especially with youngsters, the very prospect of help partially reorganizes denial defenses. I might encounter the Alfred E. Neuman smile and attitude: "What? Me worry?"[i] Or a Mr. Resistive. Or a litany of vague complaints such as "stressed out" or "upset" or "unhappy" or "depressed." I know I am in for a workout when it comes to entrenched denial. Here is where an item-by-item review of a symptom inventory may be helpful since kids (and adults) will occasionally endorse items or provide marginal comments that reveal issues too touchy to openly address (for example, Owen above).

Denial of this sort, of course, reflects a hidden distrust of

---

i. For the younger generation of my readers, the goofy gap-toothed figurehead of *Mad Magazine*, famed for his motto, "What? Me worry?"

authority. Or, to put the matter differently, a belief that accepting an offer of protection and understanding can only hurt rather than help. It is therefore critical not to directly confront the evidence of distrust, for this only serves to increase anxiety and reinforce denial defenses. For example, if youngsters endorse an inventory item that they worry about something awful happening to their parents, but deny it when face to face with them, I do not challenge the discrepancy, and especially do not go further and question their inability to trust. Such insensitivity not only validates their perception of authority as hurtful, but also proves I am just another clueless adult. Case closed.

Rather, I might want to inquire of the adults present—still another reason to have grown-ups in the room—if they have noted such behaviors or concerns. Regardless of whether they affirm or deny, the issue is now on the table. Another denial-softening and anxiety-reducing technique is to make use of a strategy we devised at the St. Peter Regional Treatment Center: "Third Person Invisible (TPI)." The idea is to structure communication as if it were directed to a nonexistent (invisible) third party, the effect of which is to relieve the present (visible) party of the burden of responding.

For example:

[Case Study]
Justin: Mirroring Detachment

Just yesterday I see in consultation a high school senior boy who is referred from a crisis center because of suicidal thinking, alcohol abuse, and physical abuse by his father. There, he was restarted on Antidepressants he had discontinued several months before in order to qualify for army reserve boot camp. He now reports that once again the medications are helping

Clarification

improve sleep and reduce ruminations. Also, he is seeing the therapist to whom the crisis people had referred him.

It turns out he had done well in boot camp, in fact agrees with my comment that he must have thrived on the order and discipline of military life, understandable in view of the crisis center report of childhood turmoil, which included witnessing and experiencing physical abuse.

Nonetheless, in high school he had performed so well that he became eligible to sit college level courses by the time he was a junior, and subsequently earned twenty-three college credits. Later he was started on Antidepressants, which he found helpful, but which he did not resume after boot camp (although they would be not be prohibited when he begins basic training after graduation). Subsequently he was found sitting intoxicated on a railroad track and later had no memory of it—hence the crisis center evaluation that brought him to me.

In the company of his mother, he presents as a lanky, cooperative, compliant youngster dressed in clean sweats. At first he engages, but as I go through the referral documents and past history he seems to withdraw a bit; he is not resistive but needs prompts to elicit information. Even when he agrees with my suggestion that some of his "depression" might very well reflect residuals from his abuse experiences, he remains inward and does not volunteer details. Obviously he prefers his doctors somewhat detached and impersonal.

Accordingly I segue into TPI mode and begin discourse on the history of Antidepressants, the belated discovery of their mode of action ("antistressant"), side effects, length of treatment, and so on. The idea is to mirror his detachment with a somewhat pedantic, dry approach, figuring he is more comfortable with facts than interpretations. At the same time I swivel toward the window as if I were peering at a classroom audience, minimizing eye-to-eye contact. His mother listens, nodding approval. I conclude by renewing his medications, suggesting he return in a month, with longer follow-up intervals thereafter if things seem to be going well. I also encourage him to continue with his therapist.

This vignette illustrates that when it comes to denial dynamisms there is no one-size-fits-all interview technique. Be prepared to conform to the comfort level you perceive your client can tolerate. Here, as the interview progressed I began to feel somewhat rebuffed in my attempts to engage him, to promote more spontaneity. But, emulating Dr. Searles by listening to my countertransference, I distanced myself a bit by delivering a canned Antidepressant lecture, which, in fact, he needed to hear because of his noncompliance. I'm pretty sure he will return at least once; his mother will see to that. But his history of noncompliance suggests his denial may well be entrenched. Time will tell. Should he, however, commit to a regular follow-up schedule, it would be important to retain the TPI protocol until his behavior encourages a less impersonal approach.

Denial Masquerading as Compliance

Here the denial is subtle but tenacious. Its hallmark is a failure to improve.

[Case Study]
Samantha: The Tenacity of Denial

She is sixteen, seen with her mother, referred by her therapist for follow-up of an Antidepressant recently prescribed by her family doctor.

There is a history of conflicts with peers, cutting, death thoughts, and possible Attention Deficit Disorder. She has been "depressed" since the death of her stepfather, an alcoholic with "rage outbursts," two years ago. She is a talented artist and good

Clarification

student—perfectionistic, according to the therapist. There was a bullying incident three years ago and—reading between the lines—issues with lateness and truanting ever since. Her mother works at home giving art lessons and providing day care.

At direct examination Samantha is composed, placid, opaque, deferring to her mother, complaining of difficulties concentrating and following through.

I suggest the basic issue is not "depression" but "hidden fears" and recommend she work on abandonment and entanglement issues with her therapist. Thereafter she continues with her therapist, and with me for medication management. She drives herself to her appointments and elects not to include her mother by taking advantage of my emancipation escape clause.

Over the course of twenty visits, unaccompanied by her mother, we tinker with various psychotropics including a trial of Adderall, without any sustained benefit. A pattern of partial school avoidance becomes apparent. When I inquire, she fluctuates between denial and global admissions of anxiety. Either she is blasé and bland—"Things are going good at school"—or "I worry about everything." When I suggest her avoidance behavior hints of success or rejection fears, she minimizes, attributing the problem to "feeling tired" or "lack of energy."

As graduation draws near, however, she more consistently reports anxiety. Another contributing factor may be her mother taking full-time employment out of the house. The first clear-cut signs of peer entanglement appear: "I feel I have too many friends … I feel bad if I don't hang out." Later she is quite bitter about not being invited to a prom party arranged by a friend. "I've done a lot of crying … I've wasted my high school on other people." Again I identify the issue as one of entanglement and suggest she discuss it with her therapist.

On the positive side she reviews her plan to find a summer job and enroll in a community college.

The next visit she at first denies anxiety: "I try to forget about it." She then proudly announces she is resisting the critical comments of her ungrateful "best friend." I congratulate her on improved boundaries.

This turns out to be her last visit.

Managing Samantha was wandering in a swirling fog: one meeting providing glimpses of her emotional landscape, the next obscured by mist. Had her mother been present, the collateral data from their spoken and unspoken interaction might have been sufficient to erode Samantha's denial and promote clarification. However, when Samantha took advantage of the emancipation option to come alone, I greeted this as welcome evidence of developing maturation and attachment. Perhaps it was in some respects.

Nonetheless, only after a year's work did the issues with peer relationships, obvious from the beginning, frankly emerge. I can only guess what sustained her denial so long, but after I strongly reinforce her assertive behavior, her dropping out provides a clue. It suggests that she played Cinderella to her (ugly stepsister) peer group: a scapegoat for their putdown gossip, counseling them when forlorn over boys, sharing her homework, things of that sort. Moreover, she had to risk their jealousy if she were too proficient academically or musically. But if she were too forthright with them she also risked rejection. On the other hand, if she were too frank with her therapist or me, she would be in danger of feeling pushed into some type of confrontation. Her "solution" when things got too hot was to avoid and minimize, at school via irregular attendance, at my office by bland denial.

In retrospect it is clear I made a mistake with my frank recognition of her assertiveness. I forgot to practice my usual shtick of qualified approval (chapter 10). I think that, in the midst of my hunger for progress, I forgot that Samantha was still an adolescent.

Denial Masquerading as Resistiveness

I do not recall the information provided by Mr. Resistive after Dr. Searles's capitulation, probably because I was so charmed by his performance that I stopped paying attention to the ensuing proceedings. Mr. Resistive's defenses collapsed once Dr. Searles acknowledged his power. Since all defensive maneuvers are variations of denial, we can ask what type of denial invigorates resistiveness.

In my experience it has something to do with pessimism about the possibility of a relationship devoid of exploitation and loss. Resistive youngsters view others through a prism of cynicism and distrust: *relationships are manipulative, entangling affairs with but one outcome—I lose.* They don't deny the pain of loss; they deny it can ever be rectified. My hunch is that when Mr. Resistive encountered Dr. Searles's one-human-to-another posture, it ignited an explosion of hope. *Things can be different; the future is not written.*

It is important not to mistake adolescent resistiveness to engagement—not uncommon in this age group—with inattentiveness. Resistive clients are quite alert, even hypervigilant, because of their concerns that any form of cooperation, even responding to a greeting, will again expose them to manipulation. Recall that in the face of Dr. Searles's capitulation, Mr. Resistive's silent impassiveness would not have collapsed so abruptly had he been distracted or daydreaming or hallucinating.

Denial Masquerading as Provocativeness

In chapter 4 and elsewhere I discussed acting-out behavior as a technique by the client to manage Attachment Ambivalence, as a way to get close but not too close. This behavior is used to construct a boundary and protect against entanglement.

Thus management consists of teaching youngsters to construct boundaries with words, not behavior.

Provocativeness is watered-down acting-out. In contrast to Jackie (chapter 4), whose acting-out transfixed an entire psychiatric community, provocative behavior is more limited, tending to be confined to a particular setting: at home, in therapy, at school, or with a peer group. Hostile, snotty, cutting, defiant language is used—usually without conscious intent since, after all, we are dealing with a defense here—to keep the other off balance, irritated, disgusted, at a distance. However, if you ask younger children if they get a kick out of irritating their parents or teachers, often as not the response is a guilty smile, which confirms the presence of an attachment issue. Older youngsters, however, tend to confess they have no idea why they say such things; they may even express guilt and seek forgiveness. And not everyone is a target. Some relationships are seen as safe, others less so.

Since the difference between the two denial techniques is only one of degree, not substance, the same principles of understanding and management apply. Which is to say, teachers and sponsors need to:

- Avoid the notion of Oppositional Defiant Disorder (ODD)
- Remain aware of the fear of loss behind the behavior
- Teach youngsters to use words rather than behavior to negotiate boundaries

With respect to the first item, I will inveigh once more against this pernicious label that, in my experience, is utterly destructive when it comes to understanding adolescent academic and social difficulties. Earlier I termed it the "empty calorie diagnosis." I apologize for this unwarranted calumny since calories do have some nutritional value. I should have labeled it the "cotton candy diagnosis": looks good, smells

Clarification

good, tastes good—no substance whatsoever.

Let me put it this way. Most studies of the factors contributing to adolescent academic achievement cite teacher training and parental involvement as the most important. That's right: quality of teachers and quantity of sponsors. Therefore every parent, every sponsor, every teacher, every psychiatrist should begin the day with a "Pledge of Attachment Awareness" to banish the brain fog that the ODD label elicits in the unwary. And the pledge should be repeated every time the label is encountered. In the life of an adolescent, secure attachment equals success and achievement and (hopefully) satisfaction. The role of adult authority is to "fund" attachment.

Now, this may appear to contradict what seems so true of today's adolescents: peer authority is what counts, not adult authority. Where does the latter fit in if, as I will discuss later in volume 2, the ruling emotion among today's adolescents is anxious ruminations about peer-group acceptance?

Well, if adult supervision were so oppressive, we might conclude that adolescents would welcome teachers' strikes. In fact, they do ... for a day or two. Then they become discontented without the structure and security that the routine of school life provides. Plus school is where the drama is, where their buddies are. Otherwise life is pallid, pale, and aimless. Schools guard their exits not to keep students in but to keep dropouts and truants from other schools out.

True, kids en masse might test the limits of adult surveillance because the very presence of a limit provokes the energy and feelings of security to challenge it. But if adults demonstrate reliable and predictable leadership, the testing is evanescent and occasional. Most youngsters accept the boundaries that their testing at some level is intended to elicit. They desire the security of rules; testing helps define what they are. Boundaries morph and constrain adolescent anxiety into a creative force.

But consistently provocative behavior signals shaky attachments and the presence of an anxiety that separates and divides.

The peer group is not safe. Safety resides not in the group but in isolation. To be connected is dangerous because it risks further loss and abandonment. Therefore, while you take note of whatever provocative or defiant behaviors might be apparent, your mind must avoid the cotton candy diagnostic dead end. You must think *attachment, attachment, attachment*! You must think *this youngster is using words and behavior to keep people at a distance.*

Fortunately, provocative kids are generally easier to engage than resistive ones. You, the audience, offer them a risk-free chance to declaim, beef, complain, blame, and bully.

It is important to remain aware that such provocativeness is *always* fueled by hidden worries. They wish to remain attached but untangled. Hence deploying a certain amount of stagecraft—manipulation—will keep them engaged without frightening or provoking them. Since such kids tolerate a direct question well—it gives them the chance to remain on their soapbox—there are two I like to ask, carefully formulated as inquiries, not accusations. (Again, this is where having a parent or sponsor in the room is very helpful because you can demonstrate how to manage a dialogue without attacking or collapsing.)

One is "Does it ever make you feel in charge when you upset Mom (Dad, Teacher)?" Even the youngest of children, if they don't respond verbally, will nod with a guilty smile. This sets the stage for the follow-up: "Do you every worry about Mom?" Usually the response is a more vigorous nod. Much more often than not, parents express amazement that their recalcitrant child worries about them.

But a few parents, unfortunately, refuse to accept the notion. This suggests a less favorable prognosis, one sign of which is when the sponsor yanks the child out of treatment just when it seems to become effective. It signifies that the parents have attachment issues of their own, that they cannot face the loss that is an inevitable part of their youngsters' growing up. This sets the stage for an enduring angry-parent/provocative-child entangled relationship that has the potential to endure for years, even into adulthood. As adults, usually daughters, they describe an endless series of intensely frustrating, reciprocal angry rejections and reconciliations with their aging mothers. Such patients are usually described as hostile-dependent, which is a very superficial assessment, about as enlightening as ODD, the likely diagnosis of their childhood. For counseling to be helpful, therapists must promote clarification to enable their clients to recognize the separation and abandonment fears that nourish the anger of both parties.

In volume 2, I will examine the dynamism of the security/authority dyad from the opposite point of view when I discuss William Golding's influential but pessimistic parable of youth *Lord of the Flies*.[4] As he sees it, adolescents—and by extension, society—when offered an opportunity to choose between tyrannical versus democratic authority, prefer the former and inevitably revert to savagery. As I will argue, however, there is no need to be pessimistic about today's adolescents as long as we provide them with unflagging leadership.

Promoting Insight

The other goal of clarification is promoting the development of *insight*. In contrast to some public awareness of the notion of denial, the idea of uninsightfulness rarely crashes the headlines except perhaps in the form of entertaining media accounts featuring "dumb crooks" or in accounts of particularly brutal or cold-blooded crimes where you might find reference to the perpetrator's "lack of empathy." Otherwise it is safe to say that the idea of an impoverished emotional life posing a burden or threat to anyone escapes popular concern. However, psychiatrist and psychologists find that lack of insight is a familiar therapeutic roadblock. In extreme form we call it *alexithymia:* a state of *no-words-for-feelings.*

The paradox is that we now live in a tell-all society where personalities, both eminent and obscure, compete to overwhelm us in numbing detail with intimate accounts of their experiences. We are so far removed from the late 1950s—when the novelty of Oscar Levant confiding his manic-depressive/alcoholic escapades to Jack Paar transfixed a national audience—that in some respects I find it odd to put in a word or two about the need for clients to establish greater clarity of felt emotions. Yet when it comes to attachment issues, this is exactly what is required.

Why?

Because as denial softens, feeling states that have been dissociated begin to surface. But their shape is typically vague, amorphous, fleeting, unlikely to be crisp and exact, particularly with adolescents. Adults are generally more adept at giving form to their concerns because a natural part of maturation is, regretfully, to relinquish pretending; to be older is to recognize that not all endings are happy. But as kids try to come to terms with their inner world, we are more likely to hear statements such as "I feel funny … things aren't right … weird feelings come over me … stress … I'm depressed … thoughts run through my mind …I think about death." And even here, such complaints are less likely to be spontaneous, more likely needing prompting to be elicited.

This does not mean that on average youngsters with attachment issues are alexithymic. The issue is not a lack of feeling or empathy but rather, too much: suffering, and suffering so intense it has to be denied and buried, which creates disability. It is when disability can no longer be ignored that youngsters come in or are brought in to your office. As denial defenses—hopefully—erode, the misery and pain that emerge will frequently be too intense to bear to openly reveal pell-mell, which means a good deal of patience will be required as their story emerges in bits and pieces. Recall it took Samantha, discussed earlier in this chapter, a year. And what comes forth is now precise, then vague, here detailed, there opaque because it is the job of denial to protect from insights that are too painful to accept. Kids and young adults will need help to grapple with pain and suffering that no longer can be ignored.

What insights are likely to help adolescents (and their parents and sponsors) the most? Three of the most important are:

- Distinguishing "depression" from anxiety
- Distinguishing death preoccupation from suicidal intent
- Identifying the fears that lurk behind anger

The First Consideration: Is It "Depression" or Anxiety?

Earlier I spent some time proposing an understanding of the terms "anxiety" and "depression" derived from my years of work with adults and youngsters. Consequently I approach this question with the assumption that most "depression" is a manifestation of separation anxiety, loss, and attachment trauma *until proven otherwise.*

This requires that I begin by accepting statements at face value. For the record, I conscientiously chart verbatim complaints such as "depression" or "stress" but make a mental note to return to such statements, either then or later, to inquire about their referents. The idea is to determine if possible the particular behaviors or feeling states or events to which the words refer. Further, I might even prompt some patients not to use the word "depression." I ask them instead, "Tell me more about what your 'depression' is like without using the word." I explain that much of treatment is "like a landscape emerging from a fog, but here the fog is in your mind and the landscape is the details of your life."

Denial yields to clarification but resists tenaciously. Thus an investigative attitude must invigorate every contact and extend throughout treatment even in those infrequent situations where it is clear that the "depression" refers to a bona fide Endogenous

Depression. Recall Rose (chapter 9), who, in the midst of years of struggling to survive an unquestionable Bipolar Disorder, once again called for an emergency appointment, mired in an enervating "depressive" experience of sudden and apparently mysterious onset. But when prompted to investigate the matter further, in her next visit she returned to report that not only had she experienced abandonment, but she clearly realized it was only the latest of a series dating to her childhood. After ten years of management, finally clarification.

The Second Consideration: Is It Death Rumination or Suicidal Intent?

Perhaps a half dozen times a year I am referred youngsters whose behavior reflects a preoccupation with death. Generally the referrals come from therapists or school officials whose motivation is, understandably, purely a playing-it-safe legal strategy. But occasionally I detect a certain confusion about the significance of the behavior: does it represent suicidal intent or not? And if the referral comes from a youngster's parents, there is no confusion; their anxiety is palpable.

Preoccupation with loss and death is an essential feature of high school life in fact and fiction.

In *Staggerford,* Jon Hassler's touching account of small-town life, we encounter Staggerford High School teacher Miles Pruitt, now in his twelfth year of teaching senior English, as he wearily contemplates corralling the energies and attentions of his students. He then skips faculty lunch to lounge outside in the bleachers, refreshed by the delights of a fine fall day. Then he conscientiously takes up the task of grading 114 essays on the topic *"What I wish."*

> Losing. That was the melancholy strain running through dozens of papers every year. Parents lost in death and divorce, fingers lost in corn pickers, innocence lost

behind barns and in back seats, brothers and uncles lost in Vietnam, friends lost in drug-induced hallucinations, and football games lost to Owl Brook and Berrington.[5]

To this list of fictional deaths and disasters let me add the two youngsters, discussed in vignettes herein, killed by trains and diving accidents, plus others reported by my patients: a girl run over by a truck, suicides by hanging or overdose, parents and relatives and friends killed by the police or gangs, friends killed in accidents or dead from cancer. Add parents and relatives or siblings with serious disability—think of Maddie (chapter 10), the girl with an entangled heart whose foster sister was severely disabled and foster father unemployed because of health issues—or aging and increasingly enfeebled grandparents. And consider this is just their direct experience and doesn't include media accounts of local or national or international disasters, current or looming. Or school shootings. To which we must add climate change.

Is the adolescent use of drugs and alcohol any mystery?[ii]

Because adolescence is a transition from the relative security of childhood to the insecurities and excitements of adulthood, death comes into view even for those youngsters fortunate enough to have thus far escaped abuse and trauma.

Death, in Fact, Creates Meaning

To illustrate, consider a literary classic, *The Magic Mountain*, Thomas Mann's search for meaning in the wake of the catastrophe of World War I.[6]

---

ii. In volume 2 I will discuss David Riesman's notion that due to economic forces social conformity is now driven by anxiety rather than the shame and guilt that historically regulated social behavior. I conjecture that attempts to manage pervasive anxiety is a major cause of the recent explosion of adolescent and young adult substance use and substance overdoses, as well as an increasing rates of youthful suicide.

We first meet Mann's protagonist, Hans Castorp, as he travels to spend a few weeks with his favorite cousin, Joachim, who has retired to the Sanitarium Berghof in the Alps for treatment of tuberculosis. Castorp ends up staying seven years. We come to know him well for Mann gives us extended descriptions of the impressionable Hans—"life's delicate child"—especially his "inborn attraction to death."

Having experienced the loss of both parents by the age of six, he is taken in by his rather remarkable, even mesmerizing grandfather. And Hans finds inexplicable delight in endlessly inspecting an engraved silver christening bowl, a family heirloom stored in a locked glass case in his grandfather's office amid a litter of intriguing castoffs. As he listens yet again to the old man's stately recitation of the generations of Castorps christened with the bowl,

> Religious feeling mingled in his mind with thoughts of death and a sense of history, as he listened to the sombre syllable; he received therefrom an ineffable gratification—indeed, it may have been for the sake of hearing the sound that he so often begged to see the christening basin … a familiar feeling pervaded the child: a strange, dreamy, troubling sense: of change in the midst of duration, of time as both flowing and persisting, of recurrence in continuity—these were sensations he had felt before on the like occasion, and both expected and longed for again, whenever the heirloom was displayed.[7]

Young Hans is also fascinated by a full-length portrait of his grandfather, which to his mind's eye comes to represent the real appearance of the old man, since it presents him in the full formal garb of his former office as councilor and senator. And this is his last earthly appearance when Hans is called to view grandfather in death:

Thus he was glad from his heart that it should be the authentic, the perfect grandfather who lay there resplendent on that day when he came to take last leave of him ... lying in a silver-mounted coffin, upon a begarlanded bier... there he lay, with a stern yet satisfied expression, on his bed of state ... thus for the third time in so short a space and in such young years did death play upon the spirit and senses—but chiefly on the senses—of the lad ... in three or four months after his father's passing he had forgotten about death; but now he remembered, and all the impressions of that time recurred, precise, immediate, and piercing in their transcendent strangeness.[8]

Much later during his years-long sojourn at the Sanitarium Berghof, Hans, fatigued by talk and starved for solitude, skis high into the mountains where he becomes lost—perhaps deliberately—in a snowstorm. Intoxicated by fatigue, oxygen starvation, and wine, he falls into a trance in which he witnesses a succession of images: first joyful children at play, then an oppressive and menacing temple, finally two dreadful hags dismembering and devouring a baby. He struggles to escape, awakens with great relief, then tries to understand what he has experienced. Is it, he wonders, a dream of man's state as a courteous veneer of civilized behavior hiding blood sacrifices that must be consummated? *Or does it mean that life can only be understood in the context of death and disease?* "The recklessness of death is in life, it would not be life without it." He realizes he has acquired some understanding of his lifelong fascination with death, which, he vows, will no longer dominate his thoughts. True, death is a power that must be respected, but it is goodness and love of humanity that must have sovereignty over one's spirit, he concludes.

Elated, he bounds down the mountain back to his companions, no longer suffocated by the Berghof's "highly civilized atmosphere," thereafter possessed by his "dream of love."

The Magic Mountain ends when Castorp, increasingly dismayed by reports of the great struggle taking place in the flatlands, throws off the spell of high places and rushes off to cheerfully fling himself into the "desperate dance" of World War I trench warfare. As he vanishes into the turmoil of battle, Mann bids his "delicate child" good-bye with soaring affection but "without great concern" and offers him a blessing that the "dream of love" Hans Castorp once experienced when lost on the mountain will one day come to pass for all humanity.

A similar preoccupation with death appears in accounts of the lives of saints, mystics, prophets, and existentialist philosophers such as Kierkegaard and Camus.[iii] Of course, our average adolescent is not a Hans Castorp or existentialist philosopher, obsessed with death in the midst of life. On the other hand our average adolescent is observant and intelligent enough to become aware of and contemplate that life is not forever. In other words, thinking of death is not pathological. Rather it is part of our human condition, as Holden Caulfield finally realizes. To be alive is to live with risk of loss.

Death Preoccupations

Death preoccupations may represent a developmental stage, part of normal maturation, or something more ominous.

For example, Peggy, whose stormy adolescence is an admixture of both.

---

iii. In fact, Styron quotes from Camus's *The Myth of Sisyphus*: "There is but one truly serious philosophical problem, and that is suicide. Judging whether life is or is not worth living amounts to answering the fundamental question of philosophy."

[CASE STUDY]
Peggy: The Risks of Attachment

I first meet Peggy after psychological testing suggests "depression." When she could not promise her physician that she would stay safe, she was sent to the hospital via ambulance. She was placed on an Antidepressant, now is feeling calmer and less depressed. According to her mother, "I think she's really good now." She has started to see a therapist, Beth.

At direct examination she presents as a cautious, wary, cooperative girl who is somewhat inhibited by her mother's presence yet seems comfortable with her, soliciting her feedback. There is no evidence of Depressive signs or symptoms.

I make a diagnosis of an adjustment disorder and start to follow her for medication management combined with limited supportive therapy.

Over the following years she comes in for a few visits—never more than six, typically just two or three—then disappears, only to return months later for a few more. Several trials of Antidepressants are without sustained benefit. Interestingly, she is always accompanied by her grandmother, but asks that she not sit in because she doesn't want to involve her in her problems. I agree since Peggy is frank, forthright, and mature beyond her years. She continues to see her therapists regularly.

At age seventeen she reappears after another hiatus, reporting that a friend had been run over by a car while crossing a street listening to her earphones. Since then she had been troubled, "by thoughts that people I love might die." She has nightmares of drowning. Tearfully, "I try to make other people happy ... and then I'm stuck like this." And finally, "I would like my family to care."

We discuss—see principle 2, chapter 12—her need to accept problems such as these without blaming, either herself or others.

I assure her she is doing her very best to help the people in her life, a difficult task even for experts like myself.

Here's how the next visit goes:

> *Peggy: Reports more tragedy. The mother of the girl who was killed by a car had died of cancer:* "She didn't want to get help … knowing that she passed away, feel sad." *Moreover just last week she learned that a coach had died in his sleep. Gloomy:* "I just don't know how to deal with death well."
>
> *Dr. C, attempting to undermine her self-blaming:* "Who does? It is hard to ignore!"
>
> *Peggy:* "Right!"
>
> *Dr. C:* "How is school?"
>
> *Peggy (each of her worlds—home, school, dance line— has its problems):* "It never ends … stressful …"
>
> *Dr. C: Describes his experience with patients who fear death:* "The issue is not hell but being alone."
>
> *Peggy, choking up, crying:* "If something happened to me … would anyone care …. they never ask me … I'm always asking them …"
>
> *Dr. C: Discusses the need to accept the risk of love, that one has to weigh the pains of aloneness versus the pains of connectedness. Then adds:* "Your grandmother unquestionably loves you, she's always with you when you come here."
>
> *Peggy, collapsing into tears:* "If anything happened to her I would go into complete shock."
>
> *Dr. C:* "To think about death is human."
>
> *Peggy: Silence.*
>
> *Dr. C: Suggests it is natural to be troubled by the thought of something happening to a person so important to her.*
>
> *Peggy: Leaves visibly distressed. Later she reports she*

Clarification

is on the outs with her grandmother, but her mother is now more supportive.

She returns a year later at the request of her mother, gloomy, subdued, listless. "I need to come."

There have been many developments: her grandmother doesn't want to talk to her and she had a "huge argument" with her mother. But on the plus side, she's found part-time work, she will be graduating with a GPA of 3.0, she's been accepted at a private college, and she's seeing a school counselor as well as her longtime counselor, Beth.

She is close to tears, irritable, tense, tight, ventilating at length about her boyfriend, Bart: "Broke up with me ... alcohol ... he says that alcohol at least can make him happy ... I believe it ... I try to make him happy, not good enough ... booze comes first ... I feel sad all the time, not even worth my own time ... it's hard for me to focus on myself when I'm in love ... especially with an alcoholic." When I inquire she denies any death thoughts. Despite her complaints, she strikes me as improved.

She does not return for sixteen months, then calls for an appointment.

> *Dr. C, opening with my usual question after a long absence: "Tell me about your adventures."*
> *Peggy: Provides a serious, mature, blow-by-blow of a tumultuous interval. But now she is back on an Antidepressant, has reconnected with her therapist Beth. Bart is back in the picture. But her anger is more noticeable.* "I still get very emotional ... also, my anger, coming out more ... one day excited and confident, the next angry and upset ... Bart is the one I usually lash out at."
> *Dr. C:* "It sounds like you have fears of closeness."
> *Peggy agrees, but not only with Bart:* "Also with my friends ... I don't know why." *Silence, then expresses*

> *her ethic:* "There is something out there that is worth living for ... I was put here for a reason."
>
> *Dr. C: Respectfully agrees, then suggests she return in two weeks to work on verbal skills to manage intimacy without needing to create a boundary by lashing out.*

She returns two weeks later.

Peggy has broken up with Bart because of his lying. She has started a new job, third shift at a convenience store, plus she has just started server training at a restaurant.

> *Dr. C:* "It sounds like a lot of good things today to balance off the loss of your boyfriend."
>
> *Peggy ignores the comment at first, then:* "I don't feel tied down ... feel more stable with my job and family ... But I don't like the feeling of being lonely ..."
>
> *Dr. C: Silent.*
>
> *Peggy suddenly remarks. She's:* "talking to my grandmother again ... she didn't approve of Bart."
>
> *Dr. C: Silent, thinking, Good for you, grandmother.*
>
> *Peggy, wondering how to handle being alone:* "It's like I'm noncompassionate."
>
> *Dr. C: Silent.*
>
> *Peggy:* "Is it time to focus on my own needs?"
>
> *Dr. C:* "Yes."
>
> *Dr. C: Discusses her need for an inanimate project,* "to manage noncompassion feelings."
>
> *Peggy listens, finally remarks as we prepare to stop:* "I'm nervous about my grandmother ... she's eighty-three."
>
> *Dr. C: Clarifies that her task now is to find a balance between her need to fix people and her need to*

fix herself. Suggests she return in two weeks to discuss the issue.

But again she vanishes.

The Significance of Peggy's Behavior

As I prepared this summary, I wondered if her experiences were too complex to use as an illustration of the difference between death thoughts as a developmental stage versus as a harbinger of suicidal behavior.

One the other hand, this case illustrates the complex issues involved in assessing the significance of adolescent preoccupation with death. Any assessment of danger requires, at a minimum, the following database: a face-to-face interview, information from collaterals, and, if available, a review of medical, psychiatric, and counseling records. In order to determine whether or not hospitalization is indicated, many factors must be taken into consideration, the most important of which are *hopelessness, opportunity, intent, impulse control,* and *support*. Most important, if any of the above, either alone or in combination, suggests a crisis, my practice is to always refer to an emergency room, for two reasons: Emergency room personnel are more highly qualified than the average mental health practitioner, including me, to assess dangerousness simply because they see more of it. And a trip to the emergency room plus the waiting to be seen frequently defuses the situation because it mobilizes support.

With respect to Peggy, she first elicits concern at age fourteen when a mental health screening questionnaire scores positive for Depression. Her therapist alertly refers her to her physician. In that encounter I suspect she does reveal some of the components of authentic, potentially deadly self-destructive behavior. Fortunately she is not without support.

Hence when she refuses to contract for her safety, she is

hospitalized. A few weeks later she arrives in my office much improved, without any signs or thoughts of suicidal preoccupation. Her Antidepressant has kicked in and she is now the beneficiary of enhanced support from her mother and a therapist. So I decide to focus on the present and the future, while allocating to her therapist the detective work of clarifying her previously unendurable pain.

She demonstrated a good deal of maturity in refusing a safety contract. Safety contracts have dubious validity, in my opinion, especially when it comes to adolescents. Such a contract is a request to predict the future, a questionable matter under most circumstances, and particularly with troubled adolescents at greater risk of impulsive behavior than your average flighty youngster. Refusing to commit, as Peggy did, probably has more predictive value than an agreement to commit. I am always on guard to not request of youngsters more than they can provide. It is better to avoid safety contracts altogether in favor of safety arrangements that enhance social support.

Despite recurrent frustrations with immature boyfriends, nonetheless Peggy is not troubled by death thoughts again until age seventeen when a contemporary is killed by a train. She begins to recognize that relationships are contingent, that nothing is forever; she grieves and is sad, but not suicidal. Now aware of the risk of connectedness, she yet longs to be comforted and protected as she has tried to comfort and protect others. And she does not minimize the suffering that the sickness or death of her grandmother might precipitate: more evidence of her maturity. Thoughts of death have returned, but not as a "solution," theoretical or immanent. Such thinking is not pathological but rather reflects the tragedy of the human condition. It also reflects the ambiguity of intelligence, that insight and foresight are a mixed blessing. Later we will see that Peggy chooses to live with it despite the pain.

A year later she returns, now on the outs with her grandmother and her mother. While entangling tendencies have always been a background personality trait, now she is deeply enmeshed with Bart, a jerk who is impervious to her attempts to rescue him. Of course, it is all her fault, thus she is "depressed"; that is, blaming herself for something over which she has no control. But there are pluses. She is moving ahead academically, she continues to see her counselor, there are no death ruminations, and she is willing to try another Antidepressant. She improves, disappears again, this time for sixteen months.

There has been a lot of turmoil in the interim, no surprise since the jerky Bart is back in her life. Eventually she sloughs off Bart. It turns out her grandmother did not approve of him, which is why she stopped talking to her for a while. Again, she frankly expresses her worries about grandmother, who is now eighty-three.

Rather than "depression," she now finds herself prone to another emotion: anger. A troublesome development this, something new. Up to now others have been the angry figures in her life, she the supportive and nurturing one. More troubling yet is that the target of her "lashing out" is those close to her—friends and especially Bart, who floats in and out of her life. She resists the impulse to rescue him, which leaves her feeling lonely, "noncompassionate." Fortunately her years of therapy now bear fruit for she's quite insightful. She's quick to accept the notion that fear of closeness is what drives her anger, that therefore she needs to find a way to use words to protect herself without going on the attack. Also, she understands she needs to find a somewhat more impersonal outlet for her "compassionate" nature, one that avoids entanglement.

For now, therefore, we can conclude it seems that risk of suicide is less. And it appears she has a better grip on what at times makes her pain seem so hopeless: powerlessness in the face of suffering and death. It is clear she was entanglement prone when she entered adolescence. And most likely she is at greatest risk of suicidal behavior when a rescue mission fails, so to speak. I suspect she figured that somehow she could protect

Bart from his immaturity by becoming his guardian angel, of course a hopeless project as she eventually recognized.

More generally, this dynamic is at work in ping-pong adolescent suicides, a phenomenon totally mischaracterized in the media as "copy-cat" suicide. When teenagers suicide, either overtly or by incredibly reckless stunts—think of the forlorn *Saturday Night Fever* character, Bobby[iv]—among the peers left behind may be a few who had some awareness if not outright knowledge of the impending tragedy. Like Peggy, they are simultaneously angry and guilty, feeling betrayed and rejected. And to the extent that any had become entangled with the suicidee, say as a confidant or go-between, the failure to foresee or forestall the deadly behavior may provoke a sense of powerless too much to bear.

School officials must address this dynamic at convocations by firmly recognizing the limits of assistance. More importantly, school officials—and parents—must avoid invoking guilt as a motivation not to suicide. That is, they must not make an appeal to how bad people would feel were another child to commit suicide. To youngsters already overburdened by a sense of responsibility for the happiness of others, this is simply another crushing weight.

I have never been called on to preside at a convocation prompted by the suicide of a student, but in my role as psychiatric consultant I have on occasion served as an advisor at psychological autopsies convened because of the suicide of a clinic patient. Officially the function is designed to review the history and treatment of the suicidee to determine if signals were missed or if the treatment plan could have been more responsive—things of that sort. Unofficially, however, we are called together to offer support to the therapist because we know it can, and will, happen to everyone in this business.

---

iv. Only marginally accepted by his peers, he slips off a bridge girder and falls to his death while trying to impress them with a daring stunt.

I usually conclude the proceeding with a "prayer" that goes something like this:

> We must remember we are perched on a rock in the river of life, surrounded by souls drowning in its burdens, crying for help. So we reach out and try to pull some to safety. But we are never to reach with both hands, otherwise we will be pulled in. We must remember the adage of seaman from the days of sail. "One hand for the ship, one hand for yourself. You are no good to anyone if you go over the side." We try to do the best we can for our clients, but we must be realistic; some will go under no matter what. We must not let our guilt suck us in after them, or resign our perch. Learn from this experience, reaffirm your commitment, focus yourself because when this conference ends and you go to your offices, you will certainly again have to cope with a chorus of needy souls pleading for assistance. Our mission is not that of the lone hero or heroine. Be not afraid to ask for help.[v]

To close this chapter in her life, one can feel somewhat optimistic about Peggy. And she has returned to her trusted therapist, with whom, hopefully, she can sort out her guilt. Better yet, despite her fears of connectedness, she seems ready to test the support proffered by her parents. And even better, she accepts the love and regard of her dear grandmother, perhaps because she no longer shrinks from the knowledge that their days together are numbered. And it seems she is better able to resist the temptation to blame herself for feelings and emotions over which she has marginal control.

---

v. Because my private practice was solo, I had no colleagues to turn to in situations like this. However, for years I shared and referred patients with a therapist, Ken, who also served as a sounding board when I needed feedback.

In contrast to Peggy, who in the course of her struggles to recognize the dangers of entanglement remained firm in her belief that there was purpose in her life, let me present someone seriously contemplating Camus' "fundamental question" and Hamlet's "To be or not to be."

[CASE STUDY]
Lindsey: To Suicide or Not

She is a twenty-three-year-old law student referred by her therapist: "depression, anxiety … suicidal ideation … I think about self-harm and cutting a lot … but I don't cut." Recently she was started on low doses of Prozac and propranolol at a crisis center, and now needed follow-up. The latter is helpful: "Calms me down." She's had eight sessions to date with the therapist, reports good chemistry. Yet she still thinks about throwing herself off a freeway overpass.

Other problems include low energy, increased naps, reduced appetite, trouble concentrating, critical self-talk, and feeling hopeless about ever getting better. These have been present off and on since age sixteen, when she discovered she could not trust a beloved relative, more intense in the last six to eight months.

Her therapist's referral letter provides additional detail. Lindsey first contacted her therapist after a "relationship stressor" precipitated a bout of suicidal thoughts. She reported dependency feelings on others, particularly her boyfriend. She tended to ruminate about cutting or suicide, typically following incidents when she judged herself a failure, either socially or academically. Worse, she viewed such negative thinking as an indication that she was "bad" and that she was "using my mind to torture myself." After a recent painful incident, for which she blamed herself, she developed a plan to go to the overpass "with a lot of alcohol and jump." This scared her enough to consider starting the medications. Another problem was anxiety about her grades, feeling they would never be good enough despite considerable evidence to the contrary. She would use alcohol or marijuana to feel better. Finally, just one week previously she broke up with the boyfriend.

On the plus side, her therapist enumerated much strength, including a powerful commitment to continue therapy after the counseling center closed for the summer.

At direct examination she presents as a quiet, compliant, alert, focused, attentive, serious, intense, attractive, personable, intelligent young woman who has little to say unless prompted. She is just a bit resistive to engagement, so I maintain some distance by making the usual inquires. She reports a quite uneventful childhood, having been raised with her younger brother by her biological parents. She denies trauma, either witnessed or sustained, yet the therapist's letter says otherwise. There is no history of prior psychiatric contacts, although she did obtain some counseling in high school and again last year in college. She denies any history of euphoric episodes. (On the other hand, the letter states she was alarmed by what sounds like an overnight hypomanic episode after the crisis center evaluation, which made her hesitate starting the medications.) Finally, my routine inquiry about spiritual beliefs or practices prompts the unequivocal reply: "Pretty nonexistent."

I agree with prior diagnoses of Depression and Anxiety, concluding she is stable at that moment. I also note with starred emphasis, "Big Boundary Issues."

But I focus on the implications of hopelessness, that she is at significant risk of suicide because two of its four prerequisites of motivation (hopelessness) and opportunity (multiple freeway overpasses nearby) are present, while the third (intent) and fourth (support) are shaky. But I do not recommend hospitalization at present, I continue, because she has a "life issue" that a hospital cannot solve. Hospitals are for emergencies. Should she begin to feel she is losing control, that's the time to go to the hospital; don't even wait to talk to me. "Tell them to examine you, then call me. You'll probably be feeling better by the time you get there anyhow."

Then I continue, just a bit didactically to maintain some distance. Her history and her preoccupation with cutting and rumination about suicide strongly suggest that her "life issue" is an intense conflict about relationships, "a boundary problem … sort of a confusion about whose needs are primary." Her inability to discover an immediate solution is stirring up anxiety. This anxiety is binding her down, her productivity is dropping along with her self-esteem, she's blaming herself—"depression"—and feeling hopeless because she can't find an answer, and she's used to finding answers. Now's the time to be patient and sort things out with therapy and medications.

I conclude by suggesting she continue her medications, continue to see her therapist, then return in two weeks. I give her a copy of my notes to present to her therapist if she wishes.

Two weeks later:

Dr. C: Medication?
Lindsey: "Not much … no side effects, no benefits … I feel about the same."
Dr. C: Wonders what's been happening.
Lindsey: Reports she is medication compliant, using the propranolol as needed: "calms me down right away." She continues to see her therapist. She continues to feel "sluggish … lack of motivation … negative self-talk … thinking about self-harm, but not suicide." She still feels anxious.
Dr. C: Silent.
Lindsey: Silent, then: "I wonder if it is hopelessness …"
Dr. C: "Are things getting better?"
Lindsey: Silent, reflects, then the ambiguous reply: "I would say I'm agnostic …"

> *Dr. C: Not sure what to make of this, agnostic about belief? About improvement? So decides to make a more structured inquiry, wonders about the idea of boundary issues.*
>
> *Lindsey:* "It really fits ... I just read a book on codependency, really fits ..." *Then suddenly, spontaneously confesses that she is a perfectionist.*
>
> *Dr. C: Concludes things are about the same, that the situation is stable, that she increase the Prozac a bit while continuing the propranolol. Then another somewhat didactic discussion of how "what if" thoughts drive perfectionism. Then recommends she look into a Behavior Therapy technique known as Exposure/Response Prevention (E/RP).*[vi]

I explain that the idea is for her to practice "antiperfectionism" to counter her hidden belief that she can control life, prevent disaster, banish the pain of life by "being perfect." I suggest she return in a month.

Two weeks later:

> *Dr. C: ??? Makes an inquiring gesture.*
>
> *Lindsey:* "In the last week ... more suicidal than ever ... the worst was Wednesday (five days ago)," but things have been "fine" the last four days since discontinuing the Prozac."
>
> *Dr. C: Refers to the calendar, wonders if the recent increase in the Prozac could be a factor.*
>
> *Lindsey: Ignores me, instead remarks she has not taken any propranolol recently, no need to because she feels "calmed down."*
>
> *Dr. C: Silent, observing she is somewhat minimizing.*
>
> *Lindsey, continuing: School is over, therefore no counsel-*

---

vi. Discussed at greater length later in chapter 13 on the third principle: Focus on What Can Be Changed.

ing for now, but she does have an appointment ten days hence with another therapist, DC. Also, she will be starting work thirty hours per week as a personal care attendant. Then volunteers that the outburst of suicidal feelings was different from usual: not late at night when she was alone before sleep, but in the middle of the day when she was not alone.

Dr. C: Notes this is a very significant observation, but decides to postpone discussion of it until later in the interview. Instead wonders what she thinks of my previous comments that her perfectionism is, in effect, an attempt to deny that suffering is an inevitable part of life for which no one is to be blamed.

Lindsey: Disagrees. "If there is pain, someone is at fault!"

Dr. C: Disagrees. "To be human is to experience pain!"

Lindsey: Disagrees. If she causes pain, it is her fault and she deserves to be punished, and suicide is her punishment!

Dr. C: Disagrees. "Anyone with half a brain thinks about suicide now and then, and you have more than half a brain. Sooner or later everyone wonders if life is worth living."

Lindsey: Silent, tight lipped.

Dr. C: Tense silence. Finally: "My goodness, you are a stubborn one."

Lindsey: Still silent, then a burst of laughter: "You are right!"

Both: Enjoy a good laugh, tension relieved and Lindsey much less resistive.

Thereafter we wrap things up. I tell her it is very likely the Prozac caused the abrupt return of her suicidal thinking—a rare event, but I've had at least two other similar cases. So she should avoid Antidepressants from now on but continue the

Clarification

propranolol as needed. For now she should follow up with the new counselor and return to see me as needed.

Two weeks later she fails an appointment. I have had no word of or from her in the five years since.

Did she kill herself? If she had, I would have heard about it. Saint Paul is, after all, a largish small town. A death by a fall from an overpass is always reported in the media, and suicide is always considered. The medical examiner routinely inquires about signs of suicidal intent from family, friends, and physicians. So Lindsey is still out there dealing with life's pain.

You may also wonder why my comment about her stubbornness made such a difference. I think I was responding to her power, a discussion of which leads off chapter 10. She felt validated and lowered her guard.

In truth there was no reason to return to me. She had a therapist lined up and a new job to engage her that suited her personality by giving her the opportunity to provide to others the care and comfort that were lacking in her childhood. Hopefully she will experience some healing of her attachment issues without becoming too entangled, as well some relief from her tendency to be so self-critical. Moreover, I suspect that the sudden collapse of her resistiveness at the third meeting in retrospect was somewhat disturbing, stirring up conflicts of becoming dependent, which is why I left things open ended as we finished our session. And she has a lot to think about, in fact a lifetime's worth, because the meaning of suffering-amid-existence is never really settled. But she is in a good place to start on that journey.[vii]

In short, while suicidal thinking may be a sign of emotional disability, it may also be a sign of mental awareness—certainly true here. There is no question that the anxiety associated with

---

vii. Consider that it took some twenty years for me to completely come to grips with Dr. Kolb's conjecture, and I still test it on patients. Also, as our professors would remark, no valid interpretation is ever wasted. It penetrates whether we realize it or not.

her boundary conflicts induced a progressive paralysis; hence treatment with psychotropics was indicated. A much more critical issue, however, was her growing awareness that no relationship is conflict free, that a clash of needs is inevitable even between two loving individuals. This undermined her perfectionist belief that suffering could be controlled if she did things "just right." In other words, to live is to suffer—probably Camus' point—and suffering would always be her "fault"; thus her suicidal ruminations and planning.

The Third Consideration: Is It Anger or Fear?

By now I hope the idea of *anger-masking-hidden-fears* is a firmly embedded concept. Now I would like to reverse the polarity here and present the opposite notion: *fear-masking-hidden-anger.*

Anger and fear, apparently polar opposites, actually are different manifestations of one underling dynamic: concerns about separation and loss. Another way to conceptualize the dynamism is to think of it as the energies associated with unmet needs. We fear to assert our needs because we anticipate, based on our experiences, retaliation in the form of punishment or abandonment, perhaps both. So we inhibit our assertiveness and seethe at the injustice of it all. Thus when anger is apparent, as I have learned, look for the underlying fear and vice versa, where fearfulness dominates the picture, think of hidden anger. Come to think of it, this dynamism is an obvious corollary of Dr. Kolb's dictum that all anxiety is related to the prospect of separation.

For example, recall that Lindsey reports much anxiety but little if any anger. If we are to follow Dr. Kolb's dictum and its corollary, her anxiety is a signal of pressing separation and abandonment concerns due to her unmet needs for comfort and protection, which she despises because they make her feel weak and vulnerable. She turns to substances and doing so only incites more self-loathing. Hence the anger associated with her anxiety is deflected inward, which elicits the belief that she deserves punishment. Why can't she be happy and satisfied? But to attend to and assert her unmet needs is too dangerous because this risks the retaliation and punishment she sees as an inevitable part of life. Thus she panics when the energy associated with her unmet needs begins to worm its way into consciousness. Her tentative solution—suicide—is so alarming that she is forced to seek help.

My insistence that pain is part of life and no one's fault releases some of her anger in the form of her stubborn denial. My recognizing her stubbornness, which she knows to be true, validates her anger by communicating that I am not offended by it. If pain is part of being human, so is anger—and stubbornness. Hopefully this will set the stage for further exploration of these issues with her therapist.

In short, the above dichotomy is only apparent: it's both. I have found that patients more easily accept the notion of a duality when their anger is foremost. Generally, their lurking fears of separation and abandonment are not that hidden. But working with fearful and timid souls is a different matter. Their denial is tenacious, yet their anger and its perceived dangerousness must be addressed. Generally I go about this by wondering about their life experiences with anger, whether witnessed or experienced. Was their childhood one of an angry, vengeful parent? Or a household of a terrifying parental cold-shoulder rejection to temper tantrums? In time I lead up to the interpretation "In other words, in your experience, anger kills … either you or someone else is destroyed?" Occasionally what then emerges is the memory of a nurturing figure clutching her chest while gasping, "Oh, you'll be the death of me!" A few patients, on the other hand, will just drop out of treatment. Most continue to deny and change the subject. So I postpone further discussion of the issue until later.

We need to begin our management of attachment-disabled youngsters and adults by focusing on clarification of their issues. Otherwise they are at risk of developing an additional, more pernicious disability: self-blame for feelings and behaviors they are unable to change or control. The self-blame tends to isolate them, leading them to ignore or reject otherwise supportive life interventions. As therapists, parents, and sponsors, it is vital that we also practice clarification; that is, recognizing as we attempt to assist these unhappy sufferers what we too are unable to change or control today. As they and we benefit from clarification, we all also need to learn and practice *acceptance*. This I will discuss in the next chapter.

12

The Second Management Principle: Acceptance

To survive the pain of trauma we need to learn to accept the pain without blame.

Recall that the three principles of management are not sequential. Management is a struggle, a knotted, looping, arduous search of a maze that, hopefully, will clarify the difference between: 1) the trauma that precipitated the Attachment Disability with its injured trust and 2) the cognitive consequences of the disability: that is, the disability about the disability. As denial melts and insight flourishes, it is important to accept the trauma without blame. In other words, as adolescents and adults learn to clarify and identify their attachment problems—"owning the pain" in therapist-speak—it is critical they also learn "no blame for the pain." That is, they need support and encouragement to accept the lost trust without searching for an agent to blame for the loss. The "what" of the loss is important, not the "why."

Forgive? Or Forget?

In a sense, *acceptance* addresses the venerable but dubious saying "Forgive and forget." In my view, however, it should be "Forgive but *never* forget." Even if we succeed in both forgiving and "forgetting" the loss, even if we somehow are able to massage our consciousness into a state of amnesia, the trauma of the loss and its potential for disability remain embedded in our neurons. Consequently, when circumstances either in fact or in symbol later signal a potential for separation and loss, we cannot resort to previously learned adaptive strategies. In short, there is no "bag of tricks" to fall back on. We again are more or less helpless. This is when the temptation to blame emerges.

To be sure, blaming has a certain survival function. If projected, it creates meaning in a world that otherwise would appear meaningless. And it permeates our society. Look again at this morning's headlines; you will rarely find a problem without a search for a villain to blame. This is what makes blaming so seductive. It allows us—society—to shift and evade responsibility, to project it onto an external agent. It promotes inertia, which is why it takes a crisis to alter society's trajectory—and not always then.

We live in a culture of blame. In the West, whenever human affairs involve an unhappy ending, we look for someone or something to blame. Contrast this to other cultures, where tragic outcomes are "fate" or the "will of Allah." But with us the trend is to shift responsibility for the consequences of our behavior to someone or something else. In my years as a psychiatrist I have seen the concept of free-floating anxiety disappear from popular culture, to be replaced by "depression" as the "explanation" of personal problems. "Depression," no matter how painful, is easier to "own" than anxiety because we are told that "depression" is a *disease* and therefore not under our control. But anxiety ... a different story. Who do we blame but ourselves for what appears to be a moral defect, a lack of willpower?

Children, adolescents, and adults with attachment issues are particularly burdened by blaming. Their lives have been scarred by lost or abusive relationships, frequently both. Moreover, children are especially vulnerable to interjecting blame when it comes to dealing with the loss of a loving figure. The only way they can comprehend a world in which such a meaningful and powerful entity can completely vanish is to conclude it must have been their fault. So they cling tenaciously to their blame. Even Peggy, despite possessing a maturity beyond her years, tells me she would go into "complete shock" were something to happen to her grandmother. What must it feel like for a child?

Whether introjected or projected, blaming is destructive. We transfer power to an external agent. Our power to change and our power to replace what has been lost are diminished and distorted. We—children, adults, society—are tempted to wait for forgiveness or rescue or punishment. Or we go out of control.

Even in the absence of a lost relationship, youngsters who have been abused or exploited are still especially vulnerable to self-blame because, inevitably, the perpetrator blames them for the abuse. Thus they are double victimized: both by the trauma and, arguably what is worse, the responsibility for it.

Acceptance

Opposed to blaming is the notion of *acceptance*. A stance of acceptance focuses on *what is*, not *why what is* or *what should be*. It seeks facts, not explanations or solutions. Not that the latter are inappropriate inquiries; it's just that inquiry without a solid grip on *what is* slithers into speculation or fantasy. The scholastic philosophers defined truth as *the mind conformed to reality*—they distinguished between the facts and what you make of the facts. To the extent that your thinking conforms to the facts, and only to the facts, to that extent you possess the truth. Facts are "out there"; truth is in your head. Which makes fact prior to truth. And one of the most important of all facts for all of us is the fact of separation and loss.

We must not conclude, however, that we are somehow diminished or enfeebled by grabbing the pain of loss by its throat and holding on. To the contrary, a realistic awareness of loss, real or symbolic, impending or distant, unlocks our creative potentials because to accept *what can't be replaced* means to recognize *what can be.* This is what is meant by the old saying "The truth shall set you free." We recognize what can be changed, and that is where we concentrate our efforts. So the mantra for us and our adolescents is *accept the pain—no blame for the pain.*

Acceptance Includes Learning to Describe

In a sense blaming comes naturally because we humans are profoundly moral creatures. From the instance of birth we register both experience and its significance to our well-being. No experience is processed free of an implication for its survival significance. Human morality begins as the infant nervous system assigns survival value to the stimulus situations it encounters. By the second year of life, toddlers display a powerful capacity for a primitive but urgent labeling of life's options; that is, what is "good" or "bad" for them. If the latter, parents will surely encounter the nightmare that haunts the early years of child care: a screaming eighteen-month-old shouting, "*NOOO!!*" The task of teaching and parenting is to transmute this energy into an adaptive, resourceful, motivated, considerate, productive human being who takes into account the rights and needs of others when evaluating the goodness and badness—a moral keenness—of its actions.

Attachment-disordered adolescents bring to school the same moral keenness. Unfortunately, they do not bring with them a modulated, balanced moral sense. It tends to be harsh and punitive and judgmental, no doubt a reflection of their nurturing or lack thereof. Their moral filter is crude and extreme, especially when it comes to how they feel and think. Thoughts, feelings, and emotions are never experienced as such, in isolation. Instead they are experienced with a moral valence that is colored by an overpowering sense of someone being at fault.

Latent Self-Blaming Drives Adolescent Cutting and Self-Mutilation

Such behaviors, in my experience, are always—always!—a signal of a harsh and vindictive self-critical inner voice that the mutilation is designed to relieve. These suffering children, if they should come to your attention, are deceptive because of their blandness. While the mutilation may seem—and on occasion may very well be—a cry for attention, its greater significance is the extremely entangled personality structure beneath the placid Alfred E. Neuman benevolent smile. These youngsters are guilt-frozen.

They are especially challenged by their sensitivity to others' unhappiness. They come to perceive life as an endless procession of suffering souls needing rescue. They are the "catchers in the rye" to the whole world of unhappy or demanding parents, relatives, and, particularly, peers.

The sight or prospect of a sad or lonely or disappointed expression on a parent's or chum's face is unbearable pain to them. They are highly motivated to assume the problem-solver/peacemaker role within the family and between peers. Their role is that of "good" student, "good" child. Not infrequently they become quite adept in this role, which brings satisfaction and smiles to their parents, highly reinforcing for the youngster because it meets their need to please and satisfy others. So the next unhappy face is even more likely to elicit enabling behavior. For example, recall Samantha, chapter 11.

But there is always more suffering than they can manage. Slowly but inevitably, life appears to yield a bitter slogan: *first you work hard, then you die.* Life becomes an endless chore of figuring how to make happy a constant parade of unhappy faces. We know, for example, that it is precisely from such concerns that so many youngsters with sexual identity issues deal with their problems by concealing them. These children correctly assess the unhappy responses that a frank revelation of their doubts and feelings would be likely to provoke, unhappiness that could only be relieved by them promising not to have such doubts and feelings.

Eventually life comes to mean being alone—you can't confide because it will make someone unhappy if you complain—or being a slave to the happiness of others. More guilt.

As these children battle their isolation or servitude, they reveal their suffering in anonymous notes left in public places, or sometimes in quite unambiguous essays in response to school assignments, or sometimes via the more ambiguous signal of self-mutilation.

Such youngsters are uniquely susceptible to the drama of high school life, and are at risk of becoming deeply responsible for the miseries of their peers, especially if they cannot rescue them. Peer deaths by suicide or misadventure can elicit echoing self-destructive behaviors. Such extreme sensitivity to the concerns of others complicates their management because it contaminates connections with their teachers, counselors, and therapists. Healthy and secure therapeutic boundaries are a must when you engage such adolescents. Their blank façade is, after all, a defense against allowing you, a stranger, a peek at their unhappiness. You might become concerned, and they don't need another soul worrying about them. So you get stiffed, pleasantly and discreetly to be sure, but stiffed nonetheless. It is important to respect the boundary and emulate Dr. Searles's perceptiveness.

Hence, when a youngster is referred to me for a medication evaluation, I always inquire whether there is a therapist and, if there is, how things are going. "How is the chemistry between you?" I ask. If it seems to be okay, I might just nod or, perhaps, make a vague recommendation that they consider working on what strikes me as an unexplored but relevant issue: entanglement or abandonment, for example. But sometimes I find things are not okay: "He asks too many questions" or "She gets too upset when I tell her how I feel, so I just keep quiet." When I hear this I always take pains to validate the report. I note that the discomforts accompanying any treatment process, whether the problem is physical or mental, are part of owning the problem. Then I clarify that trust is the solvent of effective therapy, and if the youngster and sponsors determine that trust is lacking, they need to consider obtaining a second opinion.

Occasionally the self-mutilation is concealed not by a façade of blandness but by one of acting-out. Yet the self-injurious behavior is always a tip-off: behind the furor lurks an entangled soul. Recall the situation with Maya (chapter 4), whose cutting was the first sign of her worries about her father's behavior. Would he survive his mania for extreme sport? Were something to happen to him, she was convinced it would somehow be her fault. Fortunately her perceptive mother was able to earn her trust and share her anxieties about his reckless behavior.

Promoting Acceptance

So, how do we manage self-blaming? The first step is to recognize it. Usually this is obvious; for example, Lara (chapter 13), a habitual apologizer for anything that did not turn out as expected, including lack of benefit from medications. But not infrequently the self-criticism is occult, its presence nonetheless revealed in statements accompanied by slight changes in posture (slumping), or tone of voice (lowered), or gaze (averted). And not infrequently when you make note of the changes and their possible significance, the response may be one of indignation or frustration, perhaps even outright denial. So it is important to gently explain your observations.

Our task, then, is to *rebalance* the inner life of such youngsters by teaching them how to describe their world without judging the experience. As I tell my patients, "You already are pretty good when it comes to opinions about the stuff of your life. Let's see now if you can learn to experience the 'stuff' without deciding whether it is good or bad." Not unexpectedly, since we are dealing here with an ingrained lifelong pattern of thought and speech, this is not immediately accomplished. I first model for patients an example of descriptive language and then use a Behavior Therapy technique of *repetitive prompts* and *redirection* to promote its acquisition.

The operant word here is "repetitive." By the time youngsters or young adults take their seat before you, you are confronted with individuals who have been crippled by years of judging the worthiness, the goodness or badness, of their inner world of thoughts and feelings. It will be difficult for them to learn how to be descriptive rather than judgmental, but ownership of that world is vital if they are to learn to focus on what can be changed, which is topic of the next chapter. Without ownership of the thoughts and feelings that otherwise would trigger self-blaming, it is unlikely that any change strategy will be effective. On the other hand, as ownership develops, a potential for change is created, the many aspects of which I discuss in the next chapter.

13

The Third Management Principle: Focus on What Can Be Changed

... and recognize what can't be changed ... today.

This principle is familiar to anyone who has been touched by AA and its Serenity Prayer. The gist of it is that change is difficult. In one sense, addiction issues are "easy" to address because both the disability and corresponding corrective techniques are clear cut: practice sobriety. What needs to be changed is apparent. The path to travel is also clear, albeit arduous.

Things are murkier when it comes to attachment and entanglement disability. This is why it is not unusual to encounter addicted adolescents who frankly and knowledgeably speak of their sobriety and its challenges; for example, Peggy (chapter 11). On the other hand you will probably rarely or never meet kids who talk of their struggles with attachment or entanglement issues as such. I can recall only one youngster who at her initial consultation referred to attachment problems, and then she was quoting her therapist. More commonly, what you will hear is attachment *consequences:* the anxieties, the frustrations, the "depressions," things of that sort.

This is why I recommend focusing on pieces of the problem—in particular the piece most likely to yield to intervention, what Dr. Schiele termed the "target symptom," or what I now think of as "target behavior." "Focus" is the relevant word here. I have encountered formal treatment plans that cite and attempt to address multiple problems simultaneously, on one occasion as many as thirteen. Rather than adapting such a scattershot approach, I find the odds of success are much improved by targeting the one issue that seems most susceptible to change and maintaining a steady aim. If I am fortunate and that problem starts to crumble, other problems have a way of dissolving as well.

Identifying susceptibility to change includes its inverse: identifying insusceptibility to change. Some adolescent problems are not immediately responsive to office-based management. More is required.

The Third Principle: Limits

Conduct Disorder

These youngsters manifest a pattern of repetitive behaviors such as running away, curfew violations, felonious assaults, burglary and car theft, lying, and dealing drugs. Such a pattern signals a youngster whose abandonment issues are so profound that he or she has given up on adult leadership. Conduct behaviors are frequently misidentified as "oppositional" or acting-out. In truth, the latter, no matter how irritating or frustrating, still represents a hidden desire to remain connected with adults—but at a "safe" distance. They can be managed in the office by a therapist or school counselor adept at recognizing and dealing with boundary issues.

But authentic conduct issues are different. They require much more than office management. They need the comprehensive, impersonal support and supervision provided by a treatment center or juvenile detention facility. *It is a serious mistake to think that schools can provide such support.*[i]

Unendurable Pain

This is an anguish both intense and—of much greater significance—without the prospect of relief. Whether besieged by the physical or the psychological, eventually sufferers become consumed by a progressive feeling of hopelessness. Death seems the only way to end the suffering, to obtain peace. To emphasize this point yet again: depression disables; hopelessness kills. This is why suicide so often comes as a surprise, out of the blue.[ii] And bystanders may remark that the suicidee didn't seem "depressed"; on the contrary, they sometimes appear unusually serene before death. Or, as was the case of the woman who stepped in front of a train (chapter 10), immersed in life's routine to the very end without a skipped beat.

---

i. I will discuss this issue at length in volume 2 of this series, the thrust of which is *prevention* of AD rather than its *understanding* and *managing*, the focus of this volume. One strategy I recommend to avoid provoking or aggravating abandonment issues is discarding the venerable but outmoded policy of mandated school attendance.

ii. For example, note the totally unexpected suicide of the outstanding psychiatrist, Dr. Robert A. Woodruff, Jr., one of the pioneering psychiatrists and psychologists who labored to promote the revision of *DSM-III*. He had marital problems, was under treatment for depression, yet "all his colleagues were shocked—no one had thought he was anywhere near such an action. He had not appeared to be brooding, had not been reclusive, and his intense involvement in the revision of the manual had not slackened." Decker, Hannah S. *The Making of DSM-III: a diagnostic manual's conquest of American psychiatry*. New York: Oxford University Press, 2013, 118.

On the other hand, hopelessness can appear as an essential component of an obvious Endogenous Depression. Recall Styron's description of a mental suffering so intense it takes on the guise of a physical malady, culminating in a "state of unrealistic hopelessness." Also, consider the case of profound recurrent melancholic misery described by Dr. Yager.[1]

In adolescence, a major contribution to hopelessness is that the pain is unspeakable; that is, cannot be shared. Subjects not to be spoken of commonly include incest, rape, betrayal, gender identity, bullying, and more. It is guilt that seals the lips; not only is there pain, but that pain is the sufferer's fault. Such adolescents are remote, preoccupied, unengaged, distracted, obviously in the grip of an inner voice. The crisis places them beyond the reach of management for the time being. What they need is ongoing support in the form of day treatment, perhaps even hospitalization.

The primary task of such support is not to exhume the circumstances that precipitated the pain—abuse or betrayal, for example—but to relieve the *guilt about the pain.* Relating to another the details of a violation is not necessarily therapeutic and in fact may be experienced as a second violation if the violated person feels coerced. Administrative or criminal investigations thus risk aggravating the trauma. The pain will always have its tender residuals; it is the blame for the pain that must be addressed to mitigate its deadly burden of guilt and looming hopelessness. Hopefully, such support will also revive sufficient trust to provide for later management.

There is a paradox here. In some adolescents, death ruminations can signify hope rather than hopelessness. Here *plan* and *opportunity* are present but intent is not. When confronted by the prospect of unending pain, these sufferers console themselves with thoughts such as *This does not have to go on forever. I can always end this. I am not helpless.* Correct management in such circumstances is to focus on reducing guilt while accepting and acknowledging the autonomy of the client; for example, as with Lindsey in chapter 11.

The Third Principle: Focus on Change

The following list of change options is by no means exhaustive. Neither is it exclusive in the sense that deploying one option precludes any other.

Medication

For those who wish a more extended, theoretical discussion of psychotropic medications, I recommend consulting one of the standard psychiatric texts. Here I will limit my discussion to Antidepressants and to two antihypertensive agents best known these days for treatment of Attention Deficit Disorder: the alpha-2 agonists clonidine (Catapres) and guanfacine (Intuniv, Tenex). I and others have found the latter also helpful in the management of trauma residuals.[2]

Both Antidepressants and the alpha-2 agonists offer rich possibilities for change. If such treatments relieve a selected symptom, especially one burdened with extensive disability, the result is frequently a cascade of improvements. Second, most "depression" that comes through my office is of the Reactive variety; that is, accompanied by significant stress and anxiety, not infrequently the unrecognized manifestations of trauma. Here both Antidepressants and alpha-2 agonists can be notably effective. Finally, if administered prudently and supervised closely, their toxic potential—as opposed to side effect potential—is low. In other words, both have a very favorable benefit/risk ratio.[iii]

---

iii. My experience with Endogenous Depression, on the other hand, agrees with the literature. Antidepressants are not especially helpful in such circumstances. More support

Here, however, I will focus on the issue of what happens after a medication is prescribed: does the patient actually comply with treatment?

It is estimated that patients comply with medical recommendations perhaps 50 percent of the time at best.[3] While studies have identified a host of reasons for noncompliance, in my experience two of the most important are *context* and *content*.

By "context" I mean the symbolic significance of a medication. "Content" refers to the description of its potential risks and benefits. I will discuss each factor separately, but in practice the two are not separable. The very idea of taking a medication activates a bias that filters my presentation of its potential effects. However, bias is part of all therapeutic procedures, whether medical or alternative. Whether the recommendation is, say, for surgery, medication, counseling, or mindfulness exercises, the information is not received by a mind devoid of prior experience. It is the evaluation of information according to experience that creates *placebo* and *nocebo* phenomena, both of which powerfully influence outcome, and which I discuss at greater length in an appendix to volume 2.

For example, many trauma victims fear the night for obvious reasons. Tornadoes can strike at night or destroy the power grids that illuminate the night. Alcoholic parents stumble home long after nightfall, primed for violence. Gang shootouts are more frequent at night as are assaults and rapes and murders. Sexual abuse, whether sustained or overheard, is more likely during the sleep hours. Or victims awaken to find that a relative or parent has expired overnight. Reckless peers and friends kill themselves in nighttime crashes. Ominous news always seems to arrive via midnight phone calls. Is it any wonder, therefore, that victims become conditioned to fear sleep? The

---

is needed: Antipsychotics, day treatment, perhaps even hospitalization and electroshock treatments. See the volume 2 chapter discussion of Antidepressant efficacy for a more in-depth review of this issue.

result is a reversed sleep cycle: fatigued or catnapping by day, overstimulated by night: "I just can't go to sleep ... my mind is always racing ... and when I do sleep I keep waking up ..."

Such patients respond poorly to sleeping pills, and the more powerful the nominal sedating properties of the agent, the more intense the negative response. Their bodies—this is what Dr. van der Kolk has in mind in his book *The Body Knows the Score*—have become organized to maintain a state of constant alertness and awareness.[4] With them, any medication that reduces or dulls such scrutiny is dangerous, so they may report, "Your pill made things worse ... I was more awake than ever." They are describing a conditioned negative reaction, the *nocebo* phenomenon. The alpha-2 agonists are more likely to evoke a nocebo response of this sort, inasmuch as they tend to be more sedating than the average Antidepressant.

Context

Medications are never prescribed in an interpersonal vacuum. They represent power, a power that some recipients wish to borrow, others to escape. Youngsters are no exception. As they develop greater independence of thought and action, their motivation to accept or resist authority becomes both more intense and complex. Indeed, unmanaged emotional activation is a hallmark of Attachment Disability. We are confronted with oil and water here: on the one hand, individuals who are conflicted about the trustworthiness of power; on the other hand, a pill—the very symbol of power.

Occasionally an adolescent will refuse the offer of an Antidepressant because of concerns about its presumptive dangers, its power to damage. In the late 1990s the media headlined psychiatric research that suggested Antidepressants accentuate suicidal feelings. Note that the concern was about suicidal *feelings,* not suicidal *behavior.* Nonetheless, the FDA and pharmaceutical manufacturers recommended guidelines so restrictive that there was a decline in the prescribing of Antidepressants for adolescents. Later research demonstrated the prescribing vacuum was correlated with an increase in the teenage suicide rate. The conclusion: obviously Antidepressants play an important role in the treatment of the potentially suicidal adolescent.[iv] The restrictions on prescribing were relieved, but the fallout from this fiasco lingers both among adolescents and their sponsors.

Therefore the offer of prescribing must include a careful discussion of the risks and goals of treatment, including the option—and consequences thereof—of choosing to decline the offer. If declined, it is important to note that the offer is always on the table. If accepted, it is just as important to clarify that should the recipient experience a change of mind, frankness is called for. *"Be up front about your decision to stop,"* I say. *"Don't claim to have 'forgotten' to take the medication, or that you 'lost' it. Own your decision. Then you can learn from it."*

Antidepressants can evoke a nocebo response when they cause adolescents—and adults—to feel "flat-lined." They feel numbed rather than sedated, living a life that is colorless, without savor, dull (for example, Maddie, chapter 10). Youngsters of a more resistive bent, relatively secure in the midst of their edginess, feel threatened when their anger is replaced by an unfamiliar impulse to cooperate and agree. They feel underpowered. Threatened by a growing sense of vulnerability, they discontinue the medication and retreat behind a wall of irritation and sarcasm, now safer with boundaries reestablished. On the medication they did feel more relaxed, less stressed out, less angry, more inclined to cooperate, mellower. But life without a barrier of resistiveness leaves them feeling vulnerable, too

---

iv. Again, it is important to recall that the Antidepressant benefit does not arise from "treatment" of so-called "Depression," but from relieving the stress and anxiety that disable so many youngsters. Which is why they must always have the support of a therapist to manage the self-blaming—the disability about the disability.

easily co-opted by authority, too agreeable, too inclined to relate, which stirs latent fears of abandonment or exploitation. In short, improvement itself can evoke a nocebo reaction.

Such youngsters, in contrast to Carla, whom I will discuss later in this chapter, are usually quite forthright about their reservations, and accept responsibility for their determination to suspend treatment. Typically I applaud their frankness, note that their position is reasonable, and then suggest a follow-up appointment to see how things are going. We are now in a position, I note, to compare the risks and benefits of treatment versus those of no treatment. I do not lecture or cajole; this both ignores their power and risks provoking their resistiveness.

I owe it to Darrell, who, years ago, provided me with the opportunity to learn how to constructively manage this rather unusual response to treatment.

[CASE STUDY]
Darrell: The Dangers of Improvement

I'm sitting across from Darrell, a surly sixteen-year-old, and his grandmother. He has just informed me that he's not going to take the medication I previously prescribed for his resistive and defiant behavior. Not because it's not helping or its side effects are intolerable, he says, but because he has lost his "anger." He's becoming too inclined to agree with people, which is scary. Grandmother, who says he's mellower these days and attributes this to the medication, just shakes her head in disgust as she listens to him.

This is a lad who has been more or less abandoned by both parents, although I imagine they found him rather hard to love, given his attitude. Now his grandmother has taken him in. She has not given up on him, although you can see she finds him trying.

His concern is understandable. If he continues to agree, build trust, develop connections, he is more vulnerable to abandonment and loss, which in his experience are inevitable. Better to remain safe behind a wall of sulky, irritating, and provocative behavior.

There are two ways to go with this, I think: insist on it, or accept it. One way is the more traditional way: with adolescents you set limits and stick to them. This is how you convey that you care, which, according to theory, is what they need. This is how you build trust. The other way is game theory, the gist of which is that if you can neutralize or defeat the patient's attempts to be sick, the only option remaining is to get well. I go the gamesmanship way: it's more interesting. Besides I'm getting too old to be a cop.

"Okay," I say, "not such a bad idea. Let's have you stop taking the medication and then return in a month and let me know how things are going. This way you'll have a chance to compare how you do with it and without it."

To my mild surprise he shows up in a month, without his grandmother in tow. "I want to take the pill. Things went better in school with it." I notice he is definitely less sulky, looks lonely in fact. Eventually what comes across is an immense sadness. I rewrite the prescription, resisting the temptation to celebrate the return of the prodigal. "Come back in a month," I say, "and we'll see how things are going."

What is going on here? The games model of therapy, exemplified by Gregory Bateson and Jay Haley,[5] would suggest that as long as the lad feels powerless—not in charge, losing—he will continue to resist. To resist is to feel empowered, in control, a way of maintaining identity. Therefore take away the need to resist by giving him nothing to resist against. Moreover, let him "win"; let him make the treatment decisions, gaining a new identity. And in the process of winning he will experience what it is like to be a free agent—gratifying, perhaps, but also lonely, even terrifying.

Another way to conceptualize this is to say he simply exercised the control he already possessed, since if he is really against medications, no one has the power to make him take them. What has happened is that he has been allowed to experience choice, giving him the opportunity to learn.

For him to accept a medication was dangerous because it symbolized depending on an external agency to obtain control: a surrender of autonomy. When I gave the lad the option of taking control himself, he discovered he lost freedom because his disabilities returned. But he also learned about himself. He learned the fact—and I think this was one reason for his sadness—that to be safe meant not to be free. It meant always to be alone. So he returned to resume the medication to help him tolerate the anxieties of relationships. A paradox here: by exercising his choice to not be "free" and to take medications, he began to travel the path to freedom—not freedom from anxiety but freedom bestowed by having options with which to manage anxiety and relationships, and, by extension, life's challenges and adventures, a freedom that emerges as maladaptive learning is displaced by adaptive learning.

Not every instance of medication avoidance follows this scenario.

[Case Study]
Carla: Street Drugs Safe, Medications Dangerous

She is fifteen, accompanied by her aunt. "I'm on medication for anxiety ... getting more depressed, not doing anything for me ... so I stopped it ... it was causing depression." Nonetheless she remains "depressed."

Other problems include low motivation, life seeming pointless, death ruminations, fears of being alone, and, most significantly, many worries, especially something "awful" happening to her family or her friends. She uses marijuana and alcohol. Her aunt says it is becoming a "problem."

Ever since her parents separated a few years ago, she sees a therapist off and on, more frequently recently, who says she has an "attachment problem." There are no prior psychiatric contacts. She does not cut.

At examination she proves to be a cooperative, compliant, forthright girl who is charming, outgoing, restless, frequently looking to her aunt for support.

I say I agree with her therapist's diagnosis of attachment issues, of which her fear for her family and friends is an unmistakable indicator. I suggest a trial of clonidine, explaining it is an anti-anxiety agent with no addictive potential. She balks and instead, according to my notes, "argues persuasively for an Antidepressant." So we agree to do it her way, and I prescribe one.

She returns two weeks later to report she started the medication, took it for approximately five days, and "then I misplaced the bottle." Her affect is variable, smiling one minute, irritable the next. Nonetheless she's very active, attending soccer practice for three hours two days a week, besides working at a pizza restaurant ten hours a week, where she gets along with her boss and coworkers. She has stopped seeing her therapist. Her aunt says she's smoking more and more pot and wants her to attend an outpatient chemical dependency treatment program. The girl becomes tearful at this suggestion. I agree with her aunt.

No surprise she fails a follow-up appointment.

Obviously the girl is "treating" her anxieties with marijuana and alcohol—no mystery here. Also, it is clear she finds street drugs "safer" than prescription medications because street drugs come without burden of an attachment. On the street, no questions asked, just hand over your money. But for her, the office is a different matter. Regular visits to a therapist—or doctor—threaten to bring another relationship into her life, and she already has too many entanglements to worry about: parents, sibs, step-sibs, and friends. She doesn't need another soul to prop up. Her job is to keep people happy, to be a cheerleader, which is why she is running so hard and why she uses. This may sound like a bizarre concern, yet she worries that if she were to really open up about her miseries, it would be of no benefit other than to simply upset the other party.

This is not a fanciful concern, as I have discussed before (see Amy, chapter 3). In fact, it is such an important consideration in working with attachment-disabled youngsters (and adults) that I will address it again here.

To reiterate, kids who have experienced separation and loss have learned the hard way that life inevitably involves death, about which they ruminate as they struggle with risking further attachments. But one paradox of therapy is that participating means risking attachment. Should a youngster like Carla take the risk and reveal the dimensions of her inner turmoil—for example, death ruminations—it is critical that her therapists and counselors not panic and misinterpret them as suicidal thinking. An entangled youngster will sense the panic and either start to minimize or drop out. However, in this instance, since Carla has seen her therapist off and on for several years, I suspect she will eventually drop back in after things have cooled down at bit, in effect managing a comfortable distance in the relationship.

Generally I manage such disguised fears of entanglement with a bit of stagecraft. My favorite is to manifest obtuse bewilderment, expressing regret that the youngster is not able to agree to the offer of medication, then brightly continue, "Well, let's carry on anyhow without medication for now and see how things work out." The idea is to not let myself be manipulated into the position of the rejected one, as well as to model for parents and sponsors how to deal with being stiffed by their youngsters. I like to have the last word, even if it is only to say *see you later*.

On the other hand, sometimes I decline to prescribe even in the face of urgent requests to do so.

For example, were Carla and her aunt to later return to beseech me for yet another prescription, I might graciously decline the request. Instead I might deploy another bit of stagecraft, nominating her as *"my mystery patient of the day—I need more time to figure you out."* Older patients are usually charmed by this shtick: it tickles their grandiosity, sucks them in a bit, and disarms their distrust since it identifies them as the more powerful figure in the transaction. And it moves things along. It identifies conflict—entanglement in Carla's case—rather than obscuring it via another spurious treatment gambit.

However, an entangled youngster like Carla would find such an offer rather threatening because when it comes to "figuring things out," what defines boundaries between figurer and figuree? In our prior contacts there was always between us—apart from her aunt—another familiar entity: medication. A medication in the room brings with it an inexhaustible menu of boundary-building opportunities such as requests for information about alternative medications, complaints of lack of effectiveness, and apologies for noncompliance, all of which serve to define a dance quite familiar to her: doctor to patient. But when it comes to "figuring things out," roles become nebulous, power diffuse. It's hard to say how Carla would react to such as offer.

I also refrain from prescribing when there is a history of overdosing with prescription medications. In my experience, such acting out is not so much an attempt to escape unendurable suffering—although elements of such may be present—but rather a message that the patient is experiencing suffering that the medication regimen is not addressing.

More often than not, the suffering is a secret that can no longer be silently endured. In short, prescription overdoses are always a call for help. The motivation here is not death, or even escape, but help. Of course, sometimes death results from such overdoses, but by miscalculation, not intent. The intent is to announce that more needs to be done.

Just recently I evaluated a young adult with a history of two such overdoses, both an apparent response to her boyfriend of several years breaking up their relationship. In the course of obtaining her history, I ventured the opinion that he would be back, that she had not seen the last of him, whereupon her mother allowed that, indeed, he was already calling. I concluded the workup by saying what she needed was not resuming medications, but learning to cope with an entangling relationship that showed every sign of continuing indefinitely. Previously withdrawn and a bit sulky, she brightened up at the offer and seemed to consider a follow-up appointment. However, a few days later her mother called, angry that I had not re-prescribed, making it clear her youngster would not be back. What secret was the mother protecting?

Some instances of prescription overdose will, nonetheless, call for a resumption of psychotropics because of a return of disability in their absence. If the patient is willing to start or resume counseling, if there is someone to supervise administration of the medications, and if both patient and supervisor agree to the dispensing of just one week's supply at a time—which can be pricey—then I will resume.

Content

Antidepressants

The traditional presentation of Antidepressant efficacy is based on two principles: 1) they relieve Depressive symptoms, and 2) it takes weeks, sometimes a month or two, for relief to appear. In my experience these are dubious concepts: Antidepressants actually relieve stress and anxiety symptoms, and often quite promptly at that. Nonetheless, for those who wish a traditional understanding of Antidepressants and their indications and limitations, I again recommend perusing a standard psychiatric or pharmacologic text.

Here, however, I offer an alternative interpretation of their unquestionable benefit based on conceptualizing them as *antistressants*. I touched on this briefly in chapter 5 during my earlier discussion of Depression as a spectrum, a gradient of phenomena from Reactive to Endogenous, rather than a collection of categories. One benefit of this approach is its non-exclusivity with respect to anxiety, since it is very unusual for Depressive phenomena to present without concurrent anxiety symptomatology. Now I will expand the discussion.

Anti-Anxiety and Antistress Properties

To begin with, it is now recognized that Antidepressants have the potential to suppress and minimize the damage caused by a normally protective fight/flight response gone haywire, a finding that has emerged from decades of research on their effectiveness. The consensus explanation is that they tone down the hypothalamic/pituitary/adrenal response to fear and anxiety that threatening situations generate in the limbic lobe of the brain. This accounts for the effectiveness of Antidepressants in the treatment of several categories of anxiety.[v]

This is the subject of a recent review of the medical management of anxiety disorders in children and adolescents.[6] The authors note these disorders not only impact relationships and school performance, but also promote suicidal thinking. Three of the disorders—Generalized Anxiety, Separation Anxiety, and Social Phobia—tend to occur together and respond similarly to

---

v. See volume 2 for a more extended discussion of Antidepressant action in the context of recent questions about their worth. I realize I am repetitive, but how else to question decades of dogma?

Focus on What Can Be Changed

both medical and cognitive therapy. The authors recommend Antidepressants as the preferred pharmacological treatment, more effective when combined with psychotherapy, with perhaps 75 percent response rate.

This review roughly corresponds to my experience. I always emphasize the *antistressant* properties of Antidepressants when discussing their use with youngsters and their sponsors. In particular I outline their benefits when it comes to dealing with life changes and the anxieties and stresses they may evoke.

To be sure, I do say that not all change, whether actual or symbolic, whether present or impending, always precipitates a stress response. That is, the brain/body does not inevitably react to the prospect of change by transitioning into a combat (fight/flight) mode. Moreover, the combat mode over the short run is *enabling* for it prepares us to strive against and overcome the adversity that change, with its implication of loss, always entails. We are energized to repair or replace that loss. But the combat mode can backfire over the longer run. We remain overenergized. We become frozen or out of control, experience anxiety, complain of "feeling depressed." Regardless of its dimensions the loss becomes daunting. Over us looms the potential of a collapse into disability, more likely and more profound if there is in our background a lurking distrust inspired by past trauma, abandonments, or betrayal.

Thus, when I prescribe an Antidepressant I note we are not actually treating "depression" but rather *stression*. I emphasize that the medication's target is anxiety, tension, and stress relief, that we hope to improve concentration, sleep, emotional stability, and energy. I recommend we establish improved cognitive functioning as an indication of improvement. I say we are going to pay attention to how often "what if" thoughts intrude, whether "Igor's" background mutterings and dronings are less intrusive and less discombobulating.

Inviting the patient to view the medication as an *antistressant* not only serves to clarify the issue, but it focuses counseling.

Identifying a problem as "depression" is vague and promotes passivity in the sense that it implies one has to wait for improvement. But if the problem is characterized as *stress,* this is a tangible that invites inspection, a more active and engaged posture. It promotes collaboration and makes room for therapy. It sets the stage for investigation and identification of the change that the stress signals.

No treatment, medical or otherwise, is risk free; hence my presentation always includes a discussion of the complications of Antidepressant therapy, including lack of effectiveness. The three-out-of-four response rate cited in the above review is a bit more favorable than my experience, which I would estimate as three out of five. Unfortunately, some youngsters and young adults become so dominated by obsessive ruminations of inadequacy and the inevitability of rejection that they slide toward an Endogenous paralysis. In such cases Antidepressants need to be supplemented with or replaced by a more vigorous and supportive approach such as referral for day treatment or hospitalization, or the addition of Antipsychotic.

Promptness of Effect

The *antistressant* interpretation of Antidepressant efficacy also offers an explanation for the delay in response commonly ascribed to Antidepressants: two to four weeks according to the textbooks.[vi] In fact, many youngsters and adults report improvement in days rather than weeks: "Things don't upset me so much … I'm not so irritable … I don't worry so much … Little things don't bother me so much anymore … I don't go so up and down during the day … My thoughts don't race so much at night … I don't get so angry." They are less frozen and more in control, less disabled, more adaptive. And as they become more effective in meeting their internal standards and

---

vi. In volume 2 I will present a more extended discussion of this widespread misconception.

expectations, they become less self-critical. They begin to like themselves again. Life is enjoyable again. Thus, upon their return three or four weeks later, they tell me they are less "depressed."

The above review notes that research on the comparative merits of Antidepressant versus cognitive therapy consistently points to the same conclusion: each helps, but the combination helps more. This is why when prescribing an Antidepressant I always recommend it be combined with counseling: the former to reduce the stress component, the latter to confront the erroneous cognitive interpretation of the stress-induced disability. In other words, the academic or social underperformance was previously interpreted not as an anxiety issue but as a moral issue; that is, as an issue of fault or blame. Typically, but not always, the blame is introjected. This increases the anticipation of rejection, which aggravates the stress, increasing the disability. No psychotropic known to the mind of man can undermine negative cognitive judgments of this sort.

True, such thinking and the disability it promotes may slip into the background if a psychotropic happens to relieve the precipitating stress, but the potential for self-critical thinking smolders on, liable to flare anew at the next stress. Recall Julie (chapter 8), who, having firmly convinced herself that it was her "fault" for ever risking marriage in the first place, sabotaged her recovery from an Endogenous Depression whenever her improvement signaled a return to everyday life with its social roles and expectations.

Therefore, apart from recommending concurrent counseling, I also provide adjunctive elementary cognitive therapy to supplement my medication management of *stression*.

This is necessary because, in my experience as I note above, the odds of an Antidepressant being tolerable or effective are about 60 percent. In large part this is because physicians are not likely to refer Antidepressant responders for psychiatric follow-up—it is the nonresponders who cross my threshold. So when I recommend an Antidepressant and review its *antistressant* potential benefits and complications, I never fail to mention the possibility of a lack of benefit—for medico-legal reasons, of course, but especially to promote compliance with concurrent management suggestions and to promote trust.

In my experience the patients who report the medication did not work or had to be discontinued because of side effects—what seems to be a therapeutic failure—typically will include an apology, either via word or behavior, for the misfire. The averted gaze, the change in tone of voice, the slumped posture all signal that guilt and self-blame are at work. But here an apparent treatment failure provides an opportunity to practice therapeutic alchemy. That is, such behavior offers an opening to initiate *generic cognitive therapy and redirection* to undermine a self-destructive attitude that typically infects their entire world: accepting blame for things over which they have no control.

For example, consider Lara as the exemplar of an individual who habitually apologizes whenever things do not work out as expected. In our previous meetings I have noticed and perhaps commented on this very habitual but unrealistic worldview. Now she's back, troubled by a lack of benefit after trying another *antistressant*.

[CASE STUDY]
Lara: Everything Is My Fault

Lara (subdued tone, eyes averted, apologetic gesture): "It's not working."

Dr. C, recognizing opportunity: "Hold it … there you go again, apologizing."

Lara, puzzled, evidently forgetting our previous discussions: "What?"

Dr. C: "Why are you apologizing? You tried the pill. You can't control how it works."

Focus on What Can Be Changed

Lara, with a hint of irritation: "I'm not apologizing!"

Dr. C: "Yes you are! Look at your tone of voice, how you are sitting."

Lara, confused: "What?"

Dr. C: "Here, look straight at me and repeat louder, 'It's not working.'"

Lara, weakly: "The pill is not working."

Dr. C: "Louder!"

Lara, timidly assertive: "It's no good."

Dr. C, pointing out the window at a ridge across the freeway: "Pretend I'm standing way over there and you have to shout to make me hear."

Lara, struggling, embarrassed: "NO GOOD."

Dr. C: "Again."

Lara, distinctly annoyed, perhaps a bit sarcastic: "NOOO GOOOD!!"

Dr. C: "Very good." *Explains the reason for the shtick: to demonstrate again to Lara that she has the habit of accepting fault for things she has no power to control.*

Lara: Dubious agreement.

Although this rudimentary behavior modification technique seems rather trivial, if used consistently it is capable of powerful effects with "depressed" patients. Sometimes I supplement it by giving them a prescription to post on their bathroom mirror, such as: *"Describe your life, don't judge it,"* for a daily reminder of the mental state they need to develop. With others, I designate a gesture I will use to prompt them to reframe an apologetic behavior or statement. I explain, "You are pretty good at judging the goodness and badness of your thoughts and feelings. Now let's see if you can develop another habit—simply describing them to yourself, 'owning' them without labeling them."

And if there is a concerned partner, sponsor, or parent, I might suggest they come along at the next visit in order to have me to demonstrate the technique. Frequently such supportive parties have become somewhat demoralized themselves by having to cope with the negative talk and demeanor of their loved one, who often becomes unresponsive to their encouragement and expressions of caring. Rebuffed and discouraged as they are, it is inevitable that despite their best wishes, irritable and impatient feelings well up and consume energy to restrain, a fatiguing process and a prelude to burnout. Having the above technique to fall back on not only protects them, but also reinforces what is happening in treatment.

This approach has its limitations. Older patients might find both my behavior and the assertiveness I advocate too threatening if they are not prepared. Timing is critical. And a few are simply afraid of raising their voice; they fear they or others around them might lose control. They understand the rationale of the tactic, but to emit assertive vocalizations is threatening. Any hint of energy in their own voice recreates past abuse experiences, so they freeze up.

And with some youngsters, their blaming may be so deeply entrenched and wired in that they are not conscious of it. To address the blaming directly—for example, via the technique I just described—not only sails right over their head, but risks aggravating the problem. Here is yet another situation that, as they appraise it, is their fault. They are so bogged down by anxiety that they will simply find this technique incomprehensible. In fact, it will feel like more punishment because their world is always one of fault and retaliation. Such youngsters require different management techniques, perhaps play therapy or role-playing. The goal is to promote the idea of a world that is not always a jungle, not always cruel or exploitative, but rather a world in which lost pets and children are sometimes rescued.

And sometimes it is not necessary. When Peggy (chapter 11) reappeared after a sixteen-month hiatus characterized by a good deal of turmoil, she was frank and descriptive, owning her behavior and its consequences without apology. She recognized she had to learn from her behavior, not apologize for it. In another sense this also was true of Lindsey (also chapter 11). Despite her belief that she deserved suicide for the pain she caused—the specifics of which remained murky—her behavior never signaled apology, neither for her presumed misdeeds nor for her belief. Indeed, it signaled defiance. In contrast to Peggy, who was self-forgiving, Lindsey was unforgiving, which had to be challenged; hence our debate.

Alpha-2 Agonists

Clonidine and guanfacine can be very helpful in managing children and adolescents with anxiety, sleep, temper, or focus issues, either alone or in combination, with or without a trauma history. And they are often useful with adolescents and adults who demonstrate the trauma triad of wounded trust, dissociation, and maladaptive learning. They present a handy alternative when standard psychotropics have not been helpful, or when there is a history of substance abuse or addiction that disqualifies the use of medications that have an addictive potential, such as the benzodiazepines. In such cases, the alpha-2 agonists may be quite helpful since they have practically no addictive potential.

Their major drawback is dizziness or feeling faint when suddenly sitting or standing up—postural hypotension—due to their antihypertensive properties.[vii] It is important to fully describe this phenomenon prior to prescribing, start with a low dose, and cautiously adjust the dosage depending upon benefits and side effects. Uncommon complications of either medication include chest pain or ankle swelling, at which time it should immediately be tapered and discontinued.

Their sedating effect is rapid, clonidine more than guanfacine, which is why I prefer the former if disturbed sleep is

---

vii. In fact, they were first marketed years ago as antihypertensive agents and are still occasionally prescribed as part of an antihypertensive regimen.

a prominent problem. If I suspect the patient may be nocebo prone, I may start with a miniscule dose, explaining, "Your body needs to get used to this medication, so it needs to be trained, just as people with an allergy are given shots to desensitize them to the allergy."

Other Change Tactics

Cognitive Behavioral Therapy (CBT)

If pharmacotherapy can be conceived as a "bottom-up" approach to Attachment Disability management, CBT is "top down." In essence, medication promotes emotional stability by modulating the emotion-generating circuitry deep within the brain. It works on the "bottom" of the brain, so to speak. Cognitive therapy, on the other hand, focuses on the cerebral cortex, the "top" of the brain, by training patients to "own" emotional thoughts and investigate their (non)logical consequences. The idea is to replace "all-or-nothing" catastrophic conclusions with "maybe–maybe not" assessments. CBT and pharmacotherapy complement each other nicely. A fine example of CBT at work can be found in Dr. Jeffrey Lieberman's book *Shrinks: The Untold Story of Psychiatry*.[7] Also, a lucid summary supporting the effectiveness of CBT in adolescent anxiety appears in the June 2015 issue of the *American Journal of Psychiatry*.[8] Moreover, a recent meta-analysis of primary data from sixteen clinical trials of CBT versus Antidepressant medication found no differences between the two regardless of baseline symptom severity.[9]

Here are examples of two cognitive techniques that may seem elementary but in fact are a fundamental component of effective counseling. No therapist's toolkit is complete without them.

Reframing Judgmental Thinking

I briefly referred to this earlier. Here is a more extended presentation of what makes this technique so vital. Briefly, it is designed to enhance survival thinking. The idea is to encourage patients to look at *what* they feel and think with less preoccupation about *how* they feel and think. In order to manage their disability, they need to figure out the survival content of their mental activities while avoiding contamination by moral concerns: notions of goodness or badness. They need to distinguish the actual moral world—the world of behavior and its consequences—from the inner moral world, the world of threat and retaliation and separation. The goal is not to erode the capability to make moral assessments—most patients are pretty good at this, perhaps even too good—but to create a cognitive balance by enhancing their capability to make survival assessments as well.

The technique is deceptively simple. After patients make a statement with an implied—typically by a change in posture or tone of voice—or verbally expressed self-critical assessment, I might occasionally encourage them to say the same thing but without an apology. "Let's see if you can say that without apologizing for what you feel or think or did." Some catch on quickly. Others react like Lara above: puzzled, confused, even irritated, unaware of the guilt beneath the message. On such occasions I will call attention to their body language, encouraging them to be more forthright, perhaps even modeling their very words assertively. It is important to implement the technique according their ability to tolerate and learn from it. But this is true of all coaching.

Redirection

Not all patients are like Mr. Resistive (chapter 10). Some, in fact, bury me with words, ignore feedback, change the subject, and interrupt until I begin to feel like Dr. Searles. Verbosity of this sort has many causes: mania, psychosis, manipulation, dementia, attentional deficiencies, or some combination thereof. But the most common is an underlying *Attachment Disability with marked abandonment concerns.* These unhappy patients are driven by a need to get everything in before the meeting ends because, in their experience, there is no guarantee of another. They have learned that a medical relationship is fragile; it can disappear overnight without warning, especially in our modern era of group rather than solo practice and annual changes in insurance coverage. They have developed what therapists call "rejection sensitivity."

It does not serve patient interests to allow them to endlessly ramble and digress. If the so-called "talking therapy" is to be beneficial, learning must take place. The idea is for them to become the detective of their own life. Otherwise it is a waste of time and resources for both parties. Both are frustrated. Patients feel ignored, therapists burned out. Hence I cannot overemphasize the importance of what might seem a rather minor behavioral tactic.

For their sake and mine, I manage such verbosity by redirection. After listening for a while, I might ask, "Let's see if you can boil down what you just said into six words or less." Some are able to do so. In fact a few, after a moment or so of silent concentration, can not only deliver the requested summary but triumphantly tick off each word finger by finger as they do so.[viii] Others are perplexed and need help. To them I might say, "Well, in six words, is this what you were trying to say?" and then make a stab at boiling it down for them.

Of course, I have to manage my own verbosity as well. The idea is to tailor my statement to fit the patient's attention span. Not that I am always successful. To guard against running off

---

viii. Recall Helen's pleasure with her successful performance of this task at her graduation party (chapter 2), a double graduation of sorts, in fact.

at the mouth myself—driven by my own need for attention—from time to time I will ask patients to repeat what I have just said. This focuses the two of us. I clarify that the important thing is for them to hear my feedback and correct it if I have misinterpreted them. Whether it fits or not is another thing; that is up for them to decide. But without listening—and it is my job to promote their ability to listen—they are deprived of the opportunity to learn.

One of the more startling instances of lurking rejection sensitivity is when the feedback is exactly the opposite of what I propose. For example, when treating chronic pain patients I include a detailed review of their (often extensive) medical records, which typically reveal no indication that they have a life-threatening or tangible medical condition. After reporting such a conclusion to them, I've learned to carefully double-check what they heard because often they hear me saying, "It's all in your mind!" This is understandable since before they've been erroneously told their problem is "psychological" or "somatoform" when, in fact, the more accurate statement is that the cause of their pain is "unknown."

Astute readers will realize that redirection incorporates Management Principle One (clarification) components, which is not unusual since the three steps interact and are mutually reinforcing. Also, this example of a redirection tactic is by no means exhaustive. Creativity is the only limit when it comes to designing programmed learning within a counseling format.

A final comment about redirection: It is important to proceed cautiously. The wise coach does not always critique every misplayed ball or catch or shot. The same is true of the attentive therapist. Too much feedback risks fight-back.

Exposure/Response Prevention (E/RP)

This is well-known behavior modification technique. In essence, it involves creating an explicit schedule of incremental exposures to successively greater degrees of the threatening situation, while delaying withdrawal from it. Wikipedia (access *exposure/ response prevention*) provides an excellent introduction.

It can be self-designed and administered, which avoids the Catch-22 conundrum of social avoidance. Any parent, teacher, or coach who has experience building skill-sets in children will find the concept quite familiar. The interesting thing about the process is that it has the potential to change the behavior of the party on both sides of the schedule, as it were, because conforming to its terms promotes patience and self-restraint.[10]

For certain youngsters, the threatening situation is fear of making a mistake, either on tests or homework, which has the potential to release a torrent of self-blame. Typically they admit to perfectionism. Their homework and school work have to be perfect, their tests 100 percent correct, their grades all As. Since this is impossible, they usually arrive in my office anxious and discouraged, the personification of dejection and failure.

When I try to engage them, I avoid pointing out that no one is perfect, that perfection is an impossible dream, and so on. Instead I wonder what makes a mistake repugnant, and encourage them to think about what for them is the unthinkable. Generally what emerges is a vague notion that being perfect is a way to control life and protect against the catastrophe of someone getting upset. Again I avoid discussing the reality that one can't go through life without being upset. Instead I propose a test: why not make a deliberate mistake, a teeny one, say end a sentence without a period or fail to capitalize a proper noun, just to see what happens. Such youngsters struggle with the idea because it evokes fears of a teacher or sponsor becoming unhappy, which in their experience means someone will be rejected and abandoned. Occasionally sponsors may also struggle with the notion of a mistake, deliberate or otherwise, because of their need to present perfect children to the world in order to escape criticism of their parenting. Some may decide not to return.

For those sponsors and youngsters willing to give this strategy a try—which I call *learning antiperfectionism*—the next step is to negotiate a "mistake," the performance of which youngsters find tolerable. Its magnitude is inconsequential, of course, because to the intimidated soul all performance imperfections risk fatal consequences. So I explain we will follow an E/RP format because it gives the youngster control of the pace of what is a step-by-step treatment process. I invite everyone to research the technique on the Internet. Finally we agree on a follow-up interval. Usually no more than two or three visits are necessary because with these kids and their parents a direct confrontation with the specter of the imperfect serves to exorcise it. They learn the world does not invariably go up in flames should you make a mistake.

Eye Movement Desensitization and Reprocessing (EMDR)

EMDR is a therapeutic technique that can be uniquely effective in the treatment of patients disabled by trauma residuals: for example, flashbacks or intrusive thought. I have found that patients who are otherwise unresponsive to psychotropics or conventional cognitive therapy report significant benefit, sometimes after only a few sessions.

The therapy springs from the introspective experience of its originator, social worker Francine Shapiro, who noticed that some of her troublesome memories were accompanied by involuntary eye motions.[11] When she voluntarily exerted control of them, her anxieties diminished. Eventually she evolved a highly structured therapeutic technique that trained patients to first elicit troublesome thoughts and then couple them with rhythmic gestures or motions; for example, observing a pendulum. Since, as we all know, it is practically impossible to maintain simultaneous fully conscious awareness of our inner and exterior worlds, one awareness will evaporate, hopefully the former. Through repetition of the exercise under direction of the therapist, the troublesome thoughts extinguish.

Shapiro's conjecture is that sensory flooding of a brain unprepared for trauma inhibits normal memory processing. The terrifying cacophony of sights, sounds, feelings, and thoughts is dumped into isolated memory network. The brain becomes frozen or stuck in a replay mode—dissociated—until the walled-off circuits are "reprocessed" into standard memory modules.

Both the effectiveness and the theory of EMDR are questioned. I am not qualified to debate its theory, but I can say I have seen it work in traumatized individuals who are unresponsive to standard anxiety treatments. It is certainly worth considering in child, adolescent, and adult survivors, whether witnessed or sustained, of family or civilian catastrophes such as murder, assault, rape, motor vehicle accident, fire, tornado, and so on. Moreover, a nonprofit pilot program to treat combat-related trauma, the Veteran Resilience Project, reports very positive results.[12]

The thing to remember is that, regardless of its origins, all trauma involves not only lost or impaired attachments due to wounded trust, but also the threat of subsequent loss. This is what makes trauma not only so difficult to endure but so difficult to treat as well. It seems to me the relevant issue with EMDR, therefore, is not theory but effectiveness. Does it work? Theories are cheap, facts precious. And if it can be demonstrated that EMDR "works," that is precious indeed.

Family Therapy

When I encounter attachment-disabled youngsters, part of my workup is to scrutinize their parents to ascertain whether the disability extends beyond the proposed patient. Sometimes this is quite apparent, sometimes disguised by a veneer of solicitude projected on the youngster—everyone is wounded, but only the child feels and expresses pain. This may inhibit management and block its improvement because should the child begin to heal, this risks undermining the reconstructed family structure. How will their shared misery be managed now? To whom can they turn if there is no longer a "depressed" or angry youngster serving as a vehicle to bring their own suffering to the attention of a professional? A sign of this is the interview that begins with the youngster as the target of concerns or complaints and then gradually shifts to the sponsor's issues while the ostensible patient fades into the background.

Family therapy, especially in the form of in-home counseling, may be especially helpful in such situations. It provides an opportunity to neutralize the blaming of scapegoated youngsters, for example, or the overprotection of withdrawn and discouraged kids. All participants are invited to share their understanding and feelings about the loss that intruded into their midst, or their observations about how others are dealing with it.

Dialectical Behavior Therapy (DBT)

DBT is a highly structured behavioral intervention developed to manage persisting disabilities characterized both by failure to learn from experience and unresponsiveness to conventional treatments. It has proven helpful with a variety of difficult-to-manage conditions: recurrent suicide attempts, personality disorders, eating disorders, addictions, intractable depression, and treatment noncompliance, to name a few.[13]

"Dialectical" refers to its fundamental cognitive strategy: teaching patients the habit of "opposite thinking" to deploy in crisis situations rather than collapsing into emotional paralysis or impulsivity. As a patient once put it, *"You learn not to 'awfulize.'"*

DBT principles and practices are set forth in a protocol developed by its originator, Marsha M. Linehan, PhD.[14] This requires participants attend a weekly two- to three-hour skills group as well as one hour per week individual counseling with a trained DBT therapist. Moreover they are required to maintain a day-to-day symptom journal—a "diary card"—that also incorporates skills used to promote symptom resolution.[ix] The protocol also carefully defines therapist responsibilities and behaviors and provides for "coaching calls" from patients as well as participating in weekly consultation team meetings.

One of the more interesting features of DBT is the use of group co-therapists. On occasion one therapist will disagree with how the group process is being managed, and interrupt the proceedings to voice the disagreement. Patients who witness this later report to me a combination of horror and fascination: horror because the dispute is a replay of childhood or marital traumas, and fascination because it is resolved without bloodshed or retaliation. A wonderful learning experience.

Group Discussion

Group discussion and group therapy are similar in that each is composed of individuals who have something in common. Moreover, each is based on the idea that sometimes learning is facilitated by observing how others grapple with a familiar problem—for example, disagreement between authority figures as discussed in the preceding paragraph. But group discussion is not bound by group therapy rules regarding confidentiality, fraternization, and participation. Discussions are not confidential, they take place within—not apart from—the participants'

---

ix. While it is deceptively simple, I have found that a maintaining a daily record of this sort can have profound therapeutic effects. Apparently intractable problems have a way of evaporating if I can persuade patients to keep track of them, which smothers the "awfulizing" habit. That is, the very act of putting thoughts and feelings into a record, rather than reacting to them, is a manifestation of opposite thinking. This tactic is also an example of the first principle of disability management, clarification.

social world, and not everyone in expected to contribute.

However, one of the group therapy techniques I learned during my training from my instructor Dr. Jack Sheps is very helpful in promoting group discussion: soliciting opinion. This idea here is that when an opinion or question or challenge is directed to the facilitator, he or she presents it back to the group not only to solicit feedback but to engage participation.

This was quite helpful during ward meetings at Anoka State Hospital in the 1960s and later at the St. Peter Regional Treatment Center in the late 1980s. The agenda was open ended and participation was voluntary; the only rule was civility. Generally they were well attended by staff and patients. Usually I opened the proceedings by asking if anyone had a question or comment, letting things meander until someone raised a question or had an opinion, sometimes if only to wonder why we were having a discussion, what was the worth of it, and so on—in other words, a challenge of authority. This was the kind of opportunity Dr. Sheps taught us to recognize. Rather than engaging in a debate, the proper response is to widen the discussion. "Go around the group and ask everyone what they think," he would say. We were to inquire, Who feels the same? Who feels differently?

Generally this was enough to get things going, sometimes among the staffers as well, who typically had their beefs with administration. (Anyone who has ever worked in a hospital is familiar with this chorus.) More often than not we approached a basic issue: rules. Then I asked how people dealt with rules, noting that many times issues with rules had a lot to do with why people ended up in the hospital. Sometimes the discussions finished without a conclusion, sometimes with patients (and staff) ganging up on me, demanding my opinion, an option that Dr. Sheps never covered.

From my own experience I eventually came up with something like "I think if we are going to be part of a society, we will be subject to rules and expectations. It is important for us to learn them, to realize they change, and to accept the consequences of either following or not following them."

Predictably, either then or at a later meeting, one or more of the patients would pipe up and say that once they were out of the hospital they would no longer take medications, comply with follow-up treatments, and so on. Usually this generated vigorous debate, which was easy to avoid getting sucked into. Presenting a milder version of my Mr. POP posture (chapter 10), I explained it was my job to provide leadership, information, and recommendations, but not enforcement. What they would do—or could not help but doing—with their lives after discharge was their problem and responsibility, not mine. If they did well, that was to their credit; if they did not, that also was to their credit.

Self-Help

The idea of self-improvement is ancient. Wikipedia cites a seventh-century BCE poem, *Works and Days*, as the earliest known example of righteous self-improvement. Its author, the Greek poet Hesiod, advises his brother (who might have been a bit of a wastrel) how to cultivate a life of virtue. I have no doubt, however, that inevitably an archeologist rooting in the dumps of an earlier era, say First Dynasty Egypt, will uncover a papyrus scrap coaching a son to practice equanimity and courage when confronted with the vicissitudes of life.

In our era leadership examples might include the nineteenth-century Horatio Alger paperbacks providing economic guidance to boys, while in the twentieth-century self-improvement acquired a social veneer as Dale Carnegie and Dr. Norman Vincent Peale preached enlightened fellowship and positive thinking. However, in recent decades self-improvement underwent yet another metamorphosis, shedding its social dimension in favor of an inner mindfulness: self-help.

Although the self-help literature is vast and expanding,

it can be roughly divided according to two themes: *suck it up* versus *mellow out.* Each approach has something to offer the troubled mind. However, I favor the latter because the former is a bit dicey. Failure at mind control too frequently is interpreted as the latest in a series of life failures that may risk aggravating the low self-esteem of *depression.* Instead I recommend one of the first—and still the best in my opinion—of the "mellow out" category, *Hope and Help for Your Nerves* by the Australian physician Dr. Claire Weekes.[15]

Her idea is to mentally contemplate the feared situation rather than attempting to repress it by "sweeping it under the carpet." As I tell my patients: "When it is under the carpet it is a lump you can trip over when you least expect it. Better to have it out in the open so you know what you are facing." I encourage them to read the book and practice what she recommends: floating through the anxiety and panic, then following it to the feared consequence, typically some kind of an imagined catastrophic abandonment. I also suggest keeping the book at the bedside and each night randomly selecting a few paragraphs for meditation before sleep.[16]

Diet

Assiduous readers of this book by now would not be surprised to learn that childhood abuse or neglect is likely to lead to later Depression.[17] More surprising, perhaps, is that chronic Depression not only promotes chronic inflammation, but also "feasts" on it, a ping-pong interaction that can undermine both mental and physical health.[18] Omega-3 essential fatty acids (EFA), which possess anti-inflammatory properties, have been shown to prevent Depression[19] or augment Antidepressant effectiveness,[20] and therefore should be a regular dietary supplement in the form of fish oil capsules or equivalent. In fact, I recommend EFA be a part of everyone's diet, not just those who are trauma survivors.

Pet Companionship

For over forty years a poodle or two has been a treasured member of our family, so you would think that I would be quite aware of the security pet companionship provides. But not until I shared Maggie's grief and dismay did I begin to understand the depths of a pet relationship.

I first met Maggie over twenty years ago when consulting at a pain clinic. Later she began to see me in my own practice. Her office records from both locations are no longer available, so I am reconstructing her case from vague memory except for the episode of her cat's death, which is vivid indeed.

I estimate that Maggie was in her late thirties to early forties, never married, childless, spotty work history, and currently unemployed. She was living with her father and ailing mother when she was first referred to me because of a knotty, long-standing pain/"depression"syndrome that then and subsequently defied relief. Her pain extended from her low back to her neck and head, with episodic radiation to her extremities. It could be sharp or throbbing or aching or fleeting depending on the weather or activity or stress … in other words, a not an uncommon chronic pain problem. I started seeing her while she was under consideration for placement of an indwelling neurostimulator, a then recent pain management innovation.

In the midst of these miseries, however, she was typically upbeat, with a fixed smile, chatting on impassively about her pains, her family, the obnoxious brother-in-law landlord who lived upstairs, and her one passion: 9-ball league competition. But one day she was much different: distraught, weeping, disheveled, despairing, inconsolable. Her cat was dead. "She used to sleep on my legs every night, if I had trouble sleeping I could reach over and touch her, now I can't sleep, I have panic all night, I can't go anywhere knowing she won't be there when I get home, I don't want to do anything …"

Well, the rest of her history is hazy. I wish I could remember the name of her pet. I'm not sure whether she ever did replace Cat. Later she and her folks moved. Her mother's health began to improve, as did Maggie's pains. She still mentioned them but seemed less disabled by them, began to talk about looking for part-time work, came less often, and finally dropped out—no contact since for years.

However, the acuteness of her loss must have sensitized me because later, as a return of adolescent referrals revived my awareness of attachment issues, when obtaining a history I began to ask if there was a pet in the house.

Also, I performed a mental retrospective assessment of Maggie's life situation. For one thing, I recalled what made the brother-in-law so obnoxious: his physical abuse of her sister and demeaning behavior with Maggie. And the entanglement of mother and daughter was now obvious. I think Maggie and her dad had a close and loving relationship since they were on the same 9-ball team; possibly he taught her the game. Could her mother have been jealous of their connection? Only Cat was safe to love unconditionally. Sure, she was demanding and quirky, probably even imperious on occasion. But that's the nature of true love of a pet, and what you most remember when they are gone, for that's what defined them and was such an indelible part of their not so little personality. And why they provide such security for trauma victims.

So now I mourn with my patients when their Cat or Henry or Beauty or Sparky or Tut is gone. And when I have a patient whose landlord requests a medical certificate to verify the need for a pet in the apartment, I always provide it. And I certainly hope that Maggie has decided to risk a replacement for Cat.

This is hardly an exhaustive compilation of behavior change options that have the potential to provide relief of trauma residuals. For those who desire a more comprehensive review of the understanding and treatment of trauma, I again recommend Dr. Bessel van der Kolk's *The Body Keeps the Score*,[21] because of his clarity, his breadth of experience, and particularly his presentation of multiple treatment options in chapters 13 through 20. Some of these I have noted above while others strike me as definitely innovative—a vital need in trauma management—yet all are developed at much greater length than I have and are buttressed by his extensive research and knowledge of the literature.

But notice what they all have in common: neutralizing trauma-imprinted dissociative defense processes and facilitating the learning of more adaptive behavioral or cognitive skills, including an enhanced ability to trust and explore. Therefore any technique that has adaptive learning as its goal is worthy of inclusion and consideration here.

The day may come when genomic analysis will reveal the precise cause of attachment vulnerability. But even then, the sturdiest of genetic constitutions will yet remain susceptible to the stresses and anxieties of life; in particular the reality of loss, abandonment, and trauma. In short, pharmacology cannot be expected to be the last word in managing attachment disability. It is a first step—occasionally a very vital first step—one that dampens brain static, setting the stage for learning. But learning a new bag of tricks is the ultimate goal here.[x]

By way of recapitulation, recall that the goal of this volume is to provide an introduction to Attachment Disability, a unique form of emotional disability, and to identify its causes: abuse, neglect, abandonment, betrayal, and loss. Its consequence is a

---

x. The theme of volume 2, in fact, is the prevention of adolescent dropout and addictive behaviors by developing a more comprehensive skill set—that is, learning--through eliminating compulsory school attendance.

"trauma triad" of injured trust, dissociation, and maladaptive learning. The many manifestations of the triad I have discussed at length in chapters 1 through 13 to promote its *identification* and to *mitigate* its deleterious effects. Therefore in the next and final chapter I plead for reform of psychiatric assessment practices that too frequently promote dysfunction by misinterpreting and mismanaging Attachment Disability. Dropped-out and underperforming kids and adults need more from us psychiatrists than just a label and a pill.

14

Current Psychiatric Assessment: A Plea for Reform

As psychiatrists, we need to offer our patients more than a label and a pill.

Children, adolescents, and adults with attachment issues are too often misdiagnosed and mismanaged, and then, once the therapeutic imagination is depleted, deemed "treatment resistant." I see this exhaustion as the fallout of an ideology generated by our psychiatric leadership in the 1970s. A cadre of influential researchers promulgated the notion that psychiatric illness could be captured in its totality by a descriptive terminology without consideration of the inner forces that hitherto presumably drove mental and emotional disability. All referents to unobservable, nonquantifiable psychic processes were to be discarded. Our diagnostic terminology was to be reconstructed using only verifiable, observable behaviors.

After a good deal of controversy and turmoil in the 1970s, the reform element prevailed and oversaw the birth of *DSM-III* in 1980, a categorical nomenclature that attempted to avoid reference to subjective experience. The inner world of feelings, emotions, impulses, and motivations—a world all of us are familiar with, sometimes uncomfortably so—suffered a demotion.

Subsequently, as noninvasive screening of brain function became available in the 1980s, a second initiative emerged: the reduction of psychiatric signs and symptoms to neurophysiological events and, eventually, a further reduction to "biomarkers" that could reliably identify and predict psychiatric disease.

In the midst of these dual ambitions, the notion of symptom causality was revised. What I refer to in this book as dynamic thinking—that is, cause/effect analysis—was to be reduced to strictly physiological, quantitative phenomena. Moreover we were to learn to think and communicate via a new vocabulary, both for us and our patients.

I did not directly participate in this evolution as an insider except during my few years in clinical research when I sat in on department meetings or research conferences. However, over the last fifty years as a clinician, I have observed psychiatric assessment and practice from the sidelines, and it is from this perspective, a report from the trenches, so to speak, that I will present my view of what psychiatry has gained and lost.

I will begin with my experiences as a psychiatric resident at the New York State Psychiatric Institute (PI), 1962 to 1965.

Training Experiences: Psychiatry in the 1960s

In chapter 5, I described my limited exposure as a resident to a state psychiatric hospital. Here I will focus on another, much more intensive aspect of my training: learning the art of psychodynamic assessment and therapy.

My training occurred from 1962 to 1965 during the era of *DSM-I*, which endured from 1952 to 1968 and incorporated psychoanalytic notions of psychic conflict. In other words, as residents we were presented with a system that included both classification *and* explanation; that is, both a description and an explanation of what was described. In that sense it was a "dynamic" system, which is why as residents our workups were to include a psychodynamic assessment formulated according to Freudian concepts. Not only were we to describe how our patients were, we were also supposed to "explain" why they were the way they were.

Now for me, Freudian psychoanalytic terminology, which makes use of now familiar terms such as *ego, id, superego, unconscious,* and so on, was difficult indeed to grasp. I recall spending long hours in the PI library studying a preliminary version of David Rapaport's synthesis of psychoanalytic theory.[1] From a theoretical perspective I experienced two problems. While the terminology was meant to describe common, authentic human conflict, it verged on the metaphorical and analogical. Which created the second problem: how to interpret metaphor and analogy. Subsequent Freudians could not escape the territory Freud had staked out and still claim to be of his school. But that did not prevent his disciples from later revising and modifying his language. I'm sure I was not alone in finding the terminology slippery, inconsistent, and context dependent, not "scientific." It certainly lacked the rigor and precision of, say, the scholastic philosophers I had studied in college.[i]

And then there were practical issues as well: communication and effectiveness. As a therapist I saw my role as one of making timely interpretations of patient issues to identify and clarify underlying conflicts. But translating psychoanalytic ideas that I myself only imperfectly grasped into everyday language was daunting. Moreover, even if I was successful in presenting the basis for a symptom manifestation, the symptom typically continued to manifest.

For example, fifty years later I retain a vivid recollection of

---

i. For those of you in need of a system with order and consistency, look no further!

my therapy of "Bill," a middle-aged unmarried fellow, hospitalized because he was more or less housebound due to fear of panic attacks, who was never without a fedora jammed tightly on his head. Eventually I offered the interpretation that he was afraid that he might "blow his top" if he were without the hat to control his feelings. He agreed he was afraid of his anger, but the hat was never doffed, nor did his fears abate.

Eventually he participated, fedora and all, in a demonstration interview with one of our professors, Dr. Alvin Mesnikoff, who at one point may have implied that Bill was possibly exaggerating his disability. At least that is how Bill heard it. Furious, flushed with rage, Bill accused Dr. Mesnikoff of calling him a liar. The good doctor apologized and clarified his statement, Bill simmered down, and the interview continued without incident. My next clear memory is of Bill participating in outpatient group therapy following his discharge a few months later. Never did he ever appear without his fedora, yet he was improved enough to travel to group.

So what happened? To this day I'm not sure, but I suspect Dr. Mesnikoff's intervention/provocation was more therapeutic than my lame interpretation. And when word of the incident spread among the inpatient grapevine, no doubt Bill's peers had quite a giggle imagining the takedown of a lordly professor by a lowly patient. Perhaps the support and acceptance of his behavior somewhat allayed his social anxiety, and Bill could conclude that losing control in public would not lead to dangerous retaliation. In short, even an accurate interpretation of *why* a patient is the way he is does not necessarily lead to a change in the *way* he is. More is needed.

This and similar residency experiences, although not as dramatic, had me convinced by the time I finished my training that I needed another language for patient assessment and communication, something other than psychoanalytic lingo.

To be sure, I was not without exposure to other languages. Besides more or less formal lectures on psychoanalytic psychotherapy, we were also given a reading list of other schools of psychotherapy and personality theory for further study. Included in this category, especially in view of my later professional development, must be the ideas of psychoanalyst Harry Stack Sullivan, who emphasized the commonality of interpersonal and social experience; hence his dictum with reference to Schizophrenia that "Everyone is more simply human than otherwise."

Also of great significance to my later career was my exposure to the child development theories of psychoanalysts John Bowlby and Donald Winnicott, whom I discussed in chapter 1. And of interest was the concept of Adaptational Psychodynamics developed by psychoanalyst Sandor Rado, intriguing because he did not accept the traditional interpretation of emotion arousal as necessarily disorganizing. To the contrary, he viewed emotion as bringing an organizing adaptive power to life and its challenges.[ii]

Finally, and probably of greatest influence, were my contacts with Drs. Searles and Kolb. I think Dr. Kolb's passing comment that all anxiety was related to the prospect of separation, plus my witnessing Dr. Searles's unforgettable interview performance, sensitized me to the rich clinical possibilities of interpersonal theory with its focus on the felt emotion, in other words, clarification. But I did not fully commit to this interview and assessment style, of which my interview of Amy is an example, until years later (chapter 3).

Thus somewhat bereft of theory, I suppose this explains why I was so receptive to a behavioral approach when I started work at Anoka State Hospital upon finishing my training. I was prepared for something different.

---

ii. Discussed at greater length below.

Organizational Experiences: Psychiatry in the 1970 and 1980s

Although I did not realize it at the time, my dubious appraisal of the efficacy of psychoanalytic concepts was widely shared within the psychiatric profession. This issue was partially addressed in 1968 with the appearance of *DSM-II*, which defined psychiatric categories as "disorders" rather than "reactions." Apparently an innocuous change, this was to have devastating consequences for psychiatry because it was the first step in eliminating dynamic considerations — that is, cause-effect considerations — from the terminology. Nonetheless it was felt that this change did not go far enough in banishing psychoanalytic concepts.

The second step was *DSM-III* (1980), a major change because it was cleansed of all psychoanalytic referents, with "mental disorders" to be defined by inclusion and exclusion criteria.[2] A saving grace, however, was its introduction of a diagnostic template known as the "multiaxial system." This consisted of five factors or *axes*:

Axis I	Psychiatric disorders
Axis II	Personality disorders
Axis III	Medical conditions
Axis IV	Psychosocial [environmental] factors
Axis V	Degree of disability

All subsequent editions incorporated these changes until the release of *DSM-5* in 2013.

To be sure I have always been ambivalent about the *DSM* diagnostic format. On the positive side, apart from having to deal with picky insurance companies and governmental agencies, I liked the way it focused attention on the person in the context of his or her environment. It represented an affirmation of the *biopsychosocial* ideology of mid-century psychiatry, an era in which psychiatry hoped to advance beyond mind/body and unconscious/conscious dualisms.

But on the negative side, and a major defect in my view, is the topsy-turvy alignment of the five axes: I thought it completely upside down in its emphasis. For example, in my experience, two individuals fully qualified for a diagnosis of Social Phobia can vary widely in the degree of disability. One might be totally homebound but the other able to shop, attend appointments, and the like despite discomfort. Similarly, variations in the degree and quality of social support will require hospitalization for one youngster with Endogenous Depression (see chapter 5) but not another similarly troubled. The same is true of hallucinations in Schizophrenia. At this very moment I am following a patient who is completely immobilized at home because of them, but two others who are fully functional despite them.

In my mind, therefore, I would mentally rework the formula as follows:

Axis I	Degree of emotional disability
Axis II	Social support: present vs. absent, positive vs. negative
Axis III	Medical issues (a major component of disability in the injured and aged)
Axis IV	Degree of inability to learn from experience; trauma history present or absent
Axis V	Psychiatric disorder

This revision has the advantage of emphasizing Dr. Schiele's idea of *target symptoms*. If I begin by clearly recognizing the degree of symptom disability, this naturally leads to an inquiry regarding its source and a consideration of factors that might contribute to the indicated psychiatric disorder. I am more likely to avoid detours and blind alleys. Even within the boundaries of a multiaxial approach, I find that placing disability and social support issues foremost creates better understanding and management. In short, there are certain "psychiatric" issues that need more than medication.

The final step in the demotion of dynamic formulation occurred with the appearance of *DSM-5*, which more or less eliminated the five-axis concept. *DSM-5*, in an ambiguous disclaimer,[3] appears to disavow the multiaxial notation of prior editions, yet seems to retain it in part by continuing Axes I and II. In my view this discards the best features of what I consider a dubious exercise to begin with, while including the worst. True, the manual (sort of) revives the former Axes IV and V by including, after 703 pages devoted to diagnostic considerations, some sixteen pages describing *Assessment Measures* followed by another twelve regarding *Cultural Formulation*. The meager space devoted to each is obviously an indication of their relative insignificance in the minds of the manual's editors.

In fact the (former) director of the National Institutes of Mental Health (NIMH), Dr. Thomas Insel, reportedly questioned the significance of the entire *DSM-5* diagnostic approach. He noted it is not based on objective laboratory measures but rather relies on a poorly validated consensus of expert opinion. Instead he advocated the development and support of an alternative: Research Domain Criteria (RDoC), an initiative supported by NIMH. It was based on the concept of mental disorders as biological phenomena, and investigators hoped to map relevant cognitive, circuit, and genetic aspects.[4] A spirited commentary followed the news of this apparent research 180, including a (kind of) disclaimer from Dr. Insel. But it is clear that RDoC is here to stay, and that the entire *DSM-5* nosology remains a matter of opinion rather than science.

The End of Dynamic Formulation

More was banished with the appearance of *DSM-III* than just psychoanalytic notions regarding causality: the credibility of all dynamic considerations that attempted to link observable effects—signs and symptoms—to cause was undermined. In theory designated as "disorders," in practice psychiatric categories came to be considered diseases-in-waiting, hanging suspended while researchers labored to identify their biological and neurological referents.

It seemed to me this was a consequence of a change in psychiatric leadership as department chairpersons retired in the decade preceding the appearance of *DSM-III*. It was not that their replacements were less qualified. Indeed, typically their credentials and experience were impressive … when it came to research. Thus, understandably, their major interest was in producing more researchers and professors, less in training practitioners of psychiatry. I believe this change in emphasis is illustrated in yet another Dr. Kolb anecdote from my residency years, my final memory of him.

It was his practice to hold monthly meetings with us residents, a sort of informal briefing on what was happening at PI and things psychiatric in the world beyond. Toward the end of our training, we were again assembled for what would be our last contact with him. He had some parting words of advice: "When you open your practice do not accept a patient until you encounter one with an Endogenous Depression that you can treat with electroshock therapy. When he or she recovers your reputation will be made." End of meeting.

I walked out with a warm feeling, again bathed by his avuncular concern which yet supports me these fifty years later. However, it was not until about forty-five years later when I started this book that the deeper significance of his words occurred to me—not unusual when it came to fully appreciating Dr. Kolb's wisdom.

Which is this: he viewed his goal as primarily training practitioners of psychiatry, not professors. Not that our class lacked the talent to further qualify and succeed in academia. In fact, one of my classmates, John Talbott, was later elected president of the American Psychiatric Association. Rather, I suspect Dr. Kolb believed that psychiatry needed to be clinically grounded in the trial and error of tangible patient contact as the foundation of a professional career, in the midst of which research interests would flourish.

In my view, however, his idea has withered. Teaching psychiatric residents to incorporate their patients' life experiences when assessing symptom formation is no longer a priority. Now the emphasis is fitting symptoms into disease constructs. Consequently, interest in treatment strategies based on a dynamic integration of effect to cause—in other words, psychotherapy—withered. "Treatment" became synonymous with "medication."

Only recently has psychiatric leadership begun to address this issue in the person of the very eminent psychoanalyst and Baylor College of Medicine Professor of Psychiatry Glen O. Gabbard. He and his colleague Dr. Gerald Kay, taking note of an apparent split between psychotropic and psychotherapeutic treatment modalities, call for more integration of the two in residency training.[5] Likewise, psychiatric residents, sensing deficiencies in their training, have started to request instruction in and supervision of psychotherapy.[6]

In my view, training programs will experience some difficulties responding to such requests. Compared to the art of prescribing, psychotherapy is much more difficult to learn. In my day, after four years of medical school and one year of internship, we all came to psychiatry competent in the language of tangible science—the language of chemistry, pharmacology, genes, statistics, molecules—and with some prescribing experience as well. Our professors, understanding our curiosity and willingness to learn, saw little need to motivate us about mastering the burgeoning world of psychotropic treatment. They simply told us to read about medications, as did Dr. Kolb when he nagged me about starting a patient on lithium: "Dr. Curran! Look it up!" It was not necessary for him to coach me further. I was to read and learn by doing.

But the art of psychotherapy is a different matter indeed. It's hard to find an art or skill the acquisition of which is comparably arduous. In the 1960s, when the electronic media were in their infancy, opportunities to learn by observing were infrequent. I can recall only two instances: the interviews by Dr. Mesnikoff (above) and Dr. Searles. And learning by doing was unthinkable without strict supervision. Throughout the three years of our residency, we performed psychotherapy only under rigorous scrutiny by experienced practitioners. Will the directors of today's residency programs will be able to recruit a similarly qualified staff?

Consequences of Leadership Change

The withering of dynamic treatment formulations within psychiatry in favor of pharmacological ones is most regrettable, with many unhappy consequences both for patients and our profession.

Psychotherapy Ceded to Non-Psychiatrists

First of all, by the late 1960s decades of studies of the impact on symptom formation by conscious (that is, as opposed to unconscious) emotional and cognitive events had produced reliably effective dynamic treatment techniques. Investigators such as Joseph Wolpe and Hans Eysenck in the 1950s and, later, Albert Bandura determined that many patients' fears were learned; that is, the consequences of life events. They originated *Behavior Therapy* (BT), a technique designed to *decondition* and remove such learned fears via *extinction* (see volume 2 for a discussion of this and associated terms). In the same years, work by psychologist Albert Ellis and psychoanalyst Aaron Beck evolved *Rational Emotive Behavior Therapy* (REBT) and *Cognitive Therapy* respectively, the forerunners of what is now known as *Cognitive Behavioral Therapy* (CBT).[7] Both treatment strategies are designed to correct unrealistic and exaggerated assessments of dysphoric emotions, especially fear, anger, and guilt, provoked by life experience.

At the same time other theorists proposed that symptom development could in certain instances be understood as the consequence of person-to-person or person-to-group interactions. As they saw it, the determinants of behavior included *both* conscious and social processes. Anthropologist Gregory Bateson, therapist Jay Haley, and others originated the "double theory bind" of Schizophrenia, the gist of which is that the behavioral paralysis induced by simultaneous contradictory communications can precipitate psychosis in vulnerable individuals.[8] Later, Haley was instrumental in the development of Structural Family Therapy (SFT) by child psychiatrist and psychoanalyst Salvador Minuchin, derivatives of which are widely used today by family therapists.[9]

For the most part ignored by psychiatry, training in psychotherapy derived from these explanatory (that is, dynamic) theories boomed in related professions, especially among psychologists and social workers.

Treatment Repertoire of Psychiatry Impoverished

Psychiatrists were stranded without a "therapy hat" to don when faced with a medication nonresponder such as Helen (chapter 2). Ever since the birth of the Antidepressant era in the late 1950s, psychiatry has been haunted by the patient who not only does not respond to treatment with an Antidepressant, but also to subsequent trials, sometimes three or four or more. This is a formidable issue—so-called "nonresponsiveness"—that has been addressed at length in the literature, more briefly here below.

Implied therein, the alert reader will realize, is my belief that some "Antidepressant nonresponsiveness" is actually a misdiagnosis caused by a failure of psychiatrists to realize that the "depression" of which patients complain may actually be erroneous thinking—a cognitive issue. Such patients (see Rebecca, chapter 8) blame themselves for things that are beyond realistic immediate control: for example, difficult children or partners or coworkers or relatives. Or for the minute-to-minute mood swings and anxiety that are commonly a major consequence of trauma-impaired trust. Or for the chronic pain of physical disability. Or—a major consideration of this book—for fears of making a commitment. Or, as paradoxical as this may seem, for fears of feeling happy.

The list goes on and on, which pays tribute to human ingenuity when it comes to avoiding the realization that living is a risky business indeed. More comforting is the anodyne of blame. But such comfort is not without cost. Seeking forgiveness or punishment not only cedes power to an external source, but impedes learning from experience. If as psychiatrists we fail to recognize such crippling thinking, we condemn our patients to endless suffering.

For a psychiatrist without a psychotherapy option, the only alternative is to reach for the prescription pad. The cognitive issues are not addressed and the patient is at risk of exile to the purgatory of nonresponsiveness and sustained misery.

The Illusion of Objectivity

As I noted earlier, *DSM-III* eschewed psychoanalytic concepts in favor of "objective" thinking. Mental disorders were now to be defined by inclusion and exclusion criteria, as reported by the patient or observed by others or the clinician at direct examination, a nosological convention which has endured in all *DSM* revisions to date. Take, for example, Major Depressive Disorder (MDD), a diagnosis frequently utilized in outpatient work by physicians and clinicians, as described in *DSM-5*.[10] To qualify for this diagnosis, a patient must demonstrate at least five of nine criteria, all of which are discussed at length in the manual. A careful review of the discussion, however, reveals that only four criteria (mood, energy, psychomotor activity, and cognitive activity) are susceptible to observation at direct examination by the clinician or researcher. In other words, only four criteria demonstrate the tangibility that the notion of *objectivity* implies.[iii]

The others require reporting, either by the patient or by collaterals. That is, they are *subjective*, a matter of opinion. Now, in the hands of experienced clinicians, subjective reports—after all, every history by nature is subjective—are not to be discounted if deemed authentic. No mental status examination is complete without both observed and reported behaviors, which is why all the case reports in this book include both. Thus I always begin an interview with an open-ended statement such as "Fill me in" or "Tell me about your adventures." But as necessary and as informative as such accounts are, they are not objective. They are opinions, as are statements from collaterals: informed opinions, yes; crucial opinions, yes; on occasion life-and-death opinions, yes; but still opinions and, therefore, not objective and not the stuff of science. Hence the NIMH preference for the Research Domain Criteria.[iv]

Actually I first encountered this problem soon after I joined Dr. Schiele's ECDEU research group at Anoka State Hospital in

---

iii. Of course, what might be tangible to one observer might be illusive to another, which is the bane of all research.

iv. The diagnosis of Major Depressive Disorder is further complicated by the need, according to the handbook, to consider the presence or absence of nine subcategories, that is, nine additional sets of "objective" inclusion or exclusion criteria.

1965. To assess the antipsychotic potential of the novel compounds under investigation, we used the sixteen-item Brief Psychiatric Rating Scale (BPRS). One of my several duties was to rate each study patient each week for the duration of the study, taking into account both interview and reported behavior, on a one-to-seven scale. I eventually learned I could make a rating determination based on direct mental status observation on only half of the sixteen items. For the other half, per instructions, I was allowed to solicit staff observations—and that was the rub. Not all of the staff were observant, and not all of the study subjects were easy to observe because, as a group—very characteristic of institutionalized individuals—they avoided social interaction, therefore making it difficult to assess their mental contents. In my opinion this reduced the reliability of the ratings and, consequently, the validity of our research. I suspect Dr. Schiele, no fool he, eventually took note that I was no longer a true believer, which undoubtedly also contributed to his letting me go.

It was because of the unreliability of subjective observations that later, when it came to assessing the outcome of our token economy program, we chose not to make use of rating scales to evaluate change. Instead we decided to tabulate status—for example, degree of privileges—and for three reasons:

- Status and changes in status are recorded on doctor's order logs; that is, are unequivocally "objective."
- Status is a direct measure of social competence and skills.
- Status change is a direct measure of improvement or lack of thereof.

Comorbidity

The diagnosis of patients such as Jackie (chapter 4) is complicated by the issue of *comorbidity*. This is one of the persisting issues with *DSM-5* (and earlier editions). The mental and emotional diagnostic categories compiled therein are more or less mutually exclusive in theory, but not so in practice. It is unusual to find a situation where one, and only one, diagnosis accounts for all of a patient's history, complaints, symptoms, and findings, although I have a vivid recall of an exception from some forty years ago.

At that time I served as a court-appointed consultant to the Hennepin County Probate Court. Once a month in the company of another consultant, Dr. Carl Schwartz, and referee George Adzik, along with attorneys for both the plaintiff and respondent, we all traveled from hospital to hospital to participate in commitment hearings on allegedly mentally ill patients. Prior to each hearing, Dr. Schwartz, a very experienced and perceptive psychiatrist, and I interviewed the proposed patient and then presented our findings at the subsequent hearing. On this particular day the first patient was a textbook example of Paranoid Schizophrenia. Later in the day we encountered a classic case of Acute Schizophrenia, and still later unquestionable Catatonic Schizophrenia.[v] At the end of the day I commented to Dr. Schwartz how rare it was to encounter even one textbook case, let alone three, in one day. He just grunted, in assent I think.

Otherwise the conscientious clinician typically requires two (or more) diagnoses to present a complete assessment per *DSM-5* guidelines even with patients who demonstrate a minimum of emotional disability. In many instances this is due to overlapping *DSM-5* criteria. For example, four of the six criteria for Generalized Anxiety Disorder (restlessness, fatigue, difficulty concentrating, sleep disturbance) are also among the criteria for Major Depressive Disorder. Should such anxious patients then blame themselves for the impaired functioning, a common misinterpretation of disability as I have discussed

---

v. Now no longer viewed as a Schizophrenia subcategory but as a manifestation of some other mental disorder.

above, the self-reproach may be interpreted by the unwary clinician as fulfilling yet another MDD specifier, creating the potential for a double diagnosis. I fell into this trap myself when treating Rebecca. Consequently I now prefer to coach patients to use the term "stression" instead of "depression" as they relate their issues. Indeed, in my view it is likely that all Depression coexists with anxiety; for example, the Endogenous Depression of William Styron or the Rapid Cycling Mood Disorder of Rose (chapter 9). For this reason I support the movement within psychiatry to replace categorical assessment with dimensional assessment. For example, recently investigators demonstrated that targeting Major Depression *symptom clusters* rather than *overall severity* produces more effective and predictable Antidepressant treatments.[11]

To their credit, in their preface the *DSM-5* Task Force Chairs Drs. David J. Kupfer and Darrel A. Regier recognize the comorbidity issue.[12] And they include a section that not only recognizes the potential benefits of dimensional diagnosis, but also includes sample assessment measures.[13]

Misdiagnosis of Attachment-Related Distrust

Comorbidity is more a technical than a clinical issue. It usually does not lead to serious treatment errors. At its worst it may lead to the purgatory of "nonresponsiveness" from which patients escape via clinician trial and error or by obtaining a second opinion, or by the clinician coming to his senses as I did after ten years of struggling with Rebecca's "depression."

Misdiagnosis is a different matter. If the trust issues precipitated by abuse or loss are not recognized, but instead labeled, for example, as a Personality Disorder or Mood Disorder, such individuals are at risk of treatment amplifying their attachment disability. The distrust becomes pathologized and attempts to manage it focus on hospitalization and Antipsychotics. An outstanding example of this is presented in chapter 4: Jackie and the dread and turmoil her behavior provoked throughout our psychiatric community, leading to frequent unproductive hospitalizations. But she did much better while hospitalized on our unit because one effect of the token economy was to establish boundaries for both staff and patient, thus minimizing the risk of igniting her mistrust. It was not until years later, after she had established a zone of more or less safe relationships, that she began to reveal her childhood abuse, and then only obliquely. We were lucky—as was she—that the token economy, designed to promote impulse management, had the unintended benefit of also promoting trust management.

But token strategies or their equivalent are neither feasible nor available for current psychiatrists. They will have to rely on a sensitivity to and awareness of distrust as a possible manifestation of attachment issues. Which means psychiatric training must go beyond symptom description to symptom development; that is, it must be extended to include dynamic—cause and effect—considerations. Otherwise the treatment of attachment-disabled patients will be botched.

For example, Rita.

[Case Study]
Understanding Rita

She is a twenty-four-year-old unemployed mother, seen with her two-year-old, referred by her therapist, who is concerned about her "crazy behavior." Her complaints also include anger outbursts, many fears and anxieties, "depression," difficulty maintaining regular employment, and insomnia. Most troublesome of all is emotional lability. People tell her she's immature, impulsive, critical, with no sense of humor when they joke with her. She's been this way as long as she can remember. She has heard from her mother that her childhood was "troubled." As a teenager she took psychotropics, saw a counselor, did well. But then while babysitting she discovered her sister's three-month-old infant dead from sudden infant death syndrome. To this day she still has flashbacks of the lifeless body.

She dropped out of treatment, began a pattern of hanging out with what sound like slackers, punks, and minor criminals. Eventually she met her partner, who, in contrast to the others, treats her with respect. She became pregnant. Motherhood and his support have settled her down a bit.

When I inquire about the "crazy behavior," she is quite frank. Just recently she "disappeared" for twenty-four hours, went to a biker bar, had a drink, then stepped out of the bar and deliberately provoked a group of biker chicks hanging around outside. One threatened to beat her up. "Go ahead," she taunted. Fortunately a bouncer broke things up before anyone was hurt.

Consequently I asked Rita if she had a pattern of deliberately irritating people, "bugging them … make then angry." Yes, she does that to her partner. In fact, she can't figure out why he stays with her. This is why she "disappeared." But he just won't give up on her. It turns out this is also an issue with female coworkers; she doesn't trust the ones who are nice to her and try to help her. So she gets "snappy" to push them away. If that doesn't work, she quits.

At mental status examination she is cooperative, compliant, well dressed and groomed, forthright, spontaneous, without evidence of psychomotor retardation or acceleration, negative thinking, shaky impulse control, irritability, inattentiveness, or thought disorder. She denies substance use or legal issues. She is intelligent and thoughtful, attentive to her youngster, who is very well behaved, busy playing with toys.

In short, her interview behavior stands marked contrast to her history. What is going on?

Rita's situation is a good example of a focus on developing an *understanding* of emotional disability providing more clarification than a preoccupation with making a *diagnosis* of mental illness.

At first glance it seems obvious that she is eager for help, and there is no obvious target disability. So I decide to let her tell her story, reserving for later an inquiry about the "reckless behavior," the nominal target disability.

She takes full advantage of the opportunity, needing few prompts to relate her current issues and past history. When I finally ask about the "crazy" behavior, she continues to be quite frank. Her history of trauma residuals and her mother's hints of a "troubled" childhood certainly suggest abandonment issues. Hence, based on this hunch, I finally focus the interview: Does she have trouble trusting and accepting regard? Does she push people away with her behavior? With little hesitation she endorses the concept of "using" behavior as a device to manage caring relationships, to feel safer behind a wall of provocative and irritating stunts. Here is powerful confirmation of an emotional disability due to unresolved attachment conflicts.

Management of Rita

It seems that Rita fully grasps that her "mental problems" may represent an emotional problem. That is, she has realized some *clarification*. The next step for her is to learn to practice *acceptance*, recognizing that her concerns about trusting are deep-seated, yet not blaming herself for this vulnerability. She needs to learn not to think, *Why do I have trust issues?* but rather, *I have trust issues!* In therapist-speak, she needs to *own the pain without the blame*. So I conclude by suggesting she review the idea with her therapist. Also, that she sign a release so I can send her a copy of my consultation to share with her therapist (and others) if she wishes. Finally, I recommend a follow-up evaluation in three months or so.

Rita and Diagnosis of Mental Illness Versus Understanding of Emotional Disability

In the introduction I recommended that assessment of attachment disability proceed by way of *understanding*, rather than a formal *diagnostic* evaluation, in order to cultivate trust and avoid making things worse. The obvious question is, How might a business-as-usual diagnostic interview actually create risk for Rita? Would it not, in fact, mitigate risk by focusing on a specific psychiatric disorder meriting treatment?

With Rita, a standard diagnostic exercise would begin with creating a summary of relevant findings, which might include as a minimum:

Elicited history
- Trauma residuals
- Inconstant employment
- Troubled childhood
- Prior psychiatric contacts
- Episodes of provocative behavior

Mental status
- Complaints of outbursts, fears, "depression," unstable mood
- Cooperative, compliant, forthright, affectionate with child, absence of findings

At first glance, even with reference to the five-axis template, it is hard to get your diagnostic arms around such a conglomeration of data. Rita would seem to qualify for inclusion in just about every major diagnostic category.

- Posttraumatic Stress Disorder (24)
- Attention Deficit Disorder (18)
- Unspecified Impulse Control Disorder
- Bipolar Disorder (11)
- Major Depressive Disorder (9)
- Schizoaffective Disorder (23)
- Borderline Personality Disorder (9)

The figures in parenthesis after each category are rough counts of the various inclusion and exclusion criteria to consider while determining the most likely diagnostic fit—an enervating task for even the orderly mind. For help you could consult an algorithm incorporating a decision tree based on the *DSM* criteria items. If consciously completed, the result might suggest one of the above as the most *probable* diagnosis. But also listed would be several of the others, and perhaps even one or two you had never considered, in order of declining probability. Only residents in training fully engage in this formal exercise.

In practice, however, I suspect most psychiatrists, employing Dr. Schiele's target symptom format, would find the provocativeness of greatest significance and diagnose Borderline Personality Disorder or, taking into account hints of periodicity, perhaps a Bipolar Disorder.

While the former does possess some superficial validity inasmuch as it captures her primary conflict—abandonment—it mischaracterizes her abandonment valence. Rita does not fear abandonment. Rather, she fears she will *not* be abandoned. Unless she and any therapist who works with her explicitly discuss and understand this, treatment will fail. Her confrontations will continue, not only undermining her employability but inviting potentially dangerous retaliation. She needs to learn how to negotiate boundaries with words, not provocations.

Current Psychiatric Assessment: A Plea for Reform

On the other hand, certain of her complaints—such as the emotional lability, her anger outbursts, "depression," and difficulty maintaining regular employment in conjunction with the "recklessness"—might strike some therapists and psychiatrists as evidence of a bipolar process, perhaps even Rapid Cycling. Such a diagnosis would put her at risk of treatment with Mood Stabilizers and Antipsychotics, with their attendant potential of serious side effects yet with little potential for benefit.

Compare this to my assessment, reworked as discussed above, based on just the one interview:

Axis I: *Emotional disability*—Mistrust of closeness. Degree remains to be determined; e.g., limited to coworkers and partner vs. extending to all adults.

Axis II: *Social support*—Ability to solicit/tolerate remains murky.

Axis III: *Medical conditions*—No disability

Axis IV: *Personality*—History of inability to learn from experience during later adolescence suggests notable trauma fallout. Current inability to learn less dangerous ways of dealing with closeness now suggests some persisting trauma residuals. Compliance with treatment may be an issue. Time will tell.

Axis V: *Psychiatric Diagnosis*
    Attachment Disorder
    Trauma residuals
    Rule Out Attention Deficit Disorder
    R/O Personality Disorder
    Doubt Bipolar Issue

Note how this revision of the multiaxial format leads naturally to a clinical impression and summary, which might run as follows:

> *Impression:* Of course, in the absence of collateral information and medical records this is a very tentative assessment. Nonetheless, the biker chick episode (which in retrospect now strikes her as "crazy" to an extreme), her preference for marginal characters, and her inability to trust her partner and nominally helpful coworkers taken together suggest an attachment issue. Her pattern of irritating ("snappy") provocations to defeat intimacy is characteristic. Whether this all stems from the crib death incident or in part from her prior "troubled" childhood is unclear. What is clear, however, is her trust issue. Further information will be necessary to assess the contribution, if any, of attentional issues. At present a Mood Disorder seems unlikely. Collateral information from her partner and her mother will help sort this out.
>
> Management will be problematic because of her problem with trusting. Perhaps the best way to proceed here would be a frank discussion of the trust issue plus her trauma experience.

An Idea Neglected: Attachment Theory Marginalized

Defined by Bowlby and elaborated by Winnicott in the 1950s, the concept of attachment was at first widely endorsed by health professionals. Subsequently, however, it appeared to lose significance judging from the tally of citations in the Becker-Weidman handbook (Introduction), suggesting that even among child care workers there was at first little recognition of its lingering impact on both later childhood and adult relationship development.

Only in the last three decades, as the susceptibility of emotional stability and life performance to attachment disruption have become more widely appreciated, has the literature begun to recognize Attachment Disability, by manifestation if not by name.[vi]

In my view, the awakening began with authentic accounts of posttraumatic symptoms and subsequent disability among 9/11 survivors and EMT personnel, which served to alert both the public and professionals to a problem that was previously "kept in the closet" by trauma victims. Later, however, when reports appeared that a significant percentage of Iraq and Afghanistan veterans demonstrated combat-related PTSD, veterans of other wars—Vietnam, Korea, even World War II—began to come forward with their accounts of persisting trauma. Very recently, researches have uncovered evidence of a genetic susceptibility to PTSD, which may account for the fact that symptoms appear in only 5 to 10 percent of individuals exposed to severe trauma.[14]

The question becomes, Why the decades of neglect?

There are at least two causes, as I see it.

First of all, while both Bowlby and Winnicott recognized that the quality of early childhood attachments had profound lifetime implications, this aspect of their thinking was overlooked. This was unquestionably true in my case, as I described at length. At Anoka State Hospital in the late 1960s we developed a highly effective program of managing hospitalized treatment-resistant inpatients based in part on Winnicott's notion of adolescent acting-out as a disguised plea for help. Yet subsequently I perceived attachment issues as *strictly limited to childhood*, a clinical agnosia of sorts, so to speak.

In my case this was somewhat understandable because thereafter in my clinical work, both public and private, I had little need to make use of Winnicott's powerful insights. In great part this was due to the nature of my practice. I saw very few

---

vi. This may not be true of the international literature.

adolescents because of changes in referring patterns. It was not until the early 2000s—some thirty-five years later!—that his name popped back into my consciousness as I began to see more adolescents in both my consulting work and private practice.

On the other hand, it is difficult to understand how those whose practice was focused on serving children and adolescents failed to remain aware of attachment concepts. I will leave it to historians of the American child care movement to trace the origins of its agnosia, especially its neglect of Winnicott.

A second, more obvious cause, as I discussed earlier, is the overhaul of psychiatric leadership in the 1970s that radically revised psychiatric nosology in 1980 with the publication of *DSM-III*.

To recapitulate, symptom description replaced symptom development. Consequently dynamic thinking—that is, cause-effect thinking—about symptom genesis atrophied. Assessment shrank to perusing a menu of labels, which served to paralyze curiosity, while treatment became medication focused rather than disability focused. The ultimate misstep, in my view, was the creation of the five-axis format, which was subsequently appropriated by all bureaucracies—health and disability insurance companies, state and county welfare agencies, federal agencies—as the definitive expression of case assessment. Thus did a preoccupation with five-axis terminology come to invade the awareness of all parties seeking to obtain or deny benefits and reimbursement. Unfortunately demoted to fifth place was the notion of "target symptom" disability, to employ Dr. Schiele's language, a clarifying concept for me in view of the murkiness of my residency experiences.

Thus entombed by establishment leadership, assessment in psychiatry became the rigid, sclerotic, unimaginative creature of concern to Dr. Tasman and Drs. Gabbard and Kay, as well as Dr. Insel, as expressed in his preference for the NIMH Research Domain Criteria. Fortunately there are signs that the establishment is beginning to shake off its lethargy. A recent lead editorial in the *American Journal of Psychiatry,* citing evidence of the effectiveness of interpersonal psychotherapy (ITP) in the treatment of PTSD, calls on "us" to remain aware that "there may be multiple therapeutic routes to achieve the same beneficial outcome."[15] I wonder to whom the "us" is directed.

Current Psychiatric Assessment: Whence from Here?

In my view it is imperative that psychiatry come to its senses and escape from the dungeon of *DSM* thinking. Not only children, adolescents, and young adults with Attachment Disability, the nominal topic of this book, are susceptible to its constraints. All individuals with emotional disability, especially the physically disabled and the aging, are vulnerable because their ability to trust may be compromised as their physical independence is undermined. Consequently attachment issues, previously managed and held in abeyance via a lifetime of activity and achievement, threaten resurrection.

Psychiatry must develop the capacity to recognize and understand attachment issues as well as the ability to convey that awareness to other professionals, parents, sponsors, and caretakers. As I have emphasized throughout this book, Attachment Disability stems from injured trust of trauma. Psychiatry cannot hope to prevent the abandonments, lost relationships and health, neglect, and abuses that are inevitably part of life. Its goal, therefore, must be remediation—to avoid making things worse.

In education, as I plan to discuss in volume 2, remediation takes the form of abandoning mandatory school attendance. Forcing what comes naturally—learning—risks precipitating or accelerating the distrust that wounded youngsters bring to school.

In psychiatry, remediation must take the form of revitalizing the profession and moving it away from the sterile, narrow assessments that misdiagnose and mismanage so many traumatized adolescents and adults. Dr. Tasman ends his vignette (see the introduction) wondering how many other patients are misdiagnosed. I do not wonder at all.

My Suggestions

First a historical perspective.

Today we clinicians are left traversing a shaky diagnostic footbridge between the evaporating credibility of the past and the hope of a future reduction of psychiatric phenomena to quantitative neurophysiological processes. What today we deem psychiatric "science" is actually a protoscience, a process of data accumulation the goal of which is to generate testable hypotheses. Pick up any recent issue of two widely followed psychiatric journals, *JAMA Psychiatry* or *American Journal of Psychiatry,* and you will find it crammed with data generated by original investigations of the entire range of psychiatric phenomena in an attempt to reliably identify their biological referents.

Psychiatry's effort to quantify mental and emotional processes brings to mind the career of the sixteenth-century Danish astronomer Tycho Brahe. His life was devoted to compiling precise observations of the stars, year after year diligently recording their positions as accurately as possible. Not satisfied with the relatively crude instruments of his day, he constructed his own, sometimes of massive proportions, to refine his measurements. After his death, his assistant, Johannes Kepler, derived his celebrated three laws of planetary motion from Brahe's star tables, a simplification that eliminated the need for the epicycles of Ptolemaic theory to account for the retrograde motion of the planets.

Today we have not one but a host of Tychos at work map-ping another world, the inner world of brain function, compiling and refining data. And, as with Tycho, advances in instrumentation have propelled this surging research initiative: rapid and inexpensive genome analysis, a variety of noninvasive brain imaging techniques, and the development of sophisticated statistical techniques to analyze massive, research-generated data banks. But what we need is the equivalent of a Kepler to collapse the data to a testable set of laws describing the *totality* of psychiatric phenomena.

Henry A. Nasrallah, editor in chief of *Current Psychiatry*, recently addressed this need in his editorial "Is there only 1 neurobiologic psychiatric disorder, with different clinical expressions?"[16] He cites a recent meta-analysis of nearly two hundred brain imaging studies that concludes major categories of psychiatric disorders all involve damage to the same regions of brain cortex.[17] He also notes the emergence of evidence that suggests psychiatric disorders may rise from a shared genetic foundation.[18] Surveying the universe of psychiatric illnesses, he then points out that all can be viewed as the product of fixed illogical thinking difficult to modify, despite experience to the contrary, because of cortical/genetic restrictions.[vii] Thinking it would be wonderful, he concludes: "If brain research steers psychiatric nosology in the direction of a common core, we might end up with a ten-page *DSM*." In her journal editorial, "The Neural Correlates of Transdiagnostic Dimensions of Psychopatholgy," Dr. Deanna Barch also expresses cautious hope that testable hypotheses encompassing wider spectrums of behavior dysfunction are forthcoming.[19] Citing separate journal articles investigating three different domains of psychiatric disorders — cognitive control, reward processing, suicidality — she

---

vii. In other words all psychiatric illness may be viewed as the consequence of learning failure, which, if true, would imply that our basic task as psychiatrists is to promote learning. This is why I emphasize in this book the notion of *understanding* and *managing* psychiatric disability versus its *diagnosis* and *treatment*. I will address this in volume 2.

concludes that such studies, "may give rise to core behavioral dimensions of psychopathology."

The bold speculations cited by Drs. Nasrallah and Barch require testing, of course. And while the textbooks portray science as a journey of progressive triumphs, along the trail is a litter of failed hypotheses. Kepler was no exception. In the years before he derived his justly celebrated laws, he devised elegant theories hoping to preserve traditional concepts of symmetry amid circular motion. But these failed the test of Tycho's data.[20] Whether meta-analysis or transdiagnostic investigation of neurobiologic data proves to be a reliable guide remains to be seen. Thus we remain waiting for our Kepler.

American Psychiatric Association President Paul Summerfield made reference to this when he recommended patience and playing "the long game" while waiting for advances in neuroscience and genomic analysis to produce practical clinical interventions because of the "complexity of what we are studying."[21]

I can imagine a day when it will be possible to reproducibly define the neurobiological determinants of a specific mental or emotional phenomenon, such as, say, a disabling compulsion, or panic, or hallucination. But I suspect brain function will turn out to demonstrate quantum behavior: that is, as you turn up the magnification, as you more precisely define one brain phenomenon, more and more detail appears while associated phenomena begin to fade into a smear of probability.[viii] Hence our Kepler's task is not only formidable, but it is not immediately apparent. We remain stranded on our shaky footbridge. The

---

viii. All science, not just psychiatric science, confronts the magnification issue. For example, particle physicists using the Large Hadron Collider report tentative findings that suggest the existence of a fundamental new particle not predicted by the widely accepted Standard Model. Overby D. "Physicians in Europe Find Tantalizing Hints of a Mysterious New Particle." *The New York Times*. December 16:A16, 2015.

long game may prove to be an interminable game.

Thus, what are our options?

Continue to Play the Game in Its Current Format

That is, continue to rely on the diagnostic nomenclature of *DSM-5* despite what I and others view as its very significant deficiencies. The 1980 makeover of the *DSM* nomenclature was greeted as a diagnostic triumph and subsequently was adopted as "the de facto map of mental illness for every sector of society."[22] The unexpressed hope was that the diagnostic reliability provided by this revised system of measuring and tabulating mental illness would lead to therapeutic advances as well. True, certain clarifications have emerged: for example, realizing that catatonia is not a Schizophrenia subtype, or distinguishing Bipolar II as a separate mood category. However, the successive *DSM* iterations have not featured a reductive trend, a collapse of more into less, the hallmark of scientific progress.

Indeed the opposite has taken place. Diagnostic categories have increased from 106 (*DSM-I*) to 182 (*II*), to 265 (*III*), to 292 (*III-R*), to 297 (*IV*), to 365 (*IV-R*), to the current 485 (my rough tally), reminiscent of the Ptolemaic epicycles necessary to preserve a geocentric astronomy. The *DSM-5* editors describe it as a "living document" and foresee it will be subject to "ongoing revisions."[23] Consequently, it is difficult to entertain any hope that subsequent *DSM* revisions will lead to an endgame.

Accelerate the Game via Curriculum Revision to Include More Neuroscience Content

Ross et al decry the failure of clinical psychiatry to reflect what they consider striking advances in brain science and understanding psychiatric illness.[24] Yet the practice of clinical psychiatry remains unchanged. They concede that certain barriers preclude the application of theory to clinical practice, recognizing that mastering current neuroscience requires intense investment in study time and energy because the volume and complexity of neuroscience are overwhelming. Another barrier is the orientation of most residency training faculty, which tends to favor clinical rather than neuroscience instruction. They recommend better communication between researchers and educators, collaborative curriculum development, and sharing of education strategies. A very promising development in this respect is the inauguration of an Educational Review series, a joint venture of clinician-educators and neuroscientists to promote neuroscience literacy, to be published in *JAMA Psychiatry*.[25]

Others also recognize the clinical/neuroscience gap, but rather than education deficiencies, they point to research priorities as the issue: Should biomarker investigation search for causal mechanisms or for predictive accuracy? Opposing viewpoints are presented in *JAMA Psychiatry* by well-qualified investigators, each side promoting its paradigm as more likely to meld science and practice.[26] One argues for pragmatism, that psychiatric science is not yet capable of rising to the level of explanation. The other, addressing the failure of psychiatric therapeutics to progress in recent decades, advocates for an intensive effort to identify disease mechanisms.

I have no doubt that this failure of neuroscience to invigorate clinical practice is of intense concern to academic psychiatry, of which the publication of this debate is a sign. However, as I mentioned earlier, psychiatric science remains a protoscience, a process of data collection and cataloguing. As Dr. Summerfield counsels, for now we must be content with practical measures. But this does not mean we can't propose grand, sweeping propositions to be tested because that is how our Keplers, our Watsons and Cricks will emerge. In other words, this debate is not a question of which approach is more likely to speed up the "game." The history of science tells us both the tortoise and the hare are part of the game.

Promote Collaborative Care

A third option is provided by the collaborative care model, an initiative that recommends social rather than neuroscience transformation of therapeutics through the integration of primary care and behavioral health. One of its advocates, Dr. Lon E. Raney, presents a comprehensive summary of the origins and practice of this model.[27] Included is a clinical vignette of effective collaborative care of a fifty-two-year-old divorced employed woman with depression and hypertension but without a trauma history. I recommend a careful review of the article for what is a promising development in health care as long as the reader does not equate "behavioral health" with "psychiatric expertise."

As the vignette and accompanying diagram illustrate, a professionally trained and accredited in-house "care manager" who has recourse to off-site indirect psychiatric consultation provides the greater share of behavior management and consultation. Occasionally there may be direct phone contact between the psychiatrist and primary physician, typically no more than three- to five-minute—"curbside"—consultations, regarding diagnosis and pharmacology options; less often, they may discuss other treatment alternatives including referral for formal psychiatric consultation. Otherwise most discourse is between psychiatrist and care provider. An important ingredient of this model is the formation, maintenance, and periodic review of a caseload registry that includes tracking tools to ascertain progress. "Twenty or more patients may be reviewed in an hour." It is unclear if the psychiatrist is on site or participates by phone or video conference. The process is highly informal and flexible, no notes are kept, and it allows for ad hoc contacts between scheduled reviews.

Throughout her detailed presentation, Dr. Raney makes it obvious that the psychiatric "expertise" required to promote a successful collaboration of this sort is not an extensive neuroscience background beyond providing diagnostic and psychotropic opinion. More important are certain personality traits such as flexibility, openness, clinical experience, and a willingness to educate and learn.

University of Washington (Seattle) psychiatrist Wayne Katon pioneered the idea of collaborative care; early in his career, he noted that depression frequently accompanied chronic illness. In a host of randomized controlled trials, he demonstrated that incorporating psychiatric and primary care improved treatment compliance, medical outcomes, and patient satisfaction. A more comprehensive, recent account of the model at work is his group's controlled study of 214 patients with diagnosed diabetes and heart disease, selected by high scores on depression rating scales.[28] Three part-time experienced nurses, specially trained according to the model's precepts, provided structured, individualized self-care and treatment goals. The nurses obtained weekly supervision by a psychiatrist and then conveyed the resulting recommended initial and subsequent medication changes to the treating primary physician. Analysis of the study results showed that medical and psychiatric outcomes were improved in the treatment group.

To my mind this and Dr. Katon's many other reports demonstrate that collaborative care is a medical advance that needs to be incorporated into all health care. However, here, in contrast to Dr. Raney's report, it appears there was no direct contact between the psychiatrist and the treating primary care physician. Psychiatric input seems to have been limited to providing psychotropic recommendations and options based on others' observations and ratings results. Thus again I caution not to equate collaborative care with psychiatric expertise, but to see it as the extension of behavioral health principles beyond the mental health clinic. As I discussed earlier, the behavioral health innovations of recent decades have been in great part originated either by psychologists or social workers, or by psychiatrists such as Aaron Beck, dissatisfied with traditional therapeutic techniques.

Current Psychiatric Assessment: A Plea for Reform

The vignette Dr. Raney presents is of a woman who was employable and without a trauma history. Dr. Katon's study properly excluded patients with a variety of disabilities and illnesses, suggesting the majority otherwise accepted were employed. True, both articles use symptom rating scales to confirm the presence of depression, but I have found that rating scales do not correlate well with disability. A separate rating of the Axis V Degree of Disability, which all behavioral health professionals routinely assess, would have clarified this ambiguity.

Disability is the Achilles's heel of health care. As physical disability progresses, patients are deprived of the financial and emotional security that productive activity provides. Moreover, smoldering youthful trauma residuals are prone to flare up and scorch an injured trust that never fully healed. In anticipation of rejection or exploitation, disabled patients become stressed, clingy, irritable, despondent, combative, or some combination thereof.[ix]

Therefore more, indeed much more, will be needed of psychiatry if it is to participate in the collaborative care of individuals with disability due to progressive degenerative medical illness. Simply providing what I call "label and pill" advice for this population will not do at all. Psychiatrists who choose to work in collaborative care must bring with them expertise in understanding and managing Attachment Disability as well as the personality traits described by Dr. Raney.

For example, a common complication of progressive degenerative illness is chronic pain. In my experience such patients frequently are referred out to chronic pain clinics. However, it would be much more efficient and clinically productive for a psychiatrist with some experience in group dynamics to arrange chronic pain conferences for patients and their families to teach pain management. The three therapeutic principles I presented above—clarification, acceptance, and focus—would serve as the

---

ix. The most frequent cause of 1,169 nursing home consultation requests referred to my office during 1991–2006.

basis for group discussion. Although the ostensible subjects of the group are the identified pain sufferers, the actual audience is their family support system, whose members are exhausted and discouraged by their failure to be of significant benefit. The idea is to educate them and model for them how to become co-therapists at home. In many respects this is actually an extension of consultation-liaison principles of the sort Dr. Kornfeld advocated, here with the consultation directed to the patient's family rather than the hospital staff.

Another more efficient use of psychiatric expertise would be to originate a continuous-case seminar for the clinic staff, as I did during my outreach to Elk River primary and secondary schools. Thus at weekly clinic staff meetings, a staff member recommends following an emotionally troubled patient—"depressed" or demanding or never satisfied or agitated, and so on—after presenting relevant data suitably disguised to protect the patient's identity. The behavioral health consultant poses to the assembled staff the question of whether the information supports the request and why or why not. If the staff identifies the presence of abandonment concerns, he requests suggestions regarding how the identified issue might be understood and then solicits management suggestions based on the consensus understanding. The plan is noted and the case is scheduled for review at a subsequent conference after the staff member has had a chance to interact with the patient per plan. Meanwhile in the next week another troubled patient is recommended for follow-up. Eventually the seminar reaches a limiting number of cases to review. As each one comes up for review, the prior understanding is reviewed for its accuracy and efficacy, then modified as needed, and again scheduled. Dropout patients are replaced with new cases. Of course, only a small percentage of clinic patients can ever be exposed to review of this sort. But if the proceedings are video recorded and cataloged for training purposes, all clinic staff and patients would benefit from the accumulation of expertise in identifying and managing abandonment issues.

To my mind, bringing into primary care group dynamics enhanced by consultation-liaison considerations combined with an understanding of the trauma triad is a fertile therapeutic opportunity. As our population ages, a growing share of primary clinic patients will demonstrate significant medical disability. In my experience, all physical disability, whether traumatic or degenerative, inevitably promotes or activates abandonment concerns. Our current psychiatric nomenclature and training do not adequately address this issue. How, then, can psychiatry provide leadership to primary physicians? My concern is that absent such expertise the psychiatric contribution to collaborative care is at risk of degenerating to medication management by proxy.

The Research Domain Criteria (RDoC)

Another option is to follow the lead of this NIMH-sponsored initiative and base mental health classification and treatment on genetic, neuro-, and behavioral science susceptible to dimensional quantification. The project identifies five current research "domains/constructs": negative affect such as anxiety and loss, reward learning and evaluation, cognitive systems including decision science, social processes including attachment formation, and sleep/arousal modulation.[29] I find this initiative very promising because it intersects with, as the attentive reader will note, several major themes of this book.

Moreover, according to a report from the annual meeting of the American Psychiatric Association, decision science includes exploration of nonconscious cognitive processes involved in symptom formation; that is, "the meaning inherent a person's behavior and the behavior's relevance to the patient's direct experience, just as Freud implored his disciples to do."[30] In other words, the RDoC approach does not preclude dynamic thinking. As I have argued, it is the absence of such in our *DSM* nosology that promotes assessment sterility and treatment mismanagement.

Psychiatrist and eminent authority on the genetic causes of mental illness Dr. Kenneth S. Kindler similarly supports a wider investigative stance. In his view, current studies of psychiatric disorders should focus on: 1) identifying risk factors, 2) clarifying and tracing their biological and social causal pathways, and 3) understanding how patients experience resulting symptoms.[31]

On the other hand, eminent researchers, including one of my heroes from my residency years, Dr. Donald F. Klein, question "the very scientific foundation that [RDoC] proclaims."[32] In a viewpoint the editor of *JAMA Psychiatry* solicited, the author notes that the dimensional approach obscures disability determination and lumps superficial similarities. Moreover, its validity remains undetermined. In the same issue there are two other solicited viewpoints and an editorial. The gist of the four seems to be that, yes, *DSM-5* is flawed but it is the best we have at present while waiting for a refinement that RDoC at present does not seem to offer. This also appears to be the position of the distinguished psychiatric educator and researcher Dr. William T. Carpenter, Jr. In a commentary appearing in the *American Journal of Psychiatry* he observes that the RDoC controversy is not whether it is "an alternate diagnostic paradigm," but whether its focus on neuroscience research will generate findings that sharpen "clinical diagnostic concepts."[33]

Formulate a Provisional Assessment Alternative

This brings us back to playing "the long game" as Dr. Summerfield proposed: that is, we create a provisional assessment alternative while waiting for further refinement of *DSM-5* or a valid dimensional alternative. This may endure for years, even decades. But no matter how well and how long the "game" is played, I have little hope that psychiatric science will evolve to include a depth of understanding that was discarded decades ago with the appearance of *DSM-III*.

Therefore I propose that we develop an interim assessment style, one that incorporates Dr. Kolb's dictum that all anxiety is due to separation. It might proceed as follows:

1. Begin with a clear distinction between mental illness and, as is true of all physical and mental illness, the emotional disability it generates. This recognizes that the cause of mental illness is in many cases an unknown intangible versus the real tangibility of disability. Think of signature mental illnesses such as acute or chronic dementia, or mood disorders, or Schizophrenia. Any professional who has even a passing contact with demented patients can't help but become profoundly aware of the emotional turmoil they experience as their cognitive skills decline. Mood disorders by definition exhibit profound emotional disability. And high rates of comorbid depression in Schizophrenia challenge "the validity of the traditional Kraeplinean dichotomy between disorders of thought and affect."[34]

2. Assume until proven otherwise that the emotional disability bringing patients to our attention is always anxiety related.

3. Also assume the anxiety involves abandonment and trust concerns, either overt or hidden, that are associated with the prospect of change and separation, whether immediate or pending, real or symbolic.

4. The degree of disability should be quantified. My preference is the former *DSM-IV* Axis V Global Assessment of Functioning (GAF), which is similar to the Physician's Global Judgement rating we employed on Dr. Schiele's ECDEU research unit. The editors of *DSM-5* express a preference for the WHO Disability Assessment Scale (WHODAS).[35] This is a self-rated scale and

therefore totally subjective. If it is to be used, I recommend it be completed by an observer familiar with the patient's functioning.

5. The disability is to be *understood* as the "target" (to use Dr. Schiele's phrase) of our attention. Inasmuch as if it is relieved, a host of secondary disabilities—for instance, marital or occupational dysfunction, substance use, underachievement—stand to be relieved or improved as well. The understanding is to be dynamic; that is, to include a careful historical search to ascertain its cause(s), recognizing such an investigation will always be open ended, incomplete, and subject to revision. Furthermore, its primary goal is not so much to inform *us* as to assist our patients to become self-informed. As I tell my patients, "My job is to not tell you *what* you are but to teach you to be your own life detective for you to understand *who* you are."

6. The understanding needs to *clarify* that the disability threatens the loss of relationships and therefore generates fear and anxiety about the possibility of unmet needs. These emotions are to be identified as a normal response to threat. If careful inquiry identifies the presence of trauma or the resurrection of past trauma, the loss of trust should also be identified as normal. Clarification is to include the notion that while patients are not to be blamed for their disability, they are responsible for living with its consequences. The language of clarification must be common sense, everyday, and nontechnical.

7. *Management* of the disability is to be directed toward teaching patients to *accept* their disability while avoiding making things worse. It also involves teaching patients to *focus* on what can be changed and inviting them to participate in promising therapeutic modalities. The idea is to mitigate maladaptive learning.

8. Classification of the disease may be categorical per *DSM-5*, dimensional per *DSM-5*,[36] or according to the RDoC format as it may evolve.

Of course this is just my sense of how to proceed in these uncertain times. Other concerned psychiatrists will no doubt find other promising paths to follow.

Some Implications

Dr. Ronald Pies, whose opinion I value highly, presents a fine discussion of the disease/disability dichotomy, which, as I learned, "has been a matter of contention since the dawn of clinical medicine."[37] His essay was occasioned by the appearance of a proposed disease entity, "systemic exertion intolerance disease" (SEID), aka Chronic Fatigue Syndrome. Some physicians object to the idea of recognizing SEID as a disease because its criteria do not require the identification of a specific cause or pathophysiological process. Dr. Pies questions this position.

He notes that some medical and the majority of psychiatric diagnoses are, properly, based on history and symptoms alone in conformity with our modern understanding of disease. In support he turns to *Harrison's Principles of Internal Medicine*, no doubt his favorite medical school textbook (and by chance mine as well), for a definition of disease, the gist of which is any condition that disables or limits the full exercise of our human potential and that inflicts suffering. I am certain my former mentor of years ago, Dr. Schiele, would agree. Such a broad definition of disease might well serve the treatment of medical patients, but not necessarily the management of psychiatric patients. The risk is that if psychiatric disability—the suffering—is not carefully distinguished from the disease that causes it, it may become pathologized and aggravated, especially if the disability includes angry affect, distrust, impulsivity, and so on.

For example, recall Mr. POP from chapter 10. He was nominally Schizophrenic—and I have no doubt about the validity of the diagnosis. Yet his anger was not suggestive of a disorganized psychotic but rather that of a hurt, resistive, and rejected youngster: people were against him, no one cared for him, we were going to overpower him, and so on. The correct response to this was to undermine the hidden fears behind his anger rather than to interpret it as evidence of disease requiring more medication, seclusion, and possibly extension of his commitment order.

In a similar vein, consider so-called Oppositional Defiant Disorder, which, to my dismay, lives on in *DSM-5*. I will not repeat here at length my objections to this label and the obtuseness that supports it. The *DSM-5* discussion[38] makes no mention of Winnicott or his insights regarding the unmet needs that drive the behaviors of angry youngsters—and by extension, adults—or the fears behind the anger. It is appalling to think of the mismanagement of generations of such troubled kids perpetuated by confusing disability with disease. The same is applicable to the unfortunate young adults whose glaring boundary issues not only go unrecognized but are contaminated by the "diagnosis" of Borderline Personality Disorder. In my view this is one of the more if not the most prejudicial of all psychiatric labels. It emphasizes their anger and distrust without recognizing the underlying fears of attachment and abandonment, predisposing untrained professionals to reject them.

Dr. Pies concludes his essay by stating that when patients are suffering and incapacitated, we are ethically obliged "to recognize that disease is present, and to do our utmost to treat it." One cannot disagree with this restatement of a physician's historic function, but I suggest it be amended to say that our function is both to treat disease and manage disability—and be able to recognize the difference. Earlier I stressed the need for psychiatrists to possess the flexibility to don a "therapy hat" when it appears that more is needed than a "medication hat." Another way to state this is that we need both a treatment hat for disease and, in order to facilitate learning, a management hat for disability.

What Form Might a Disease/Disability Format Take?

In considering the following examples, note that while the characterization of the disability is tangible, the putative disease that I cite is strictly provisional and awaits more precise characterization by subsequent research or perhaps nomination of another more plausible candidate causal agency.

1. For example, recall the work of investigators Swartz et al and Van Dam et al cited in the introduction regarding persisting changes in the amygdala and hippocampus of children and adolescents exposed to trauma. The disease here is the altered brain structures, the disability the trauma triad or PTSD or Depression, most likely a combination thereof.

Standard PTSD management techniques include prolonged exposure therapy, of which EMDR (chapter 13) is a variant. However, Markowitz and colleagues report that managing the disability via Interpersonal Therapy (IPT), derived from Bowlby's attachment concepts and focused on the emotional context of current relationships, is as effective as prolonged exposure therapy in relief of trauma symptoms arising from childhood and adult relationship trauma.[39] Participants demonstrated a high frequency of concurrent Axis II findings and Major Depression, limited social support, unemployment, and lack of response to prior psychotherapy and pharmacotherapy. None of these demographics should come as a surprise, especially the latter, because this is the outcome when disability becomes the disease: so-called "treatment resistance."

2. Or consider comorbid anxiety cum "depressive" disorders, discussed as "stression" in chapters 8 and 9, to which perimenopausal women are especially vulnerable. Recent work suggests that they experience increased stress because the fluctuating estradiol levels associated with menopause may change how their brain assesses the threat content of change-of-life events.[40] In my view, this, combined with hypothalamic-pituitary-adrenal axis dysfunction, represents a pathophysiological condition, but one not yet sufficiently characterized to qualify as a "disease." Nonetheless such women are more likely to demonstrate dysregulated emotions in response to perimenopausal events that symbolically or actually signal abandonment or separation. To classify this as a "mental disorder" per *DSM-5*—that is, as disease—distracts attention away from the precipitants and underlying predisposition. Treatment becomes synonymous with medication management of disease. The opportunity to learn about and manage vulnerability to emotional disability is endangered. Will it only be a rare patient who has the good fortune to be seen by a psychiatrist with the expertise of a Dr. Tasman?

3. Other candidates for the disease/disability distinction might include brain structure changes in ADHD[41] or evidence of state-dependent changes in mood regulation.[42]

4. Bleuler's division of Schizophrenic symptoms into primary (affect, ambivalence, autism, association) and secondary (hallucinations, delusions) is certainly congruent with a disease/disability format. To my way of thinking his insight represented an early intuition of the essence of the illness, the later stages of which we now identify as Deficit Schizophrenia. We now understand the earlier stages as a developmental process (suggested by neuroimaging evidence,[43] neuropsychological testing,[44] and postmortem brain examinations)[45] that cripples or

distorts sensory processing. In response, the NIMH developed the Recovery After an Initial Schizophrenia Episode (RAISE) initiative to promote both symptom reduction *and* functional recovery from first-episode psychosis. The idea is to move beyond the venerable standard of just medicating *disease* with Antipsychotics. Of equal if not greater importance is managing *disability* to prevent a slide into chronicity that culminates in Deficit Schizophrenia. Consequently through RAISE the NIMH sponsored the development of a comprehensive psychosocial—that is, learning—intervention for first episode psychosis, NAVIGATE.[46]

More than forty years ago at Anoka State Hospital, our team successfully originated a behavior modification program to enrich the social skills of treatment-resistant hospitalized "chronic" patients.[47] In it we remarked, "Mental hospitals have made relatively normal people deviant. Correctly understood and administered, mental hospitals should be able to make deviant people normal." It is reassuring to find that similarly innovative outpatient strategies are now in place to forestall the functional deterioration that otherwise predisposes to "chronicity." On the other hand, it is troubling that it took so long for psychiatry to recognize the vital role of learning in preventing disability.

5. I could continue here to cite many examples from recent issues of our major psychiatric journals to support my position. All include one if not several original investigations of putative structural or functional entities that, if not a disease state, may represent an early or contributing factor thereto. Of course, the greater share of such promising studies will flame out, but that is the nature of research on the science frontier. Of larger significance is that the research itself, regardless of its yield, defines the frontier and by doing so supports the disease/disability distinction I propose. In other words, perhaps these

studies represent our collective Tycho charting the inner world of neuroscience while we await our Kepler to meld it with the world of clinical therapeutics to produce the integration so devoutly advocated by Ross, Kindler, and others.

Notes

Preface
1. Jaynes J. *The Origins of Consciousness in the Breakdown of the Bicameral Mind* (Boston: Houghton Mifflin, 1976), 85–91.

Introduction
1. Van der Kolk B. *The Body Keeps the Score: Brain, Mind, and Body in the Healing of Trauma* (New York: Penguin, 2015), 1.
2. Vachon DD et al. "Assessment of the Harmful Psychiatric and Behavioral Effects of Different Forms of Child Maltreatment." *JAMA Psychiatry.* 2015; 72 (11): 1135–43.
3. Lahey BB. "Why Are Children Who Exhibit Psychopathology at High Risk for Psychopathology and Dysfunction in Adulthood?" Editorial. *JAMA Psychiatry.* 2015; 72 (9): 865–66.
4. Sourander A et al. "Association of Bullying Behavior at 8 Years of Age and the Use of Specialized Services for Psychiatric Disorders by 29 Years of Age." *JAMA Psychiatry* 73(2):159–65; 2016.
5. Becker-Weidman A, Ehrmann L, LeBow D. *The Attachment Therapy Companion: Key Practices for Treating Children and Families* (New York: W. W. Norton, 2009).
6. American Psychiatric Association. *Diagnostic and Statistical Manual of Mental Disorders, Fifth Edition.* (Arlington, VA: American Psychiatric Association, 2013), 265 ff.
7. Van der Kolk. *The Body Keeps the Score*, 190. The textbook he refers to is Freedman and Kaplan's *Comprehensive Textbook of Psychiatry*, an authoritative reference indeed. I had memorized it while preparing for my 1970 American Board of Psychiatry and Neurology examinations.

Chapter 1
1. Bowlby J. *Maternal Care and Mental Health* (New York: Schocken, 1951); *Attachment and Loss, vol. 1, Attachment* (New York, Basic Books, 1969/1982).
2. Werner EE, Smith RS. *Overcoming the Odds: High Risk Children from Birth to Childhood* (Ithaca, NY: Cornell University Press, 1992).
3. Salinger JD. *The Catcher in the Rye* (New York: Little, Brown & Co., 1951).
4. Winnicott DW. *The Child, the Family, and the Outside World* (London: Penguin, 1973), 43.
5. Ibid. 228. See also Winnicott DW. *The Maturational Process and the Facilitating Environment* (International Universities Press, 1965), 203.

Chapter 2
1. How our nervous system is organized to help us survive trauma, especially overwhelming trauma, is another topic too extensive for inclusion in this book. Again I recommend the standard texts on the subject. For a more focused exposition, I suggest the monograph by Bessel van der Kolk, *The Body Keeps the Score,* especially pp. 52–73, based on the premise "Dissociation is the essence of trauma."
2, I owe the notion of "Igor" to my colleague Dr. Richard Anderson, who got the idea from the wife of one of his patients. Watching him sketch a framework he used to portray the ingredients of rational vs. irrational responses to a frightening thought, she suggested using "Igor" to personify his conceptualization of the irrational as a "partially hidden, cunning enemy whose goal is to frighten and disable the self." He promptly adopted the nomenclature, which patients subsequently found helpful not to say amusing, especially in group therapy. Anderson RO. "Fighting Igor: Exposing and Resisting the Irrational Side Using Cognitive-Behavioral Principles in Group Therapy of Panic/Phobic Disorders." *Journal of Contemporary Psychotherapy.* 1998; 28 (1);5–34.
3. For a constructive response to disruptive classroom behavior, other than suspension, see Friedman M. "Suspensions don't make bad kids good. Here's what does." *Star Tribune,* February 28, 2012:A7.

4. Swendse J et al. "Use and Abuse of Alcohol and Illicit Drugs in US Adolescents."*Archives of General Psychiatry.* 2012 Apr;69(4)393.
5. Briefly, relapse programs depart from the traditional AA routine by teaching their participants to identify life "triggers"; that is, those events or experiences that in the past have preceded relapse. In other words, such programs focus on exposing the conditioned roots of addictive behavior. I will address this in detail in Volume 2 of this series as well as the notion that addiction prevention begins the very first day of school; that is, when youngsters are exposed to an environment that encourages the development of an adaptive repertoire.

Chapter 4
1. *DSM-5,* 464.
2. Twemlow SW, Sacco FC. *Preventing Bullying and School Violence* (Arlington, VA: American Psychiatric Publishing, 2012), 131.

Chapter 5
1. Curran J, Jorud S, Whitman N. "Unconventional Treatment of Treatment-Resistant Hospitalized Patients." *Psychiatric Quarterly.* 1971; 45(2), 188.
2. Ibid., 188, 207.
3. Ibid., 207.
4. Ibid., 206.
5. See for example, Weiden PJ. "Helping Patients with Mental Illness Get Back to Work." Editorial. *American Journal of Psychiatry.* 2015;172 (9): 817–19.

Chapter 6
1. Hassler J. *Staggerford* (New York: Ballantine Books,1986), 10.

Chapter 7
1. Descalzi G, Mitsi V, Purushothaman I et al. "Neuropathic Pain Promotes Adaptive Changes in Gene Expression In Brain Networks Involved in Stress and Depression." *Science Signaling.* March 21, 2017; 10(471).
2. Engel G. "'Psychogenic' pain and the pain-prone patient." *American Journal of Medicine.* vol 26 #6: 899–918,

June 1959.
3. Kross E et al. "Social rejection shares somatosensory representations with physical pain." *Proceedings of the National Academy of Sciences U S A.* 2011;108 (15):6270–74.
4. Letter, undated, posted July 28, 2016.

Chapter 8
1. Dr. Kolb was certified in medicine, neurology, psychiatry and psychoanalysis. He served as president of the American Psychiatric Association and later as chairman of the American Board of Psychiatry and Neurology. He authored a highly respected textbook of neurology. Despite his formidable credentials, as a supervisor he radiated leadership rather than authority, combined with a very dry sense of humor. I think he found our struggles to learn the art of therapy engaging for I always sensed a twinkle in his eyes. Not that he was reluctant to pull rank when necessary, as I found out one time when I had the temerity to ignore twice a rather pointed therapeutic suggestion. Finally he ordered, "Dr. Curran! Start lithium treatment on your patient! Look it up!" I did and the patient promptly improved enough to be discharged. It was an honor to know him and be supervised by him. (A rather charming vignette of him, which captures the essential man, is available from a former student. Cf. Druss, RG. "Dr. Lawrence C. Kolb: One Student's Recollection." *American Journal of Psychiatry:* 2001;58 (5):692.)

    As the years passed and as I began to grasp the wisdom involved in his conception of anxiety, I was amused by the irony of receiving it not from above high on a mountaintop, but high in PI cornered in an elevator.
2. Milrod B. "An Epidemiological Contribution to Clinical Understanding of Anxiety." *American Journal of Psychiatry.* Editorial 172 (7);2015:601–2.
3. Chapman A, Monk C. "Domestic Violence Awareness." Commentary. *American Journal of Psychiatry.* 172 (10);2015:944–45.
4. I am using "relationship" generically here to include any sense of connectedness one might enjoy beyond the tangible, immediate, and personal; for example, with forebears, class, institutions, clubs, gangs, the Almighty, Nature, and so on. The point is that even an intangible source of support and security is vulnerable to change, real or symbolic.

5. Balt S. "Assessing and Enhancing the Effectiveness of Antidepressants." *Psychiatric Times,* June, 2014:30.

Chapter 9
1. Cf. Moffitt TE, Harrington H, Caspi A et al. "Depression and generalized anxiety disorder: cumulative and sequential comorbidity in a birth cohort followed prospectively to age 32 years." *Archives of General Psychiatry.* 64, 651, 2007.Also Rapaport MH, "Prevalence, recognition, and treatment of comorbid depression and anxiety." *Journal of Clinical Psychiatry.* 62(suppl 24), 6, 2001.
2. Jureidini J et al. "Efficacy and safety of antidepressants for children and adolescents." *British Medical Journal.* 328 (April 10, 7444), 879–83, 2004.
3. Herxheimer A. "Antidepressants and adverse effects in young patients." *Canadian Medical Association Journal.* 170 (4, Feb 17), 487–91, 2004. Similarly a meta-analysis of thirty-four studies of fourteen different antidepressants involving 5,260 nine- through eighteen-year-olds concluded that only Prozac was better than placebo. Cipriani A and Zhou X. "Comparative efficacy and tolerability of antidepressants for major depressive disorder in children and adolescents: a network meta-analysis." *The Lancet.* 2016 June 8. doi: 10.1016/S1040–6736[16]30385.3. In an accompanying editorial, "Antidepressants fail, but no cause for therapeutic gloom," Dr. Jureidini concludes the adverse benefit/risk ratio of antidepressants in the young only rarely favors their use in adolescents, "in children almost never." *The Lancet.* 2016 June 8. doi: 10.1016/S1040–6736[16]30385.2
4. I will discuss this report at greater length in volume 2 with my review of the psychotropic management of attachment disability.
5. Nemeroff CB et al. "Differential responses to psychotherapy versus pharmacotherapy in patients with chronic forms of major depression and childhood trauma." *Proceeding of the National Academy of Sciences of the United States of America.* November 25, 2003, v.100 (24).
6. Belden AC et al. "Anterior Insula Volume and Guilt." *JAMA Psychiatry.* 2015;72(1):40-48.
7. Arnow BA et al. "Depression Subtypes in Predicting Antidepressant Response: A Report From the ISPOT-D Trial." *American Journal of Psychiatry.* 2015; 172 (8): 743–50.

8. Balt S. "Assessing and Enhancing the Effectiveness of Antidepressants."
9. Parker G et al. "Issues for *DSM-5:* Whither Melancholia." *American Journal of Psychiatry.* 2010: 167, 745.
10. Jureidini et al. "Efficacy and safety of antidepressants for children and adolescents."
11. Kindler K. "The Phenomenology of Major Depression and the Representativeness and Nature of DSM Criteria." *American Journal of Psychiatry.* 2016;173 (8):771–80. This is a wonderful example of constructive critical analysis, a truth-seeker's delight.
12. Styron W. *Darkness Visible: A Memoir of Madness.* New York: Vintage Books, 1990. It is a must read for anyone interested in a deeper understanding of the paralysis of emotional disability and the hopelessness that propels one into suicidal thinking and behavior. The memoir does not celebrate the benefits of psychiatric intervention; indeed, the insensitive ministrations of his psychiatrist occasion a dry and lengthy commentary. Styron's decision to seek hospitalization and the banal tranquility he found there proved critical: "For me the real healers were seclusion and time." And the life-saving support of his loyal wife and friends, even the relentless cheerfulness of his hospital art therapist.
13. Styron, *Darkness Visible,* 81. Readers, please excuse this lengthy quotation but I can find no better words to express in such touching fashion the devotion of a lost parent and the eternal if unrecognized longing for its restoration. So wonderful for all of us that Styron survived.
14. Stanley IH et al. "Acute Suicidal Affective Disturbance (ASAD): A confirmatory factor analysis with 1442 psychiatric inpatients." *Journal of Psychiatric Research.* 2016 September: 80, 97–104.

Chapter 11
1. Ford R. *The Grim Reaper.* New York: Sarpedon, 1996, 123.
2. Diamond J. *Collapse: How Societies Choose to Fail or Succeed.* New York: Viking, 2005.
3. Twemlow SW, Sacco FC. *Preventing Bullying and School Violence.*
4. Golding W. *Lord of the Flies.* New York: Penguin, 1999.
5. Hassler. *Staggerford,* 10.
6. Mann T. *The Magic Mountain,* H. T. Lowe-Porter, Tr. New York: Vintage, 1969.

7. Ibid., 22–23.
8. Ibid., 26.

Chapter 13
1. Yager J. "Addressing Patients' Psychic Pain." *American Journal of Psychiatry* 172:10, October 2015, 929–43.
2. Arnsten AF et al. "The effects of stress exposure on prefrontal cortex: Translating basic research into successful treatments for Post-Traumatic Stress Disorder." *Neurobiological Stress*. 2015 Jan 1;1(1):89–99. PMID 25436222 In emergencies the brain's power to increase attention and focus is activated by "fight-or-flight" molecules produced in the body. The alpha-2 agonists help balance—and block if necessary—an excessive amount.
3. World Health Organization (2003). Adherence to long-term therapies: evidence for action (PDF). Geneva: World Health Organization.
4. Van der Kolk B. *The Body Keeps the Score*.
5. Bateson G et al. "Toward a Theory of Schizophrenia," *Behavioral Science*, vol.1, 1956, 251–64. (Reprinted in *Steps to an Ecology of Mind*.) Cf. also Haley J. *Strategies of Psychotherapy*. Crown; Bethel (CT), 1990.
6. Strawn J, Sakolsky D, Rynn M. "Psychopharmacologic treatment of children and adolescents with anxiety disorders." *Child and Adolescent Psychiatry Clinics of North America*.2012; 21:527-539. See also Culjpers, C. "Combined Pharmacotherapy and Psychotherapy in the Treatment of Mild to Moderate Major Depression." Editorial, *JAMA Psychiatry*, 71 (3), July, 2014, 747.
7. Lieberman. *Shrinks*, 226–28.
8. Kendall PC, Peterman JS. "CBT for Adolescents with Anxiety: Mature Yet Still Developing." Review and Overview. *American Journal of Psychiatry*. 2015;172 (6):519–30.
9. Weitz ES et al. "Baseline Depression Severity as Moderator of Depressive Outcomes Between Cognitive Behavioral Therapy vs. Pharmacotherapy: An Individual Patient Data Meta-analysis." *JAMA Psychiatry*. 2015;72 (11):1102–09.
10. For a more technical treatment of the topic, see Himle M and Franklin M. "The more you do it, the easier it gets: Exposure and response prevention for OCD." *Cognitive and Behavioral Practice*. 2009;16:29–39.

11. Shapiro F. "EMDR and the adaptive information processing model: integrative treatment and case conceptualization." *Clinical Social Work Journal*.39: 191–200.
12. Brunswick M. "New PTSD therapy ruffles feathers, but shows results." *Star Tribune*. May 30, 2016 A1.
13. A concise review of DBT is featured in the April 2013 issue of *Psychiatric Annals*, "Dialectical Behavior Therapy: A leaning theory-based treatment shown to be effective if difficult-to-treat patients." Nelson, K. et.al.
14. Linehan M. *Cognitive Behavioral Treatment of Borderline Personality Disorder*. New York: Guilford, 1993.
15. Weekes C. *Hope and Help for Your Nerves*. New York: Signet, 1969.
16. See the Wikipedia article for a concise summary of her understanding of the panic-mental cascade. It corresponds to what collapsed Dyllen's classroom performance and is rather similar to Dr. Anderson mental ogre, Igor.
17. Nanni V et al. "Childhood maltreatment predicts unfavorable course of treatment outcome in depression: a meta-analysis." *American Journal of Psychiatry*. 169; 141–51: 2012.
18. Kiecolt-Glaser J et al. "Inflammation: Depression Fans the Flames and Feasts on the Heat." *American Journal of Psychiatry*. 172 (11); 1075–91: 2015.
19. Su KP et al. "Omega-3 fatty acids in the prevention of interferon- alpha-induced depression: results from a randomized, controlled trial." *Biological Psychiatry*. 76; 559–66: 2014.
20. Sarris J et al. "Adjunctive Neutraceuticals for Depression: A Systematic Review and Meta-Analysis." *American Journal of Psychiatry*. 173 (6); 575–87: 2016
21. Van der Kolk. *The Body Keeps the Score*.

Chapter 14
1. Rapaport D. *The Structure of Psychoanalytic Theory: A Systematizing Attempt*. Madison, CT: International Universities Press, 1967.
2. In her definitive account of this revolutionary cleansing of psychiatric nomenclature of all psychoanalytic referents, historian Hannah S. Decker includes a fascinating chapter, "The Psychoanalytic Awakening to DSM-III," which details the ultimately fruitless struggles of the psychoanalytic establishment to derail the descriptive

insurgents. As she concludes, "Almost no one surrenders power voluntarily." Decker HS. *The Making of DSM-III: a diagnostic manual's conquest of American psychiatry* (New York: Oxford University Press, 2013), 223–50. Her book is of more than just historical interest to me, first of all because I got to know Dr. Decker during my medical school years at P&S, secondly because later at PI Dr. Robert Spitzer—without question the "father" of *DSM-III*—haunted our lunch hour impaling us even then with his "subversive" views.
3. *DSM-5*, 14.
4. Lane C. "The NIMH Withdraws Support for DSM-5." *Psychology Today:* May 4, 2013.
5. Gabbard GO, Kay J. "The Fate of Integrated Treatment: Whatever Happened to the Biopsychosocial Psychiatrist?" *American Journal of Psychiatry*. Volume 158;2001:1956–63.
6. Faden J, McFadden R. "Use PRESS to craft a concise psychodynamic formulation." *Current Psychiatry*. Vol 14; 2015 May(5):12.
7. An informative discussion and illustration of CBT is presented by Dr. Jeffrey Lieberman, the current director of my psychiatric alma mater, the New York Psychiatric Institute, in his book *Shrinks*, 223–29.
8. Bateson G. "Toward a Theory of Schizophrenia," reprinted in Bateson, *Steps to an Ecology of Mind*.
9. Minuchin S. *Families and Family Therapy*. Cambridge, MA: Harvard University Press, 1974.
10. *DSM-5*, 160–68.
11. Chekroud AM et al. "Reevaluating the Efficacy and Predictability of Antidepressant Treatments: A Symptom Clustering Approach." *JAMA Psychiatry*. 2017; 74 (4):370–78.
12. *DSM-5*, xii.
13. Ibid., 733 ff.
14. Ressler KJ. "The Intersection of Environment and the Genome in Posttraumatic Stress Disorder." Editorial. *JAMA Psychiatry*. 2016; 73 (7):653–54.
15. Roy-Burne P. "Improving Relationships in Trauma Victims: The Case for Interpersonal Psychotherapy and PTSD." *American Journal of Psychiatry*. Editorial. 2015;172 (5);303–5.
16. *Current Psychiatry*, July 2015, 10.
17. Goodkind M et al. "Identification of a common neurobio-

logical substrate for mental illness." *JAMA Psychiatry.* 2015; 72 (4):305–15.
18. Cross-Disorder Group of Psychiatric Genomics Consortium. "Identification of risk loci with shared effects on five major psychiatric disorders: a genomic-wide analysis." *Lancet.* 2013;381(9875):1371–79.
19. Barch D. "The Neural Correlates of Transdiagnostic Dimensions of Psychopathology." *American Journal of Psychiatry.* Vol 174 (7), July 2017; 613–14.
20. Mazur J. *Zeno's Paradox: Unraveling the Ancient Mystery Behind the Science of Space and Time.* New York: Plume, 2008, 86–88.
21. Summergrad P. "The Long View." *American Journal of Psychiatry.* Vol 172 (8), August 2015, 714–16.
22. Lieberman. *Shrinks,* 147.
23. *DSM-5,* 13.
24. Ross D, Travis M, Arbuckle M. "The Future of Psychiatry as Clinical Neuroscience: Why Not Now?" Editorial. *JAMA Psychiatry* 2015; 72 (5):413–14.
25. Arbuckle M et al. "Integrating a Neuroscience Perspective Into Clinical Psychiatry Today." [Editorial] *JAMA Psychiatry* Vol 74 (4); 2017:313-14. Cf. also adjacent editorial, Heckers S. "Project for a Scientific Psychiatry: Neuroscience Literacy." Ibid., 315.
26. Paulus MR. "Pragmatism Instead of Mechanism." Pine D, Liebenluft E. "Biomarkers with a Mechanistic Focus." *JAMA Psychiatry* Vol 72 (7); 2015:631-635.
27. Raney L. "Integrating Primary Care and Behavioral Health: The Role of the Psychiatrist in the Collaborative Care Model." *American Journal of Psychiatry* 2015; 172 (8):721–29.
28. Katon WJ. "Collaborative Care for Patients with Depression and Chronic Illness." *New England Journal of Medicine.* 2010; 363(Dec. 30):2611–20.
29. National Institute of Mental Health, Research Domain Criteria (RDoC). http://www.nimh.nih.gov/research-priorities/rdoc/nimh-research-domain-criteria-rdoc.shtml (accessed 8/14/15).
30. *Clinical Psychiatry News,* July 2015, 7.
31. Kindler KS. "The Structure of Psychiatric Science." *American Journal of Psychiatry.* Vol 171 (9), September 2014, 931–38.
32. Weinberger DR, Glick ID, Klein DF. "Whither Research Domain Criteria (RDoC)? The Good, the Bad,

and the Ugly." Viewpoint: *JAMA Psychiatry* Vol 72 (12); 2015:1161–62.
33. Carpenter WC Jr. "The RDoC Controversy: Alternate Paradigm or Dominate Paradigm?" *American Journal of Psychiatry*. Vol 173 (6), June 201, 562–63.
34. Holt DJ. "A Pathway to Understanding Emotional Dysfunction in Schizophrenia." (Editorial). *JAMA Psychiatry*. 2016;73 (6):555–56.
35. *DSM-5*, 16.
36. Ibid., 12–13, 733ff.
37. Pies RW. "What is 'Disease'? Implications of Chronic Fatigue Syndrome." *Psychiatric Times*. March 2015 32(3), 1.
38. *DSM-5*, 462–63.
39. Markowitz JC, Perkova E, Neria Y et al. "Is exposure necessary? A randomized clinical trial of Interpersonal Psychotherapy for PTSD." *American Journal of Psychiatry* 2015; 172 (5):430–40. Cf. also editorial Roy-Byrne P. "Improving Relationships in Trauma Victims: The Case for Interpersonal Psychotherapy and PTSD." Ibid., 403–5.
40. Newhouse P, Albert K. "Estrogen, Stress, and Depression: A Neurocognitive Model." *JAMA Psychiatry*. 2015;72(7):727–29. Also, Schmidt, PJ, et al. "Effects of Estradiol Withdrawal on Mood in Women With Past Perimenopausal Depression A Randomized Clinical Trial." *JAMA Psychiatry* Vol 72 (7); 2015:714–26.
41. Greven CU et al. "Developmentally Stable Whole-Brain Volume Reductions and Developmentally Sensitive Caudate and Putamen Volume Alterations in Those with Attention-deficit/Hyperactivity Disorder and Their Unaffected Siblings." *JAMA Psychiatry* Vol 72 (5); 2015:490–99.
42. Rive MM et al. "State-Dependent Differences in Emotion Regulation Between Unmedicated Bipolar Disorder and Major Depressive Disorder." *JAMA Psychiatry* Vol 72 (7); 2015:687–96.
43. Wheeler AL et al. "Further Neuroimaging Evidence for the Deficit Subtype of Schizophrenia." *JAMA Psychiatry*. Vol 72 (5); 2015:446–55.
44. Saykin AJ et al. "Neuropsychological deficits in neuroleptic naïve patients with first-episode schizophrenia." *Archives of General Psychiatry*. 1994;51(2):124–31.
45. McCullumsmith RE. "Evidence for Schizophrenia as a Disorder of Neuroplasticity." Editorial. *American Journal of Psychiatry*. 2015;172 (4):312–13.

Notes: page 421

46. Mueser KT et al. "The NAVIGATE program for first-episode psychosis: rationale, overview, and description of psychosocial components." *Psychiatric Services*. 2015;66(7):680–90. Cf. also Carey B. "The Treatment of Choice," for a detailed account of how "Frank" benefited from a similar program, OnTrackNY, after several relapses with conventional treatment. *The New York Times*, December 29, 2015:D1.
47. Curran J, Jorud S, Whitman N. "Unconventional Treatment of Treatment-Resistant Hospitalized Patients."

Bibliography

American Psychiatric Association, *Diagnostic and Statistical Manual of Mental Disorders, Fifth Edition: DSM-5*. Arlington, VA: American Psychiatric Publishing, 2013.

Anderson RO. "Fighting Igor: Exposing and Resisting the Irrational Side Using Cognitive-Behavioral Principles in Group Therapy of Panic/Phobic Disorders." *Journal of Contemporary Psychotherapy*. 1998; 28 (1);5–34.

Arbuckle MR et al. "Integrating a Neuroscience Perspective Into Clinical Psychiatry Today." [Editorial] *JAMA Psychiatry* Vol 74 (4); 2017:313-14.

Arnow BA et al. "Depression Subtypes in Predicting Antidepressant Response: A Report From the ISPOT-D Trial." *American Journal of Psychiatry*. 2015; 172 (8): 743–50.

Arnsten AF et al. "The effects of stress exposure on prefrontal cortex: Translating basic research into successful treatments for Post-Traumatic Stress Disorder." *Neurobiological Stress*. 2015 Jan 1;1(1):89–99. PMID 25436222.

Balt S. "Assessing and Enhancing the Effectiveness of Antidepressants." *Psychiatric Times*, June, 2014:30.

Barch D. "The Neural Correlates of Transdiagnostic Dimensions of Psychopathology." *American Journal of Psychiatry*. Vol 174 (7), July 2017; 613–14.

Bateson G et al. "Toward a Theory of Schizophrenia," *Behavioral Science*, vol.1, 1956, 251–64. Reprinted in Bateson G, *Steps to an Ecology of Mind*. San Francisco: Chandler, 1972.

Becker-Weidman A, Ehrmann L, and LeBow D. *The Attachment Therapy Companion: Key Practices for Treating Children and Families*. New York: W. W. Norton, 2009.

Belden AC et al. "Anterior Insula Volume and Guilt." *JAMA Psychiatry*. 2015;72(1):40-48.

Bowlby J. *Maternal Care and Mental Health* (New York: Schocken, 1951); *Attachment and Loss, vol. 1, Attachment*. New York: Basic Books, 1969 and 1982.

Brunswick M. "New PTSD therapy ruffles feathers, but shows results." *Star Tribune*. May 30, 2016 A1.

Carey B. "The Treatment of Choice," *The New York Times*, December 29, 2015:D1.

Carpenter WC Jr. "The RDoC Controversy: Alternate Paradigm or Dominate Paradigm?" *American Journal of Psychiatry*. Vol 173 (6), June 201, 562–63.

Chapman A and Monk C. "Domestic Violence Awareness." Commentary. *American Journal of Psychiatry*. 172 (10);2015:944–45.

Chekroud AM et al. "Reevaluating the Efficacy and Predictability of Antidepressant Treatments: A Symptom Clustering Approach." *JAMA Psychiatry*. 2017; 74 (4):370–78.

Cipriani A and Zhou X. "Comparative efficacy and tolerability of antidepressants for major depressive disorder in children and adolescents: a network meta-analysis." *The Lancet*. 2016 June 8. doi: 10.1016/S1040–6736[16]30385.3.

Cross-Disorder Group of Psychiatric Genomics Consortium. "Identification of risk loci with shared effects on five major psychiatric disorders: a genomic-wide analysis." *Lancet*. 2013;381(9875):1371–79.

Culjpers C. "Combined Pharmacotherapy and Psychotherapy in the Treatment of Mild to Moderate Major Depression." Editorial, *JAMA Psychiatry*, 71 (3), July, 2014, 747.

Curran J, Jorud S, and Whitman N. "Unconventional Treatment of Treatment-Resistant Hospitalized Patients." *Psychiatric Quarterly*. 1971; 45(2).

Decker HS. *The Making of DSM-III:A Diagnostic Manual's Conquest of American Psychiatry*. New York: Oxford University Press, 2013.

Descalzi G, Mitsi V, Purushothaman I et al. "Neuropathic Pain Promotes Adaptive Changes in Gene Expression In Brain Networks Involved in Stress and Depression." *Science Signaling*. March 21, 2017; 10(471).

Diamond J. *Collapse: How Societies Choose to Fail or Succeed*. New York: Viking, 2005.

Bibliography

Druss RG. "Dr. Lawrence C. Kolb: One Student's Recollection." *American Journal of Psychiatry*: 2001;58 (5):692.)

Engel G. "'Psychogenic' pain and the pain-prone patient." *American Journal of Medicine*. vol 26 #6: 899–918, June 1959.

Faden J and McFadden R. "Use PRESS to craft a concise psychodynamic formulation." *Current Psychiatry*. Vol 14; 2015 May(5):12.

Ford R. *The Grim Reaper*. New York: Sarpedon, 1996, 123.

Friedman M. "Suspensions don't make bad kids good. Here's what does." *Star Tribune*, February 28, 2012:A7.

Gabbard GO and Kay J. "The Fate of Integrated Treatment: Whatever Happened to the Biopsychosocial Psychiatrist?" *American Journal of Psychiatry*. Volume 158;2001:1956–63.

Golding W. *Lord of the Flies*. New York: Penguin, 1999.

Goodkind M et al. "Identification of a common neurobiological substrate for mental illness." *JAMA Psychiatry*. 2015; 72 (4):305–15.

Greven CU et al. "Developmentally Stable Whole-Brain Volume Reductions and Developmentally Sensitive Caudate and Putamen Volume Alterations in Those with Attention-deficit/ Hyperactivity Disorder and Their Unaffected Siblings." *JAMA Psychiatry* Vol 72 (5); 2015:490–99.

Haley J. *Strategies of Psychotherapy*. Bethel, CT: Crown, 1990.

Hassler J. *Staggerford*. New York: Ballantine, 1986.

Heckers S. "Project for a Scientific Psychiatry: Neuroscience Literacy." *JAMA Psychiatry*. 2017 Apr 1;74(4):315.

Herxheimer A. "Antidepressants and adverse effects in young patients." *Canadian Medical Association Journal*. 170 (4, Feb 17), 487–91, 2004.

Himle M and Franklin M. "The more you do it, the easier it gets: Exposure and response prevention for OCD." *Cognitive and Behavioral Practice*. 2009;16:29–39.

Holt DJ. "A Pathway to Understanding Emotional Dysfunction in Schizophrenia." (Editorial). *JAMA Psychiatry*. 2016;73 (6):555–56.

Jaynes J. *The Origins of Consciousness in the Breakdown of the Bicameral Mind*. Boston: Houghton Mifflin, 1976.

Juireidini J. "Antidepressants fail, but no cause for therapeutic gloom." *The Lancet*. 2016 June 8. DOI: http://dx.doi.org/10.1016/S0140-6736(16)30585-2.

Jureidini J et al. "Efficacy and safety of antidepressants for children and adolescents." *British Medical Journal*. 328 (April 10, 2004), 879–83, 2004.

Katon WJ. "Collaborative Care for Patients with Depression and Chronic Illness." *New England Journal of Medicine*. 2010; 363(Dec. 30):2611–20.

Kendall PC and Peterman JS. "CBT for Adolescents with Anxiety: Mature Yet Still Developing." Review and Overview. *American Journal of Psychiatry*. 2015;172 (6):519–30.

Kendler KS. "The Phenomenology of Major Depression and the Representativeness and Nature of DSM Criteria." *American Journal of Psychiatry*. 2016;173 (8):771–80.

———. "The Structure of Psychiatric Science." *American Journal of Psychiatry*. Vol 171 (9), September 2014, 931–38.

Kiecolt-Glaser J et al. "Inflammation: Depression Fans the Flames and Feasts on the Heat." *American Journal of Psychiatry*. 172 (11); 1075–91: 2015.

Kross E et al. "Social rejection shares somatosensory representations with physical pain." *Proceedings of the National Academy of Sciences U S A*. 2011;108 (15):6270–74.

Lahey BB. "Why Are Children Who Exhibit Psychopathology at High Risk for Psychopathology and Dysfunction in Adulthood?" Editorial. *JAMA Psychiatry*. 2015; 72 (9): 865–66.

Lane C. "The NIMH Withdraws Support for DSM-5." *Psychology Today*, May 4, 2013.

Lieberman J. *Shrinks: The Untold Story of Psychiatry*. New York: Little Brown, 2015.

Linehan M. *Cognitive Behavioral Treatment of Borderline Personality Disorder*. New York: Guilford, 1993.

Mann T. *The Magic Mountain*, H. T. Lowe-Porter, tr. New York: Vintage, 1969.

Markowitz JC, Perkova E, Neria Y et al. "Is exposure necessary? A randomized clinical trial of Interpersonal Psychotherapy for PTSD." *American Journal of Psychiatry* 2015; 172 (5):430–40.

Mazur J. *Zeno's Paradox: Unraveling the Ancient Mystery Behind the Science of Space and Time*. New York: Plume, 2008.

McCullumsmith RE. "Evidence for Schizophrenia as a Disorder of Neuroplasticity." Editorial. *American Journal of Psychiatry*. 2015;172 (4):312–13.

Bibliography

Milrod B. "An Epidemiological Contribution to Clinical Understanding of Anxiety." *American Journal of Psychiatry*. Editorial 172 (7);2015:601–2.

Minuchin S. *Families and Family Therapy*. Cambridge, MA: Harvard University Press, 1974.

Moffitt TE, Harrington H, Caspi A et al. "Depression and generalized anxiety disorder: cumulative and sequential co-morbidity in a birth cohort followed prospectively to age 32 years." *Archives of General Psychiatry*.64, 651, 2007.

Mueser KT et al. "The NAVIGATE program for first-episode psychosis: rationale, overview, and description of psychosocial components." *Psychiatric Services*. 2015;66(7):680–90.

Nanni V et al. "Childhood maltreatment predicts unfavorable course of treatment outcome in depression: a meta-analysis." *American Journal of Psychiatry*. 169; 141–51: 2012.

Nasrallah H. "Is there only 1 neurobiologic psychiatric disorder, with different clinical expressions?" *Current Psychiatry*, July 2015, 10.

National Institute of Mental Health, Research Domain Criteria (RDoC). http://www.nimh.nih.gov/research-priorities/rdoc/nimh-research-domain-criteria-rdoc.shtml (accessed 8/14/15).

Nelson K. "Dialectical Behavior Therapy: A leaning theory-based treatment shown to be effective if difficult-to-treat patients." *Psychiatric Annals*, April 2013; 43 (4): 149–50. DOI: 10.3928/00485713-20130403-03.

Nemeroff CB et al. "Differential responses to psychotherapy versus pharmacotherapy in patients with chronic forms of major depression and childhood trauma." *Proceeding of the National Academy of Sciences of the United States of America*. November 25, 2003, v.100 (24).

Newhouse P and Albert K. "Estrogen, Stress, and Depression: A Neurocognitive Model." *JAMA Psychiatry*. 2015;72(7):727–29.

Parker FN et al. "Issues for DSM-5: Whither Melancholia." *American Journal of Psychiatry*. 2010: 167, 745.

Paulus MR. "Pragmatism Instead of Mechanism."

Pine D and Liebenluft E. "Biomarkers with a Mechanistic Focus." *JAMA Psychiatry* Vol 72 (7); 2015:631-635.

Pies RW. "What is 'Disease'? Implications of Chronic Fatigue Syndrome." *Psychiatric Times*. March 2015 32(3), 1.

Raney L. "Integrating Primary Care and Behavioral Health: The Role of the Psychiatrist in the Collaborative Care Model." *American Journal of Psychiatry* 2015; 172 (8):721–29.

Rapaport D. *The Structure of Psychoanalytic Theory: A Systematizing Attempt*. Madison, CT: International Universities Press, 1967.

Rapaport MH. "Prevalence, recognition, and treatment of comorbid depression and anxiety." *Journal of Clinical Psychiatry*.62(suppl 24), 6, 2001.

Ressler KJ. "The Intersection of Environment and the Genome in Posttraumatic Stress Disorder." Editorial. *JAMA Psychiatry*. 2016; 73 (7):653–54.

Rive MM et al. "State-Dependent Differences in Emotion Regulation Between Unmedicated Bipolar Disorder and Major Depressive Disorder." *JAMA Psychiatry* Vol 72 (7); 2015:687–96.

Ross D, Travis M, and Arbuckle M. "The Future of Psychiatry as Clinical Neuroscience: Why Not Now?" *JAMA Psychiatry* 2015; 72 (5):413–14.

Roy-Byrne P. "Improving Relationships in Trauma Victims: The Case for Interpersonal Psychotherapy and PTSD." *American Journal of Psychiatry*, Vol. 172, No.5, May 1, 2015, 403–5.

Salinger JD. *The Catcher in the Rye*. New York: Little, Brown & Co., 1951.

Sarris J et al. "Adjunctive Neutraceuticals for Depression: A Systematic Review and Meta-Analysis." *American Journal of Psychiatry*. 173 (6); 575–87: 2016.

Saykin AJ et al. "Neuropsychological deficits in neuroleptic naïve patients with first-episode schizophrenia." Archives of General Psychiatry. 1994;51(2):124–31.

Schmidt PJ et al. "Effects of Estradiol Withdrawal on Mood in Women With Past Perimenopausal Depression A Randomized Clinical Trial." *JAMA Psychiatry* Vol 72 (7); 2015:714–26.

Shapiro F. "EMDR and the adaptive information processing model: integrative treatment and case conceptualization." *Clinical Social Work Journal*.39: 191–200. [mo/yr?]

Sourander A et al. "Association of Bullying Behavior at 8 Years of Age and the Use of Specialized Services for Psychiatric Disorders by 29 Years of Age." *JAMA Psychiatry* 73(2):159–65; 2016.

Stanley IH et al. "Acute Suicidal Affective Disturbance (ASAD): A confirmatory factor analysis with 1442 psychiatric inpatients." *Journal of Psychiatric Research*. 2016 September: 80, 97–104.

Strawn J, Sakolsky D, and Rynn M. "Psychopharmacologic treatment of children and adolescents with anxiety disorders." *Child and Adolescent Psychiatry Clinics of North America*.2012; 21:527–39.

Styron W. *Darkness Visible: A Memoir of Madness*. New York: Vintage Books, 1990.

Su KP et al. "Omega-3 fatty acids in the prevention of interferon- alpha-induced depression: results from a randomized, controlled trial." *Biological Psychiatry*. 76; 559–66: 2014.

Summergrad P. "The Long View." *American Journal of Psychiatry*. Vol 172 (8), August 2015, 714–16.

Swendse J et al. "Use and Abuse of Alcohol and Illicit Drugs in US Adolescents." *Archives of General Psychiatry*. 2012 Apr;69(4)393.

Twemlow SW and Sacco FC. *Preventing Bullying and School Violence*. Arlington, VA: American Psychiatric Publishing, 2012.

Vachon DD et al. "Assessment of the Harmful Psychiatric and Behavioral Effects of Different Forms of Child Maltreatment." *JAMA Psychiatry*. 2015; 72 (11): 1135–43.

Van der Kolk B. *The Body Keeps the Score: Brain, Mind, and Body in the Healing of Trauma*. New York: Penguin, 2004.

Weekes C. *Hope and Help for Your Nerves*. New York: Signet, 1969.

Weiden PJ. "Helping Patients with Mental Illness Get Back to Work." Editorial. *American Journal of Psychiatry*. 2015;172 (9): 817–19.

Weinberger DR, Glick ID, and Klein DF. "Whither Research Domain Criteria (RDoC)? The Good, the Bad, and the Ugly." Viewpoint: *JAMA Psychiatry* Vol 72 (12); 2015:1161–62.

Weitz ES et al. "Baseline Depression Severity as Moderator of Depressive Outcomes Between Cognitive Behavioral Therapy vs. Pharmacotherapy: An Individual Patient Data Meta-analysis." *JAMA Psychiatry*. 2015;72 (11):1102–09.

Werner EE and Smith RS. *Overcoming the Odds: High Risk Children from Birth to Childhood*. Ithaca, NY: Cornell University Press, 1992.

Wheeler AL et al. "Further Neuroimaging Evidence for the Deficit Subtype of Schizophrenia." *JAMA Psychiatry* Vol 72 (5); 2015:446–55.

Winnicott DW. *The Maturational Process and the Facilitating Environment.* International Universities Press, 1965.

——. *The Child, the Family, and the Outside World.* London: Penguin, 1973.

World Health Organization (2003). Adherence to long-term therapies: evidence for action (PDF). Geneva: World Health Organization.

Yager J. "Addressing Patients' Psychic Pain." *American Journal of Psychiatry* 172:10, October 2015, 929–43.

Index

AA (Alcoholics Anonymous), 33–34, 337
abandonment, 5. *See also* separation anxiety
   chronic pain and, 158–59, 160
   disability and, 154, 413
   entanglement and, 73
   fear of, 46, 96
   fear of not being abandoned, 398
   inattentiveness and, 253
   loss complicated by, 149
   need to address vulnerabilities, 241
   problem behaviors and, 169
   trauma and, 181
   verbosity and, 362
Abbott-Northwestern Hospital, 135
abuse
   acting-out and, 85
   authority and, 93
   effects of, 194
   emotional, 194
   enabling, 85–87
   problem behaviors and, 169
   residuals of, 194
   self-blame and, 331
   self-mutilating behavior and, 89–90
   verbal, of psychiatrists, 144, 164
abuse survivors, xxxvii (note xiii), 181 (note xi)
abuser, attachment to, 194
acceptance, xxxi, 5, 56, 106, 329–36, 396. *See also* management
   anxiety about, 301
   chronic pain and, 161
   difficulty of, 243
   learning to describe and, 332–33, 336
   as opposite of blame, 331
   promoting, 335–36
   recovery and, 32
   without blame, 329
achievement, recognizing, 286–87, 298
acting-out, 7–11, 22, 84. *See also* provocativeness
   abuse background and, 85
   adaptive skills and, 84
   ambivalence and, 77, 78, 299
   anxiety and, 81
   boundary setting and, 77
   case studies, 77–78, 79–85
   as claim on environment, 8, 22, 44, 119, 125, 136

as cry for help, 142
cutting, 88–90
"depression" and, 81
in *DSM-5*, 103
expressing conflicts via, 137
management of, 77
Maya, 95–99, 335
misidentification of, 338
as protection against entanglement, 98
running and, 44
in secure unit, 114
self-mutilation and, 335
by students, 168–69
sudden, 95–99
token economy and, 78, 79–85, 105, 118

Acting-out Attachment Disability, case studies, 77–99
active intervention, 139–47, 163, 183
activity, productive, xxxvi, 154. *See also* work
Acute Suicidal Affective Disturbance (ASAD), 233–34
Adaptational Psychodynamics, 116 (note iv), 381
adaptive behaviors, persistence of, 80
adaptive learning, 374
adaptive skills
  need for, 84
  strategic, 248–58
  tactical, 247–48, 259–87
  trauma and, 215
addiction. *See also* substance use/abuse
  conditioning and, 124
  negative reinforcement and, 124
  parental relationships and, 64–65
  powerlessness and, 124
  recovery, 214
  as solution, 24
addiction management, anxiety and, 33–34
ADHD, 420
Adjustment Reaction, grief and, 46
administrators, medical, 198–99
adolescent referrals, 144
adolescents, xxiii (note iv), 211. *See also Catcher in the Rye*
  anger and, 94
  Antidepressants and, 219, 226–27, 344
  anxiety and, 94
  Depression in, 226–27
  entanglement and, 6
  expectations from adults/authority, 96–97
  hopelessness in, 227
  impact of loss on, 183
  increased work with, 147–48
  inpatient hospitalizations, 148
  interview participation of sponsors, 259
  manipulations and, 276–86
  needs from adults, 99
  psychiatrists for, 148, 149 (note vi)
  rules and, 147
  suicide and, 233–34
adults. *See also* parent(s); sponsors
  adolescents' needs from, 99
  in *Catcher in the Rye*, 38

Index

expectations from, 96–97

intervention by, 62

leadership responsibilities, xxiv (note iv)

success phobia, 25 (note i)

Adventures of Huckleberry Finn, The (Twain), 36

Adzik, George, 392

Affective Interference, 105, 137–39, 147–51, 170, 183. *See also* Attachment Disability

Afifi, Tracie O., xxxvii (note xiii)

Against Medical Advice (AMA), xxix (note v)

Albert, H., xxix (note v)

ALC (alternative learning centers), xxxiii, 26, 27, 105, 169–71

alcohol. *See also* substance use/abuse

    self-treatment with, 348

    stopping, Depression and, 235–36

alcoholic parents, 20

Alcoholics Anonymous (AA), 33–34, 337

alexithymia, 303–4

Alger, Horatio, 370

alpha-2 agonists, 341, 343, 359–60

alternative learning centers (ALC), xxxiii, 26, 27, 105, 169–71

AMA (Against Medical Advice), xxix (note v)

Amanda (pseudonym), 85–87

ambiguity, clarification and, 219

ambivalence, 77–78, 299

American Journal of Psychiatry, 404, 414

American Psychiatric Association (APA), xxxviii, 91, 386, 406, 413. *See also* DSM

American Psychiatric Association's Diagnostic and Statistical Manual. *See* DSM

Amy (pseudonym), 57–63, 254, 381

amygdala, xxii (note ii)

Anderson, R. O., 208

anger, 9, 61, 74, 317, 418. *See also* acting-out

    adolescents and, 94

angry dropouts, 23

angry-parent/provocative-child, 302–3

    chronic pain and, 164

    as cry for help, 195

    fear and, 164, 326–27

    masking fear of abandonment, 96

    paranoid patient and, 267

    parents', 195, 197, 302–3

    response to, 22

    suppressing, 195

Anoka State Hospital, 105, 381, 401. *See also* Jackie (pseudonym); research experiences; Schiele, Bertrum; token economy

    behavior modification program at, 421

    described, 111–14

    experiences at, 107–34

    group discussion at, 369

    locked female unit, 112–14

    personal impact of experiences at, 126–29

445

Index

professional impact of experiences at, 120–26
suspension from, 130–33
Winston (pseudonym), 130–31, 133
Antidepressants, 19, 54, 67, 341. *See also* medication
　adolescents and, 219, 226–27, 344
　as antistressants, 68, 96, 224, 295
　anxiety and, 352–357
　combined with cognitive therapy, 355
　complications of, 354
　conditions treated with, xxvi
　efficacy of, 122, 214, 219–21, 225, 226, 352–57
　entanglement and, 68–69, 70
　guidelines for, 343–44
　nocebo response, 344–45
　nonresponsiveness and, xxxvii, 389
　primary effect of, 193 (note i)
　promptness of effect, 354–56
　suicidal feelings and, 343–44
　traditional presentation of, 351–52
　treatment of panic with, 117
　utility in children/adolescents, 219
antihypertensive agents, 341
antiperfectionism, 365
Antipsychotics, xxvi, 122, 125–26, 226. *See also* medication
antisocial behaviors, 8. *See also* acting-out
antistressants, 227, 295, 352
　Antidepressants as, 68, 96, 224, 295

chronic pain and, 166
anxiety, 16, 23–24, 26, 279. *See also* emotion
　AA and, 33–34
　about peer-group acceptance, 301
　about trust, 192
　acting-out and, 81
　addiction management and, 33–34
　adolescents and, 94
　Antidepressants and, 352–57
　Attachment Disability and, 187–214
　awareness of, 97
　case studies, 15–35, 195–206, 235
　definition of, 187, 188
　"depression" and, 187, 305–306
　exposure/response prevention and, 33
　living with, 181–82
　Major Depression and, 228
　management of, 35
　medication and, 33, 45–46, 49, 54, 64
　owning, 330–331
　pervasive, 307 (note ii)
　preoccupation with conformity, 146 (note iv)
　prognosis for, 32–34
　provocativeness and, 302
　regulation of social behavior by, 307 (note ii)
　role of, 183
　seeking help for, 32–33
　self-treating, 19
　separation and, 105, 107, 188, 198 (note vi), 208, 326, 415

as signal of change, 179
substance use/abuse and, 31
unrecognized, 55
work and, 174

APA (American Psychiatric Association), xxxviii, 91, 386, 406, 413. *See also* DSM

apologizing, 356–359

appointments, missing, 202–3

approach/avoidance paralysis., 197

approval, qualified, 298

ASAD (Acute Suicidal Affective Disturbance), 233–34

assessment/workup, 117, 143, 171, 172–83. *See also* diagnosis; evaluation; interview
  chronic pain and, 162
  clarification and, 172
  collateral history, 231–32, 259–65
  current protocol, 403–4
  dynamic thinking in, xxii, 382–87, 394, 402, 414
  five-axis system, 283–84, 382, 397–98, 402
  Freudian terminology in, 379–80
  interpersonal theory in, 381
  language for, 378–81
  listening in, 172–83
  need for reform, 377–422
  provisional alternative, 414–17
  reworked format, 399–400

attachment
  age and, 5
  background and, 5
  Bowlby on, 4–7
  concept of, xix
  origin of term, 4
  persistence of, 183, 400
  risking, 349
  risks of, 311–20

attachment conflict, disability and, 154

Attachment Disability
  ignored, xix–xxiii
  misdiagnosed, xviii
  narrow vision of, xxi
  origins of concept (*see* origins of Attachment Disability theory)
  persistence of, xix, 50–51
  prevention of, 339 (note i)
  recognition of, 401
  validity of theory, 103–4

Attachment Disorders, recognizing, 4

Attachment Entanglement. *See* entanglement

attachment issues
  beyond early childhood, 106
  as limited to childhood, 50, 149, 401

Attachment Theory, marginalization of, 400–3

Attachment Therapy Companion, The, xx, 400

Attention Deficit Disorder, 341

attentiveness, 251–53

attractiveness, of patients, 251–53

Austin Hospital, xxxv

authority, xxxvii, 258
  abuse background and, 93
  avoidance and, 44–45
  dealing with, 76, 133
  defending, 76

Index

expectations from, 96–97
predictable, 94
rebellion and, 94
security/authority dyad, 303
automatic protective wired-in nervous system defense, 215–16
autonomy, 128, 347
autopsies, psychological, 318
avoidance, 6. *See also* withdrawal
   authority and, 44–45
   case studies, 15–35, 45–55
awfulizing, 208, 368 (note ix). *See also* Igor talk; what if thinking

Balt, Steve, 214, 226
Bandura, Albert, 387
Barch, Deanna, 405–6
Bateson, Gregory, 346, 388
BD (Bipolar Disorder), 92–93, 398
Beck, Aaron, 388, 410
Becker-Weidman handbook, 400
behavior
   looking beyond, 208
   modifying, 126
   in therapy, 75–76
   behavior modification techniques/programs. *See also* token economy
   at Anoka State Hospital, 421
   Dialectical Behavior Therapy, 367–68
   diet, 371
   Exposure/Response Prevention, 33, 35, 204–5, 323, 363–65
   Eye Movement Desensitization and Reprocessing, 365–66
   family therapy, 366–67
   pet companionship, 372–373
   redirection, 336, 356–58, 361–62, 363
   repetitive prompts, 336
   self-help, 370–71
Behavior Therapy (BT), 387–88. *See also* behavior modification techniques/programs
behavioral analysis, 105
behavioral health. *See* psychiatry
behavioral stability, teaching, 114
betrayal, 340
Bill (pseudonym), 380
biopsychosocial ideology, 382–83
Bipolar Depression, 226
Bipolar Disorder (BD), 92–93, 398
blame/blaming, 86, 289, 311, 330–31
   acceptance as opposite of, 331
   accepting trauma without, 329
   chronic pain and, 158–59, 160, 164–65
   owning pain without, 396
   self-blame, 312, 331, 333–36, 344 (note iv)
   for uncontrollable, 356–59
Bleuler, E., 420
blood pressure, 222 (note iv)
Bob (pseudonym), 148
Body Keeps the Score, The (van der Kolk), xxiii, 343, 374

448

Index

Borderline Personality Disorder (BPD), 91–92, 398, 418
boundaries, 321, 322
  adolescents' desire for, 301
  caretaker, 55
  establishing with provocative behavior, 75, 76
  establishing with words vs. behavior, 77, 300, 314, 398
  ODD and, 95
  physical pain as, 89
  self-mutilating behavior and, 90
  therapeutic, 334–35
  token economy and, 120, 125, 394
boundary issues, 338
Bowery missionaries, 127
Bowlby, John, xix, xx, 4–7, 11, 150, 381, 400, 401, 419
BPD (Borderline Personality Disorder), 91–92, 398, 418
BPRS (Brief Psychiatric Rating Scale), 391
Brahe, Tycho, 404–5, 406, 422
brain
  damage to, chronic pain and, 160, 163, 166
  damage to, from trauma, xxii, xxii (note ii), 419
  fetal, 138 (note ii)
brain research, xxi, 378, 404–5. *See also* neuroscience
Brief Psychiatric Rating Scale (BPRS), 391
British Psychological Society, xxx–xxxi
Bruch, Hilde, 116, 144, 164
BT (Behavior Therapy), 387–88. *See also* behavior modification techniques/programs

bullying, xviii, 340
  crowd participation in, 94
  denial of, 291–92
bystander behavior, 94

Camus, A., 310, 310 (note iii), 320
cancer, as separation, 198
cancer phobia, 197–206
care, danger of, 45
careers, 7, 50, 65–66, 85, 181 (note xi)
Carla (pseudonym), 345, 347–51
Carnegie, Dale, 268, 370
Carpenter, William T. Jr., 414
case studies
  acting-out, 77–99
  Amanda, 85–87
  Amy, 57–63, 254, 381
  anxiety, 195–206
  apologizing, 356–57
  assessments, 173–83
  attachment avoidance, 15–35, 45–55
  Carla, 345, 347–51
  Holden Caulfield, xxxii, 35–45, 150
  Charles, xxxii (note ix), 195–206
  Charlotte, 64–67
  cutting, 88–90
  dangers of improvement, 345–47
  dangers of recovery, 209–13
  Darrell, 345–47
  death preoccupations, 320–26
  denial, 294–98

Index

Depression, 228–43

"depression", 189–94

detachment, 294–96

Dyllen, xxxii, 15–35

entanglement, 57–76, 281

fear of medications, 347–51

Georgina, 67–72

grief, 35–45

Helen, xxxii, 45–55, 178, 362 (note viii), 388

Jackie, 77–78, 79–85, 87, 88–90, 272, 300, 391, 393–94

Julie, 209–13

Justin, 294–96

Lara, 335, 356–57, 361

Lindsey, 341, 359

Maddie, 281–86, 344

Maggie, 372–73

Maya, 95–99, 335

noncompliance, 254–58

Owen, 254–258, 293

paranoid patient, 269–75

parents, entangled, 72–76

Peggy, 311–20, 331, 337, 358–59

Mr. POP, 129, 133, 161, 263, 269–75, 291, 370, 418

Punker, 72–76, 77

Rebecca, 189–94, 206, 252, 289, 393

Renée, 173–83

Mr. Resistive, 177, 177 (note viii), 248–51, 293, 299, 361

resistiveness, 254–58

risks of attachment, 311–20

Rita, 394–400

Rose, 236–43, 306, 393

Ryan, 261

Samantha, 287, 296–98, 334

stagecraft, 269–75

Styron, 151, 210, 216, 228–36, 285, 310 (note iii), 340, 393

suicide, 320–26

tactics, 281–86

timing, 254–58

token economy, 79–85

Castorp, Hans (fictional character), 151, 203, 308–10

Catcher in the Rye, The (Salinger), xxxii, 6, 36–45, 105–6, 150

    authority in, 44–45

    backstory, 37–39

    insincerity in, 39–40

    protectiveness in, 40–42

Caulfield, Holden (fictional character), xxxii, 35–45, 150

cause-effect considerations, 382–87. *See also* dynamic thinking

CBT (Cognitive Behavioral Therapy), 360–62, 388

CCC (Civilian Conservation Corps) program, 127

change. *See also* focus on what can be changed; improvement; recovery

    anxiety and, 179

    difficulty understanding, 30–32

    medications and, 341–60

    potential for, 336

    separation/loss and, 208

change tactics, 360–73

Charles (pseudonym), xxxii (note ix), 195–206

Charlotte (pseudonym), 64–67

chemical dependency, xxiv (note iv). *See also* alcohol; substance use/abuse

child care services, xx

Index

child development, parental relationships and, 3. *See also* attachment

child maltreatment, xviii. *See also* abuse

children. *See also* adolescents
Antidepressants and, 219
resilience of, 5

Chronic Fatigue Syndrome, 417

chronic illness, 410–11

chronic mental illness, 122

chronic pain, 363, 372, 411–12
abandonment and, 158–59, 160
acceptance and, 161
active intervention and, 163
anger and, 164
antistressants and, 166
blame and, 158–59, 160, 164–65
brain damage and, 160, 163, 166
clarification and, 161
distrust and, 153, 160, 161, 162–63
evaluation, 155–56
hard work and, 157–58
historical perspective on, 159 (note iii)
loss and, 160
management of, 153, 160–63
misunderstanding of, 159
not listening by patients, 166–67
rambling and, 165–66
rejection and, 158
traditional theory of, 154–60

chronic pain disability, 153–67, 183

Chronic Schizophrenia, 121

chronicity, 119, 122
behavior modification program and, 421
institutional, 124–26
rural areas and, 119 (note viii)

Civilian Conservation Corps (CCC) program, 127

C-L (consultation-liaison), xxviii, xxxvi

claim on environment, 8, 22, 44, 77, 88, 91, 119, 125, 136

clarification, xxxi, 55, 86, 106, 146, 190, 289–328, 381, 396, 416
ambiguity and, 219
of anxieties about trust, 192
chronic pain and, 161
"depression" and, 305–6
difficulty of implementing, 243
goal of, 289–90
journaling, 368 (note ix)
need for, 192–93
patient assessment/workup and, 172
promoting insight and, 290, 303–27
provocative behavior and, 76
redirection, 363
softening denial and, 290–302
sponsor participation and, 261
of use of term "depression", 218–21
vocabulary for, 192–93

clinical experiences, 105, 111–14, 123–24. *See also* Anoka State Hospital

Index

clinical psychiatry, neuroscience in, 407–8
code of silence, 85
Cognitive Behavioral Therapy (CBT), 360–62, 388
cognitive bias, 193
cognitive dissonance, 273
cognitive interference, dropping out and, 136–37
cognitive therapy, 355, 356–58, 388
collaborative care, xxxv–xxxviii, 52 (note x), 409–13
collateral history, 231–32, 259–65
college
　loss of emotional support at, 51
　orientation for parents, 66
community mental health centers, 140–41
community psychiatry, 141–42
community support, 141–42. *See also* support
comorbidity, 391–93
complaints, 265
compliance, 256–58
　BD and, 93
　commanding, 279–80
　denial masquerading as, 296–98
　recognizing, 273
conditioning, 124
Conduct Disorder, xviii, 338–39
conduct issues, authentic, 339
conflict, neo-Freudians and, 3
conformity, preoccupation with, 146 (note iv)
confrontation, denial and, 290

connectedness. *See also* attachment
　fears of, 211
　risk of, 316
consequences, 84
constraints, on management, 248–58
consultation-liaison (C-L), xxviii, xxxvi
consulting experiences, 105, 123, 130, 140–41, 167–71, 172
content, noncompliance and, 342, 351–60
context, noncompliance and, 342, 343–51
contingent reinforcement, 115
control. *See also* autonomy
　medication and, 33
　token economy and, 78
cooperation, 128–29
co-option prevention, 263–64
co-therapists
　group, 368
　recruitment, 264–65
cotton candy diagnosis, 300–1, 302
countertransference, 249, 250, 252, 296
county fairs, 145
criticism
　expectation of, 164
　persistent self-criticism, xxvi
crowd participation, in bullying, 94
CTMBO (Crowd That Must Be Obeyed), 279
curbstone consult, xxxvi
Curran, J., 113 (note ii)
Current Psychiatry, 405

Index

cutting, 7, 88–90, 333–35. *See also* self-mutilating behavior (SMB)

Darkness Visible (Styron), 151, 228–36. *See also* Styron, William
Darrell (pseudonym), 345–47
DBT (Dialectical Behavior Therapy), 367–68
DD (developmentally disabled) individuals, 105, 141, 143, 168–69
death, 48. *See also* grief; loss
   avoidance and, 46
   in *Catcher in the Rye*, 35–45
   contemplation of, 203–4 (*see also* death ruminations)
   fear of, 198
   impact of, 183
   meaning created by, 307–10
   of peer, 334
   preoccupation with, 306–26
death ruminations
   as consolation, 97
   as developmental stage, 315
   as hope, 340–41
   vs. suicidal intent, 306–26, 349
decision science, 413
Decker, Hannah S., 339 (note ii)
defiance, 9 (note v)
degenerative disease, xxxvi–xxxvii
denial
   adolescent, 290
   of bullying, 291–92
   confrontation and, 290
   entrenched, 293–96
   insights and, 304–5
   masquerading as compliance, 296–98
   masquerading as provocativeness, 299–303
   masquerading as resistiveness, 299
   softening, 290–302
   Third Person Invisible, 294
denial defenses, 180
dependency, 87
Depression, 6, 419. *See also* Antidepressants
   in adolescents, 226–27
   Antipsychotics and, 226
   apparent lack of precipitant, 236–43
   Attachment Disability and, 215–43
   diet and, 371
   in *DSM*, 222–23, 226, 227
   Endogenous Depression, 151, 193 (note ii), 221–22, 225–36, 305–6, 340, 341–42 (note iii), 354
   hopelessness and, 231–35, 340
   management of, 135
   medications and, 214
   misdiagnosis of, 194
   reactive component, 241
   Reactive Depression, 221–22, 224–25
   self-assessment of, 216–17
   similarity to chronic pain disability, 153
   spectrum thinking and, 223–28
   stopping substance use and, 235–36
   subtypes, 221–23
   use of term, xxvi, 218

Index

vulnerability to, xxi
"depression", 53–55
   acting-out and, 81
   anxiety and, 187, 305–6
   case studies, 189–94
"depression", chronic illness and, 410–11
"depression"
   clarification and, 305–6
   definition of, 217–18
   as Endogenous Depression, 305–6
"depression", entanglement and, 67
"depression"
   as "explanation" of personal problems, 330
   meanings of, xxv–xxvi
   medications for, 45, 47
   vs. stress, 354
   use of term, xxvi, 54, 192, 193 (note ii), 217–21
depression, 193 (note ii), 224
   failure and, 371
   use of term, xxvi, 192–93, 218
description, learning, 332–33, 336
detachment, 295–96
detention, involuntary, 128
developmental issues, 258
developmentally disabled (DD) individuals, 105, 141, 143, 168–69
diagnosis. *See also* assessment/workup; *DSM*; evaluation
   of BPD, 91–92
   comorbidity and, 391–93
   cotton candy diagnosis, 302
   deficiencies in, 103–4
   diagnostic agnostic, 111
   in *DSM-III*, 111
   in *DSM-5*, 390
   empty calorie diagnosis, 93, 95, 300
   five-axis template, 283–84, 382, 397–98, 402
   increase in diagnostic categories, 407
   of MDD, 390 (note iv)
   objective thinking in, xxii, xxxiv, xxxiv (note xi), 389–90
   of ODD, 93–95
   in psychiatry, 223
   of PTSD, 104
   recognizing degree of disability and, 383–84
   Research Domain Criteria, 384, 390, 402, 413–14
   research experiences and, 110
   Rita, 394–400
   Schiele and, 110–11
   of Schizophrenia, 197 (note iv)
   subjectivity in, xxxiv (note xi), 390
   vs. treatment, 105
   vs. understanding, xxix, 99, 396, 397–400
Diagnostic and Statistical Manual of Mental Disorders. *See DSM*
diagnostic styles, change in, 92
Dialectical Behavior Therapy (DBT), 367–68
Diamond, Jared, 290
diary card, 368
diet, 371
disability, 399

Index

abandonment and, 154, 413
collaborative care and, 411
vs. disease, xxx, 11, 275, 415
health care and, 52, 411
impaired trust as, xxx
management of, 416, 419 (*see also* management)
medical approach and, 51–52
preventing, 421
quantifying degree of, 415
recognizing degree of, 383–84
recovery from, 32 (note ii)
responsibility for living with consequences, 416
as target of attention, 416
disability, target symptom, 402
disability triangle, 77
disease
degenerative, xxxvi–xxxvii
vs. disability, xxx, 11, 275, 415
need for treatment of, 419
trauma as, xxix
Disease/Disability Format, 419–22
Disinhibited Social Engagement Disorder, xxi, 5 (note i), 103
disorders, 385
disruptiveness, 8. *See also* acting-out
dissociation, xvii, 20, 90, 216, 366
distrust, xviii. *See also* mistrust
chronic pain and, 153, 160, 161, 162–63
connection with trauma, 123
of hospitals, 201–2
neutralizing, 163

pathologizing, xxx–xxxi, 99, 104, 393
role of, 123
as sign of emotional damage, xxxi
ditchdigging, 127
Docherty, John, 107, 112, 113, 118, 123, 130
doctor-as-cop, 257–58
doctors
fear of, 202–3, 204
role of, 52
dropout equation, 136–37
dropouts, 19–20
angry, 23
Holden Caulfield, 150
Focus Program, 106, 167–71
silent, 23
dropping out, xxiv, 18
as beneficial, 28
causes of, xix
cognitive interference and, 136–37
rates of, 139
underperformance and, 136
Work Opportunities Center and, 135–39
drugs. *See* medication; substance use/abuse
DSM
Depression in, 226, 227
diagnostic format in, 382–84
increase in diagnostic categories and, 407
Major Depression in, 228
DSM-I, 378
DSM-II, elimination of dynamic formulation in, 382–87

Index

DSM-III, 116, 159 (note iii), 415
  criteria in, 382
  Depression in, 223
  diagnostic format of, 111
  end of dynamic formulation and, 385
  objective thinking in, 389–91
  revised nosology in, 402
  revision of, 339 (note ii)
  subjective experience in, 377–78
DSM-IV, 415
DSM-5, xvii (note i), 5 (note i), 382, 414, 420
  acting-out behavior in, 103
  attachment issues in, 50
  comorbidity and, 391–93
  continued reliance on diagnostic nomenclature of, 407
  deficiencies of, 407
  diagnostic approach of, 384
  fatuous diagnostic categories in, 93
  MDD in, 390
  ODD in, 93, 418
  personality disorders and, 91
  Reactive Attachment Disorder in, xxi, 103
ducks, 41, 44, 45
Dyllen (pseudonym), xxxii, 15–35, 235
dynamic thinking, xxii, 394, 402
  credibility of, 385
  elimination of, 382–87
  RDoC and, 414

Early Clinical Drug Evaluation Unit (ECDEU), 109, 121, 122, 126, 390, 415

eating disorders, 89 (note iv)
ECDEU (Early Clinical Drug Evaluation Unit), 109, 121, 122, 126, 390, 415
education. *See also* dropouts; dropping out; learning; school
  anxiety and, 34–35
  compulsory school attendance, xxiv (note iv), 339 (note i), 374 (note x), 403
  history of, 106
  reading and, 168
  underperformance and, 168
education reform, xxiii–xxiv (note iv)
EFA (Omega-3 essential fatty acids), 371
Ehrlich, Paul, 126
electronic medical records (EMRs), xxxv (note xii)
electrotherapy, 226
Elk River School District Focus Program, 169–71
Ellis, Albert, 388
EMDR (Eye Movement Desensitization and Reprocessing), 365–66, 419
emergency room referrals, 315
emotion. *See also* Affective Interference; fear
  establishing clarity of, 304
  focus on, 381
  hidden, 138
  interaction with external events, 116 (note iv)
  learning and, 137
  no-words-for-feelings, 303–4
  as organizing, 381
emotional damage, distrust as sign of, xxxi
emotional interference, 62

456

Index

emotional support, loss of, 51. *See also* support

empathy, excessive, 49, 85

empty calorie diagnosis, 93, 95, 300

EMRs (electronic medical records), xxxv (note xii)

enabling, 85–87, 334

Endicott, Jean, 116

Endogenicity, 225–36

Endogenous Depression, 151, 193 (note ii), 221–22, 225–36, 305–6, 340, 341–42 (note iii), 354

energy, intrapsychic, 116, 116 (note iv), 117

engagement, resistiveness to, 62, 251. *See also* resistiveness

Engel, George, 156–57, 159, 159 (note iii)

enmeshment, 6 (note ii). *See also* entanglement

entanglement, 6–7, 148 (note v)
   acting-out as protection against, 98
   Antidepressants and, 68–69, 70
   avoiding, 317
   belated recognition of, 241–42
   case studies, 57–76
   defensive posture, 61
   guilt and, 62, 63
   hopelessness and, 63, 68
   Maddie, 281–86, 344
   managing fears of, 349–50
   nurturing professions and, 65–66
   parents and, 66–67, 69, 70–71, 72–76
   peer, 297
   Peggy, 316–17
   pretending ignorance, 61
   protectiveness and, 63, 65
   provocativeness and, 74–75, 302–3
   recovering from, 285
   Rose, 239
   SMB as sign of, 97
   treatment approach, 69, 72
   vulnerability to suicide and, 63
   work and, 75

entertainment business, 145

environment
   claim on (*see* claim on environment)
   good enough, xxxii, xxxiii, 7–8, 8 (note iv)

E/RP (Exposure/Response Prevention), 33, 35, 204–5, 323, 363–65

evaluation. *See also* assessment/workup; diagnosis; interview
   of chronic pain, 155–56
   consultation-liaison, xxviii, xxxvi
   sponsors in, 60 (*see also* sponsors)

experience
   in assessment, 377–78, 381
   learning from, 30, 31, 62, 91, 183, 293

exploitation, 331. *See also* abuse

Exposure/Response Prevention (E/RP), 33, 35, 204–5, 323, 363–65

externalizing behavior, 7–11, 22, 103. *See also* acting-out

Index

extrapsychic energy, 117
Eye Movement Desensitization and Reprocessing (EMDR), 365–66, 419
Eysenck, Hans, 387

failure
    depression and, 371
    fear of, 25 (note i)
    repetitive, 216
    as safe, 25, 84
fairness, 277–79
family practice, integrated with psychiatry, xxxv–xxxviii, 52 (note x), 409–13
family therapy, 366–67, 388
fathers. *See* adults; parent(s); sponsors
fear. *See also* emotion
    anger and, 164, 326–27
    awareness of, 97
    contemplating, 371
    of death, 203
    of doctors, 202–3, 204
    of entanglement, 349–50
    of revelation, 175
    of sleep, 342–43
feelings. *See* emotion
feelings, no-words-for-, 303–4. *See also* insight, promoting
fibromyalgia, 223
Fieve, Ronald, 116
Fink, M., 117 (note v)
firefighters, 126
five-axis system, 283–84, 382, 397–98, 402
flashbacks, 180, 181
flooding, 204

focus on what can be changed, xxxi, 55, 106, 337–75, 416
    chronic pain and, 161
    difficulty of implementing, 243
    limits of, 338–41
    medications and, 341–60
Focus Program, 106, 167–71
forgiveness, 330
Freud, Sigmund, xxii, 413. *See also* neo-Freudians
Freudian terminology, in assessments, 379–80

Gabbard, Glen O., 386, 402
GAF (Global Assessment of Functioning), 415
game theory, 346–47
gang behavior, 94
gender identity, 340. *See also* sexual identity issues
Generalized Anxiety, 352–53
Georgina (pseudonym), 67–72
girls, entanglement and, 7
Global Assessment of Functioning (GAF), 415
goals, of book, xxiii–xxxiii
Golding, William, 303
good-enough parenting/environment, xxxii, xxxiii, 7–8, 8 (note iv)
graduation, entanglement and, 67–72
Great Society, 127
Green, Richard, 115, 117, 122, 136, 136 (note i)
grief. *See also* death; loss
    acceptance and, 209
    Adjustment Reaction and, 46
    avoidance and, 46

case studies, 35–45
  in *Catcher in the Rye*, 42–44
  incomplete mourning, 236
  prolonged, 209–13
grief counselor, 54
group co-therapists, 368
group discussion, 368–70
group therapy, 368, 369
guilt, 28, 220, 278, 361
  about pain, 340
  entanglement and, 62, 63
  suicide and, 318

Haley, Jay, 346, 388
hallucinations, xi–xii
Hamlet (fictional character), 203, 320
Harrison's Principles of Internal Medicine, 417
Hassler, Jon, 150, 306
healing
  in *Catcher in the Rye*, 42
  failed, 10
health care
  adolescent referrals, 144
  collaborative care, xxxv–xxxviii, 52 (note x), 409–13
  disability and, 52, 411
  HMOs, 135, 139–40, 148
health maintenance organizations (HMOs), 135, 139–40, 148
Heimarck, Greg, xi, xii–xv
Helen (pseudonym), xxxii, 45–55, 178, 362 (note viii), 388
helicopter parents, 66–67
help
  accepting, 32–33
  cry for, 9, 119, 142, 195, 351
  danger of, 179, 294

  as threat, 57–63
Hennepin County Medical Center, 133
Hesiod, 370
hippocampus, xxii (note ii)
history, collateral, 231–32
HMOs (health maintenance organizations), 135, 139–40, 148
homosexuality, 197, 201
hope, death ruminations as, 340–41
Hope and Help for Your Nerves (Weekes), 371
hopelessness, 226, 322
  in adolescents, 227
  in *Catcher in the Rye*, 44–45
  Depression and, 231–35, 340
  entanglement and, 63, 68
  inattentiveness and, 234–35, 253
  signs of, 234–235
  suicide and, 210, 231–35, 321, 339–41
hospitalization
  chronic, 119
  involuntary, 128
How to Win Friends and Influence People (Carnegie), 268
human behavior, 149
Humphrey, Hubert, 127
hypertension, 222 (note iv)
hypnosis, 204–5
hypocrisy, in *Catcher in the Rye*, 41
Hysteria, 155

ideology, generated by psychiatric leadership, 377
ignorance, pretending, 61

Igor talk, 21, 208, 353. *See also* voice, irrational; what if thinking

illness, chronic, xxxvi–xxxvii, 410–11

illness, vs. disability, 275, 415. *See also* disease

impersonal approach, 62–63

improvement. *See also* change; recovery
  dangers of, 345–47
  difficulty understanding, 30–32

impulse control, 80, 129

inattentiveness, 234–35, 253, 299

incest, 340

independence, physical, xxxvi–xxxvii. *See also* autonomy; disability

inflammation, chronic, 371

inhibited attachment disorders, 4–5, 6

inner mindfulness, 370

innovation, receptivity to, 135

input, from sponsors, 62

Insel, Thomas, xxx (note vii), 384, 402

insight, promoting, 290
  distinguishing anger from fear, 326–27
  suicidal intent vs. death ruminations, 306–26

insincerity, 38, 39–40

insomnia, 16, 19

insubordination, 132

integrated care, xxxv–xxxviii, 52 (note x), 409–13

internalizing behavior, 11

interpersonal psychotherapy (ITP), 403

interpersonal theory, 381

Interpersonal Therapy (IPT), 419

intervention
  active, 139–47, 163, 183
  by sponsors, 62
  timing of, 254–58

interview. *See also* assessment/workup; evaluation
  resistance in, 177
  signal in, 176–77
  sponsors in, 69, 259–65 (*see also* sponsors)
  transfer-of-care, 176–77
  unstructured, 178

intrapsychic energy, 116, 116 (note iv), 117

"Is Chronic Pain Organic?" (Curran), 162

isolation, 334

Jackie (pseudonym), 77–78, 79–85, 87, 88–90, 272, 300, 391, 393–94

JAMA, xxxvii (note xiii)

JAMA Psychiatry, 404, 408, 414

James, Julian, xi–xii

Jepson, William, 132

Joiner, Thomas, 234

Jorud, S., 113 (note ii)

journal, symptom, 368, 368 (note ix)

judgmental thinking, reframing, 361

Julie (pseudonym), 209–13

Jureidini, Jon N., 219, 227

Justin (pseudonym), 294–96

Katon, Wayne, 410, 411

Index

Kay, Gerald, 386, 402
Kepler, Johannes, 404, 405, 406, 422
Kierkegaard, S., 310
Kindler, Kenneth S., 228, 414, 422
Klein, Donald F., 116–17, 117 (note v), 414
Kolb, Lawrence, xiv, 105, 107, 116, 188, 198 (note vi), 206, 207, 248, 325 (note vii), 326, 381, 385–86, 387, 415
Kornfeld, D., xxvii–xxix, xxix (note v), 412
Kraepelin, Emil, 228
Kupfer, David J., 393

labels, 22–23
Lahey, Benjamin, xviii
Lakeland Mental Health Center, 105, 140
language of psychiatry, xxv. *See also* nomenclature
Lara (pseudonym), 335, 356–57, 361
Large Hadron Collider, 406 (note viii)
leadership, psychiatric, 402
    change in, 385–94
    ideology of, 377
    nomenclature and, xxx (note vii)
leadership, responsibilities of, xxiv (note iv)
learning, 403. *See also* education; school
    adaptive, 374
    by adolescents, xxiv (note iv)
    difficulty with, 30, 62
    emotions and, 137
    from experience, 30, 31, 62, 91, 183, 293
    hating, xix, xxiv (note iv)
    listening and, 362, 363
    maladaptive, xvii, xviii, 290, 416
    from patients, 171–83
    prepartum, 138 (note ii)
    recovery and, 32 (note ii)
    role in preventing disability, 421
learning avoidance, xxiv (note iv)
Levant, Oscar, 304
Lieberman, Jeffrey A., 201 (note vii), 360
Lincoln, Abraham, 268
Lindsey (pseudonym), 320–26, 341, 359
Linehan, Marsha M., 367
listening, in patient assessment, 172–83
listening style, 143
locked unit, 78, 112–14
loneliness, 45
Lonely Crowd, The (Riesman), 66, 89 (note iv), 257 (note iii)
Lord of the Flies (Golding), 303
loss. *See also* death; grief; separation
    abandonment and, 149
    avoidance and, 46
    awareness of, 43, 97
    change and, 208
    childhood, Depression and, 229, 230–31
    chronic pain and, 160
    denying, 291
    disability and, 154
    energizing potential of, 236

grief and, 213
ignoring threat of, 291
impact of, 183
literary depictions of, 150–51 (*see also Catcher in the Rye*; *Darkness Visible*)
preoccupation with, 306–26
problem behaviors and, 169
of security, 104
suppression of, 97
in theory of human behavior, 149–51
threat of, 291, 366
of trust, 45–55
as unavoidable, xxxii–xxxiii
love, asking for, 10
Luhrmann, T. M., xxx (note vii)

MacKinnon, Roger, 171, 177, 179, 207
Maddie (pseudonym), 281–86, 344
Maggie (pseudonym), 372–73
Magic Mountain, The (Mann), 106, 151, 203, 307–10
magnification issue, 406 (note viii)
Major Depressive Disorder (MDD), 220, 228, 390, 390 (note iv)
maladaptive behaviors, avoiding reinforcing, 247
maladaptive learning, xvii, xviii, 290, 416
males, 19–20
Malingering, 155
management, 337–75. *See also* acceptance; clarification; focus on what can be changed; self-management; stagecraft; token economy

of acting-out, 77, 84
of ambivalence, 77
avoiding making things worse, xxx, 248
CBT, 360–62
of chronic pain, 153, 160–63
constraints on, 248–58 (*see also* attentiveness; resistiveness; timing)
of developmentally disabled, 105
of disability, 416
of eating disorders, 89 (note iv)
focus on, xxvii
impersonal approach, 62–63
need for, 419
principles of, xxxi, 55, 243 (*see also* acceptance; clarification; focus on what can be changed)
provocative behavior and, 76
of PTSD, 419
of Rita, 396–97
of self-blame, 335–36, 344 (note iv)
self-management, 51–53, 162
strategic, 247–58
tactical, 259–87
vs. treatment, 53
use of term, xxvii–xxix
Manhattan State Hospital, 107–9
Manic Depressive illness, 92–93
manipulation, 84–85, 268–75, 302
calling for stagecraft, 276–86
in token economy, 275–76

462

Index

Mann, Thomas, 106, 151, 203, 307–10
manners, learning, 276
marijuana, 18, 348. *See also* substance use/abuse
Markowitz, John C., 419
maternal care, 138 (note ii)
maturation, entangled parent and, 71
Maya (pseudonym), 95–99, 335
MDD (Major Depressive Disorder), 220, 228, 390, 390 (note iv)
meaning, search for, 307
med-check routines, 178
medical-legal evaluations, 154
medication, 45, 191. *See also* Antidepressants; treatment
  abuse background and, 93
  alpha-2 agonists, 343, 359–60
  Antipsychotics, 122, 125–26, 226
  anxiety and, 33, 45–46, 49, 54, 64
  autonomy and, 347
  Bipolar Disorder and, 92, 93
  change and, 341–60
  chronic mental illness and, 122
  chronic pain and, 166
  control and, 33
  dangers of improvement and, 345–47
  for "depression", 47
  Depression and, 214, 226, 341–42 (note iii)
  Early Clinical Drug Evaluation Unit, 109, 121, 122, 126, 390, 415
  efficacy of, 105, 122, 125–26
  fear of, 347–51
  focus on, 386–87
  med-check routines, 178
  misdiagnosis and, 183
  nocebo response, 344–45
  noncompliance and, 342, 343–51
  nonresponsiveness, 388–89
  overdose and, 350–51
  for panic, 65, 117
  power and, 343
  rejection of, 33
  relapse and, 210
  vs. street drugs, 347–51
  suicidal thinking and, 324
  taking charge of, 53–55
  tapering, 48, 49
  treatment synonymous with, 386
medication resistant patients, 217
meditation, 215
Melancholia, 226
mental health, trauma and, 220
mental illness. *See also* disease
  chronic, 122
  vs. disability, 275, 415
Mesnikoff, Alvin, 380, 387
MGH (Minneapolis General Hospital), 132, 133, 195–206
midlife crisis, 277
military service, xxxvii (note xiii). *See also* veterans
military tactics, 290
mindfulness, inner, 370
Minneapolis General Hospital (MGH), 132, 133, 195–206
Minnesota, 145
Minuchin, Salvador, 388

463

Index

misdiagnosis, xviii, 183, 193, 393–400, 404
   of BD, 92–93
   of Depression, 194
   nonresponsiveness and, 389
   Rita, 394–400
mistrust, 106. *See also* distrust
Mood Disorder, 197 (note iv)
moral keenness, 332–33
moral world, actual vs. inner, 361
Mortimer, John, 279
mother, "good-enough", 7–8
mothering, 8. *See also* parenting, good enough
mothers. *See* adults; parent(s); sponsors
motivation, 85
mourning, incomplete, 229–230, 236. *See also* grief
multiaxial system. *See* five-axis system
Murray, Charles, 8 (note iv)
Myth of Sisyphus, The (Camus), 310 (note iii)

Nasrallah, Henry A., 405, 406
National Institutes of Mental Health (NIMH), 384, 390
   Recovery After an Initial Schizophrenia Episode (RAISE), 421
   Research Domain Criteria, 384, 390, 402, 413
"need", replacing with "should", 165
need conflicts, 180
negative reinforcement, 88, 124
Nemeroff, Charles, 220
neo-Freudians, 3, 116
nervous system, peripheral, 160
neuroscience, 407–408. *See also* brain research
New York State Psychiatric Institute (PI), 105, 107–9, 116, 117, 141, 188, 378
night, fear of, 342–43
NIMH (National Institutes of Mental Health). *See* National Institutes of Mental Health (NIMH)
   9/11 jumpers, 233
   survivors/responders, 401
nocebo response, 342, 343, 344–45
nomenclature, 407. *See also* assessment/workup; diagnosis; *DSM*; evaluation; nosology
   critique of, xxx (note vii)
   leadership and, xxx (note vii)
   noncompliance, 256–57
   content and, 351–60
   context and, 343–51
   reasons for, 342
nonresponsiveness, xxxvii, 217, 388–89, 393
nosology. *See also* assessment/workup; diagnosis; *DSM*; evaluation
   brain research and, 405
   lack of dynamic thinking in, 414
   revised, 402
no-words-for-feelings, 303–4. *See also* insight, promoting
nurturers/nuturing, 3, 8. *See also* parent(s)
nurturing professions, 7, 50, 65–66, 85, 181 (note xi)

obedience, 251, 251 (note i), 256, 279–80. *See also* resistiveness

objective thinking, xxii, xxxiv, xxxiv (note xi), 389–90

obsessive thoughts, 142–43

ODD (Oppositional Defiant Disorder), xviii, 9 (note v), 22–23, 93–95, 300, 301, 418

Omega-3 essential fatty acids (EFA), 371

one-to-one doctor-patient format, 123

OOO (out-of-control) behavior, separation anxiety and, 114

operant conditioning, 115

opinion, soliciting, 369

oppositional, misidentification as, 338

oppositional behavior, as cry for help, 9

Oppositional Defiant Disorder (ODD), xviii, 9 (note v), 22–23, 93–95, 300, 301, 418

origins of Attachment Disability theory, 104–6. *See also* Anoka State Hospital; Kolb, L.; research experiences; Schiele, Bertrum; Sheridan, Frederick

    active intervention therapy techniques, 139–47

    Affective Interference, 137–39, 147–51

    anxiety's relation to separation, 105, 107 (*see also* Kolb, L.)

    chronic pain disability, 153–67

    clinical experiences, 105, 106, 111–14, 123–24

    consulting experiences, 105, 123, 130, 140–41, 167–71, 172

    Focus Program, 106

    learning from patients, 106, 172–83

    specialty training, 105

    summary of, 183

other-directed society, 257, 257 (note iii)

other-directedness, 89 (note iv)

out-of-control (OOO) behavior, separation anxiety and, 114

outpatient consulting appointments, 123

outreach services, 167–71

overdose, prescription medication and, 350–51

overprotectiveness, 63

Owen (pseudonym), 254, 293

ownership, 336. *See also* acceptance

Paar, Jack, 304

pain

    chronic (*see* chronic pain; chronic pain disability)

    disproportional, 155 (*see also* chronic pain)

    emotional, response to, 158–59 (note ii)

    escape from, 231–33

    guilt about, 340

    learning from experience and, 31

    owning without blame, 396

    as part of life, 327

    phantom, 156

    physical, 89, 158–59 (note ii) (*see also* cutting)

    psychogenic, 156–57

    unendurable, 339–41

pain management, 106

pain-proneness, 156–57
panic, 16–17, 21, 23, 31
  entanglement and, 64
  medications for, 65, 117
paranoid patient, 267
Paranoid Psychotic Disorder, xxxiv
Paranoid Schizophrenia, xxxi (note viii), 272
parenting, good enough, xxxii, xxxiii, 7–8, 8 (note iv)
parent(s). *See also* sponsors
  ability to command compliance, 279–80
  addicted, 64–65
  alcoholic, 20
  angry, 197
  angry-parent/provocative-child, 302–3
  childhood development and, 3 (*see also* attachment)
  entanglement and, 66–67, 69, 70–71, 72–76
  graduation and, 71
  in interviews, 69, 259–65
  leadership by, xxiv (note iv)
  underperformance and, 168
  use of term, xxvi–xxvii
patients
  learning from, 106, 171–83
  medication resistant, 217
Peale, Norman Vincent, 370
peer entanglement, 297
peer-group acceptance, anxiety about, 301
peers, in *Catcher in the Rye*, 39
Peggy (pseudonym), 311–20, 331, 337, 358–59
pension programs, 127

perfectionism, 323, 324, 364–65
performance anxiety, 21, 22, 25 (note i), 27. *See also* Dyllen (pseudonym)
peripheral nervous system, 160
personality disorders, in *DSM-5*, 91
pet companionship, 372–73
phantom pain, 156
pharmacological treatment. *See* medication
philosophy, 310, 331–32
phobia, cancer, 197, 202, 204
phobias. *See* fear
phobic avoidance, 202–3
  exposure/response-prevention (E/RP) protocol, 204–5
  treatment of, 204–5
phone contact, protocol for, 206–7
phoniness, 39. *See also* insincerity
physical independence, xxxvi–xxxvii
physicians. *See also* psychiatrists
  abuse background and, 93
  fear of, 202–3, 204
Physician's Global Judgement, 415
PI (New York State Psychiatric Institute), 105, 107–9, 116, 117, 141, 188, 378
Pies, Ronald, xxx (note vii), 417, 418
placebo phenomena, 342
politics, 126–28
Pollock, Tony, 195–96
POP, Mr. (pseudonym), xxxi (note viii), 129, 133, 161, 263, 269–75, 291, 370, 418

Posttraumatic Stress Disorder (PTSD), xvii (note i), 103–4, 401, 403, 419
posttraumatic symptoms, 157 (note i), 401
posture, defensive, 61
power
    abuse background and, 93
    medications and, 343
    responding to, 325
power struggle, 250–51
powerlessness
    admitting, 124
    trauma and, 181
prevention, xviii–xix
primary care, integrated with psychiatry, xxxv–xxxviii, 52 (note x), 409–13
prognosis
    for anxiety, 32–34
    for attachment acting-out, 10–11
protectiveness
    by abuse victims, 85
    of addicted parent, 65
    in *Catcher in the Rye*, 40–42
    entanglement and, 65
protocol, 206
provocativeness, 73, 74–75, 272. *See also* acting-out; Punker
    angry-parent/provocative-child, 302–3
    anxiety and, 302
    denial masquerading as, 299–303
    entanglement and, 302–3
Psychiatric Interview in Clinical Practice, The (Buckley and Michaels), 171 (note v)
Psychiatric Times, xxxiv

psychiatrists. *See also* physicians
    HMOs and, 139
    shortage of, 148
    verbal abuse of, 144, 164
psychiatry. *See also* behavioral health
    in 1960s, 378–81
    in 1970 and 1980s, 382–84
    community, 141–42
    goal of, 403–4
    integrated, xxxv–xxxviii, 52 (note x), 409–13
    language of, xxv (*see also* nomenclature)
    reform in, xxiii–xxiv
psychoanalysis, 3, 143, 378–80, 382
psychological autopsies, 318
psychological development, 3
psychology, abnormal, xii
psychotherapy
    ceded to non-psychiatrists, 387–88
    need for training in, 386–87
    psychodynamic, 143
PTSD (Posttraumatic Stress Disorder) (copy), xvii (note i), 103–4, 401, 403, 419
public health, principles of, xxxii
publication, on token economy, 124–26
Punker, The, 72–76, 77

Rado, Sandor, 116 (note iv), 381
RAISE (Recovery After an Initial Schizophrenia Episode), 421

rambling, chronic pain and, 165–66
Raney, Lon E., 409, 410, 411
Rapaport, David, 379
rape, 340
Rapid Cycling Mood Disorder, 236, 240
Rasminsky, S., xxxv (note xii)
Rational Emotive Behavior Therapy (REBT), 388
RDoC (Research Domain Criteria), 384, 390, 402, 413–14
Reactive Attachment Disorders, xxi, 4–5, 6, 103
Reactive Depression, 221–22, 224–25
Reactivity, 224–25
reading, 168
Rebecca (pseudonym), 189–94, 206, 252, 289, 393
rebellion, 74–75, 94. *See also Catcher in the Rye*
REBT (Rational Emotive Behavior Therapy), 388
recognition, as dangerous, 84
recovery, 32 (note ii). *See also* change; improvement; relapse
    acceptance and, 32
    from Attachment Entanglement, 285
    danger of, 84, 209–13
    Recovery After an Initial Schizophrenia Episode (RAISE), 421
redirection, 336, 356–58, 361–62, 363
Redlin, Terry, xxxii (note ix)
referrals
    of adolescents, 144
    medical-legal evaluations, 154

reform, education, xxiii–xxiv (note iv)
reform, psychiatric, xxiii–xxiv
reframing judgmental thinking, 361
regard, unconditional, 42
Regier, Darrel A., 393
reinforcement, 7 (note iii)
    contingent, 115
    intermittent, 7–8
    negative, 124
    selective, 126, 128
    strategies, 84
reinforcing stimuli, 142
rejection
    chronic pain and, 158
    entanglement and, 73
rejection sensitivity, 241–42, 362, 363
relapse, 124, 210–211, 214
relationships
    after trauma, xvii
    BPD and, 91–92
    difficulties maintaining, 46
remediation, xxxiii, xxxv, 403–4
"Remember That Drive-by Shooting?" (Tasman), xxxiv–xxxv
Renée (pseudonym), 173–83
repeating yourself, 270 (note v)
repetition, 293
repetitive prompts, 336
Research Domain Criteria (RDoC), 384, 390, 402, 413–14
research experiences, 105, 107, 109–11
    diagnosis and, 110

Early Clinical Drug Evaluation Unit, 109, 121, 122, 126, 390, 415
  impact of, 120–23
residency, xxii, xxvii–xxix, 171, 386
resilience, 8
Resistive, Mr. (pseudonym), 177, 177 (note viii), 248–51, 293, 299, 361
resistiveness, 248–51, 256, 266–67
  denial masquerading as, 299
  entanglement and, 62, 63
  games model of therapy and, 346–47
  vs. inattentiveness, 299
  in interview, 177
  overcoming, 325
  pretending ignorance, 61
  softening, 257
responsibility, 370
retirement programs, 127
revelation, fear of, 175, 177 (note viii)
reward, 7 (note iii)
rhetoric, heated, 265–66
Rhodes Scholarship, xii
"Richard Cory" (Robinson), 231–32
Riesman, David, 66, 89 (note iv), 257 (note iii), 278, 307
Rita (pseudonym), 394–400
Robinson, Edwin Arlington, 231–32
Roffwarg, Howard, 116
Rosary Society, 279
Rose (pseudonym), 236–43, 306, 393
Ross, David A., 407, 422

rules, 128–29, 146–47, 277–78, 279. *See also* clarification
running, 44–45
rural areas, chronicity and, 119 (note viii)
Ryan (pseudonym), 261

Sacco, Frank C., 94, 291–92
sadness, 45
safety contracts, 316
Salinger, J. D., 6, 36–45, 42 (note iv), 105–6
Samantha (pseudonym), 287, 296–98, 334
Saturday Night Fever (film), 318
scapegoating, 72, 73
Schiele, Bertrum, 105, 107, 109, 110–11, 120–23, 133, 227, 338, 383, 390, 391, 402, 415, 417
Schizoaffective, 148 (note v)
Schizophrenia, 196–207, 381, 392
  Chronic, 121, 124
  double theory bind of, 388
  overdiagnosis of, 197 (note iv)
  Recovery After an Initial Schizophrenia Episode (RAISE), 421
  symptoms, 420–21
  treatment of, 201–2
Schmidt, Ed, 105, 141–43, 145, 163
Schmidt, Mary, 105, 141, 143, 144–46, 163, 277
Schmidts (family), 279
school. *See also* dropouts; dropping out; education; learning
  conduct issues and, 339
  maltreatment at, xviii
  mandatory attendance, xix, xxiv (note iv), 339 (note i),

Index

374 (note x), 403

Schwartz, Carl, 392

Schynoll, Guido, 130, 131, 133

Searles, Harold, 116, 249–51, 296, 299, 381, 387

seclusion, need for, 118, 119

security
  adolescents' desire for, 301
  death and, 43
  loss of, 104
  sponsor participation and, 261–62

security/authority dyad, 303

seductiveness, of patients, 251–53

SEID (systemic exertion intolerance disease), 417

self-blame, 312, 331, 333–36, 344 (note iv). *See also* acceptance; blame/blaming

self-criticism, persistent, xxvi

self-deprecatory triad, 216

self-destructive behavior, 10. *See also* cutting; self-mutilating behavior (SMB); substance use/abuse; suicide

self-help, 370–71

self-improvement, 370

self-management, 51–53, 162

self-medication, 216. *See also* substance use/abuse

self-mutilating behavior (SMB), 10, 88–90, 333–35. *See also* cutting
  abuse background and, 89–90
  acting-out and, 335
  negative reinforcement and, 88
  as sign of entanglement, 97

self-respect, 127

separation
  anxiety and, 105, 107, 188, 198 (note vi), 326, 415
  cancer as, 198
  change and, 208
  effects of, 4
  fear of death and, 204
  looking for, 208
  phone contact and, 206–7
  prospect of, 208
  Catcher in the Rye, 36–45

separation anxiety, 142, 352–53
  managing, 5
  out-of-control behavior and, 114

Serenity Prayer, 337

servitude, 334

sexual identity issues, 334. *See also* gender identity; homosexuality

SFT (Structural Family Therapy), 388

shame, 278

Shapiro, Francine, 365, 366

Sheps, Jack, 116, 369

Sherburne County Social Services Department, 169

Sheridan, Frederick, xxxiii, 62 (note iv), 105, 114–15, 135–39, 147, 170

"should", replacing with "need", 165

Shrinks: The Untold Story of Psychiatry (Lieberman), 202–3 (note vii), 360

signals, 176–177

Skinner, B. F., 115, 117, 123

sleep, 19

Index

SMB (self-mutilating behavior). *See* self-mutilating behavior (SMB)

social anxiety, 18, 19. *See also* anxiety

social forces, 115

social media, self-mutilating behavior and, 89 (note iv)

Social Phobia, 352–53

social programs, 127–28

social welfare programs, 127

societies, collapse of, 290

somatization, 80

speaking to unconscious, 179, 207

spectrum concept, Depression as, 223–28

Spitzer, Robert, 116

sponsors
    as co-therapists, 265
    in evaluation process, 60
    intervention by, 62
    interview participation of, 259–65
    leadership by, xxiv (note iv)
    presence of, 257, 294, 311
    sensitivity to troubles of, 98
    use of term, xxvii

stability, behavioral, 114

stagecraft, 62–63, 265, 267–86, 302, 349–50

Staggerford (Hassler), 150, 306–7

state hospitals. *See also* Anoka State Hospital
    dynamics of, 112
    Manhattan State Hospital, 107–9
    New York State Psychiatric Institute (PI), 107–9

stimuli, reinforcing, 142

strategic adaptive skills, 248–58

strategy, for management, 247–58

street cred, 94

street drugs, vs. medications, 347–51

stress, 55, 354. *See also* anti-stressants

stress management, 49

stress response, in Depression, 224

stression, 224–25

Structural Family Therapy (SFT), 388

structure, adolescents' desire for, 301

student, responsibilities of, 52

Styron, William, 151, 210, 216, 228–36, 285, 310 (note iii), 340, 393

subjectivity, xxxiv (note xi), 390. *See also* experience, in assessment

substance use/abuse, 17, 19, 30, 216. *See also* addiction; alcohol
    entanglement and, 67
    pervasive anxiety and, 307 (note ii)
    prescription medications, 348–49
    recovery, 33–34, 214
    self-treatment with, 24
    as solution, 31
    stopping, Depression and, 235–36
    street drugs vs. prescriptions, 347–51

success
    as danger, 29–30

fear of, 25, 25 (note i)
suffering, 192, 304. *See also* pain
suggestions, 404–22
   collaborative care promotion, 409–13
   Disease/ Disability Format, 419–22
   neuroscience in clinical psychiatry, 407–8
   provisional assessment alternative, 414–17
   reliance on diagnostic nomenclature of *DSM-5*, 407
   Research Domain Criteria, 413–14
suicidal feelings, Antidepressants and, 343–44
suicidal intent, 285, 306–26
suicidal talk, vs. suicidal behavior, 285–86
suicidal thinking
   vs. death ruminations, 349
   entanglement and, 67
   medications and, 324
   as sign of mental awareness, 325–26
suicide, 320–26
   adolescents and, 233–34, 344
   attachment acting-out and, 10
   entanglement and, 7
   as escape from pain, 231–33
   guilt and, 318
   harbingers of, 315
   hopelessness and, 210, 231–35, 321, 339–41
   inattentiveness and, 235
   of peer, 334

   pervasive anxiety and, 307 (note ii)
   ping-pong, 7, 318
   psychological autopsies, 318
   as solution, 285
   Styron's plans for, 229, 285
   in Styron's works, 230
   vs. suicidal talk, 285–86
   veterans and, xxxvii, xxxvii (note xiii)
   vulnerability to, 63
   of Woodruff, 339 (note ii)
suicide risk, 6
Sullivan, Harry Stack, 381
Summerfield, Paul, 406, 408, 414
support, 8, 51, 123, 383, 384, 399
survival, vulnerability and, 11
Swartz, J. R., xxi (note ii), xxii (note ii), xxxii, 419
SWMBO (She Who Must Be Obeyed), 279
symptom causality, 378
symptoms
   target, 383, 398
   treating, 133
system, working, 276
systemic exertion intolerance disease (SEID), 417

tactical adaptive skills, 247–48, 259–87
tactical management, 259–87
   complaints, 265
   heated rhetoric, 265–66
   recognizing achievement, 286–87
   resistiveness, 266–67

Index

stagecraft, 265, 267–86
Talbott, John, 386
talking therapy, 362
target behavior, 338
target symptom disability, 402
target symptoms, 383, 398
Tasman, A., xxxiv–xxxv, xxxiv–xxxv (note xii), xxxvi, 404
tattooing, 89
teachers, as performers, 62
teacher/student interaction, 52
Teenagers, xxiii (note iv). *See also* adolescents
terminology, xxv–xxvi
therapeutic boundaries, 334–35
therapeutic relationship, 253–54
therapeutic style, 143
therapists
    availability of, 139
    as performers, 62
therapy. *See also* management; psychotherapy; treatment
    active intervention, 139–47, 163, 183
    behavior in, 75–76
    games model of, 346–47
    HMOs and, 139
    trust and, 211, 212
therapy, grief, 54
third grade transition, 20
Third Person Invisible (TPI), 294
threat denial, 291, 292. *See also* denial
threat to sign out Against Medical Advice, xxix (note v)
time-out, in token economy, 118, 119

timing, 253–58, 358
Tobian, Louis Jr., 108
token economy, 78, 79–85, 105, 268
    assessing, 391
    boundaries and, 120, 125, 394
    complaints about, 84–85
    development of, 115–18
    impact of, 82–84
    manipulation in, 275–76
    publication on, 124–26
    time-out in, 118, 119
    trust management with, 394
TPI (Third Person Invisible), 294
transitions. *See* graduation
trauma, 81
    accepting without blame, 329
    adaptive skills and, 215–16
    Attachment Disability and, 149
    brain damage from, xxii, xxii (note ii)
    changes to brain and, 419
    connection with distrust, 123
    discounting, xxxvi
    as disease, xxix
    fear of night and, 342–43
    long-term consequences of, xxi
    mental health and, 220
    powerlessness and, 181
    survivors of, xvii
    treatment of, 374
    underperformance and, xxi
trauma residuals, xxxii, 20, 365
trauma triad, xvii, 375, 419

Index

misinterpretation of, xix
vs. Posttraumatic Stress Disorder, xvii (note i)
treatment. *See also* intervention; management; medication; therapy; token economy; understanding
  approach to entanglement, 69, 72
  vs. diagnosis, 105
  integration of medication and therapy, 386
  vs. management, 53
  need for, 419
  of phobic avoidance, 204
  psychodynamic psychotherapy, 143
  of PTSD, 403
  of Schizophrenia, 201–2
  of symptoms, 133
  synonymous with medication, 386
  traditional medical approach, 51
  of trauma, 374
  understanding/management strategy, 51–53
treatment resistance, 217, 419
truancy, 27
trust. *See also* distrust; mistrust
  anxieties about, 192
  Attachment Disability and, 212
  cultivation of, 253–54
  damaged, xxv
  impaired, xxx
  injured, xvii
  loss of, 45–55
  therapy and, 211, 212
trust deficit, xviii

trust management, with token economy, 394
truth, definitions of, 331–32
Twemlow, Stuart W., 94, 291–92

unconscious, speaking to, 179, 207
uncontrollable, attempts to control, 217 (note i)
"Unconventional Treatment of Treatment-Resistant Hospitalized Patients" (Curran, Jorud, and Whitman), 113 (note ii)
underperformance, xxiv, xxiv (note iv), 19–20
  causes of, xix
  dropping out and, 136
  emergence of, 168
  parents and, 168
  trauma and, xxi
  understanding, 99, 172–83, 396, 397–400
  vs. diagnosis, xxix
  focus on, xxvii, xxix–xxx
  use of term, xxvii
understanding/management strategy, 53
unfairness, 277–79
uninhibited attachment disorders, 4–5, 6–7
unions, 126–27
unresponsiveness, in interview, 177

Vail, David, 112
Van Dam, N. T., xxi (note ii), xxxii, 419
van der Kolk, Bessel, xxiii, xxix, 343, 374

verbal abuse, of psychiatrists, 144
verbosity, 362–63
Veteran Resilience Project, 366
veterans, xxxvii, xxxvii (note xiii), 157 (note i), 401
violence, gang-related, 94
voice, irrational, 21. *See also* Igor talk; what if thinking
Voss, Pat, 131–32
vulnerability, 8, 11, 63, 344

Weekes, Claire, 371
what if thinking, 21, 31, 208–09, 227, 323, 353
Whitman, N., 113 (note ii)
WHO Disability Assessment Scale (WHODAS), 415–416
will power, failed, 216
Winkler, Julius, x, xii, 149
Winnicott, Donald, xix, xx, xxii, xxxii (note x), 6, 7–11, 22, 44, 77, 91, 98, 119, 125, 135, 136, 137, 142, 183, 381, 400, 401, 418
Winston (pseudonym), 130–31, 133
withdrawal. *See also* avoidance
   in *Catcher in the Rye*, 38–39
   response to, 22–23
WOC (Work Opportunities Center), 135–39
Wolpe, Joseph, 387
women, perimenopausal, 420
Woodruff, Robert A. Jr., 339 (note ii)
work, xxxvi
   anxiety and, 174
   chronic pain and, 157–58
   entanglement and, 75
   as solution, 28–29
   structure of, 75
Work Opportunities Center (WOC), 135–39
workers, injured, 159. *See also* chronic pain
Works and Days (Hesiod), 370
workups. *See* assessment/workup
World War I, 310. *See also Magic Mountain, The*
World War II, xix, 4, 7–8
worry, 227. *See also* anxiety

Yager, Joel, 340

Author's Note: Introducing Volume 2

My original plan was to publish a monograph on Attachment Disability in one volume. However, the loyal readers who persevered through its successive drafts were of one voice in the midst of their encouragement: the manuscript was too long. One even remarked, "... nice two or three books you have there." Eventually I addressed this issue with my indefatigable editor, Sheridan McCarthy, who diplomatically agreed: "John, it is sooo long." Thus two volumes at least, and perhaps more.

Because this volume rests on the structure of volume 1, I will provide a brief review of volume 1 here in chapter 1. But I strongly recommend the interested reader have it at hand for reference to proposed definitions and concepts therein, which I carry forward in this volume, and for convenient access to the specifics of its twenty-eight adolescent and adult case reports that I rely on to illustrate the understanding and management of Attachment Disability.

The organization of both volumes is similar. Each explores the implications of an underlying unifying concept. In the first volume it is Dr. Lawrence Kolb's dictum, "All anxiety is related to abandonment."[i]

The second volume's unifying concept is derived from

---

i. See volume 1, pages 188–89, for my introduction to this sweeping conjecture, my initial skepticism, and then my eventual capitulation because of my subsequent and continuing clinical experiences.

another dictum, this from Aristotle: "All men by nature desire to know."[ii] In other words, learning is a natural human function, akin to breathing. That is, to be human is to breathe and learn.

Nowadays we refer to all *humans*, not men. And it would be more precise to replace *know* with *learn*. And furthermore, I suggest, for reasons I will explore at greater length later, that we replace *desire* with *are activated*. Thus Aristotle's statement becomes "All humans are activated to learn." In short, while the focus of volume 1 is on the manifestations of *anxiety*, here in volume 2 the focus is *learning*.

Why the emphasis on learning? The answer is simple: attachment strength is a function of learning. If activation leads to need fulfillment, we are more likely to attach to the source of the fulfillment; that is, we undergo learning and our attachments are more likely to flourish. But whether the attachments are adaptive or maladaptive is another matter. Which brings us to a final modification of Aristotle's wisdom, which you have seen throughout volume 1: "The question is never, *Are they learning?* The question is always, *What are they learning?*"

Readers of volume 1 will recognize the source of this insight: Fred Sheridan, PhD, then principal of Work Opportunities Center (WOC), the largest of several Minneapolis high school dropout programs.

In 1982 he contacted me, requesting help to fine-tune WOC's program of dropout remediation before presenting it to a national audience. As he and his staff worked with dropout kids, he had come to realize that their academic underperformance involved more than an intellectual or cognitive disability; in many instances he suspected an emotional disability—"affective interference" is how he put it—that distorted the learning process.[iii]

---

ii. *Metaphysics*, opening paragraphs, I.1.980a21–7.

iii. See volume 1, pages 135–38, for a more complete presentation of his thinking, including his reformulation of what educators term the "dropout equation."

Introducing Volume 2

WOC enrolled former dropout students who had decided to drop back into school, so to speak, were willing to sign an education contract, and demonstrated enough impulse control to manage a classroom environment. Nonetheless some, despite good effort, did not respond to the WOC program of peer support groups, frequent student staffing, and individual student assessment and instruction. It was not enough. Some youngsters continued to fail and eventually would give up and drop out again.

Fred came up with his idea of "affective interference," an extension of the traditional explanation of dropping out as academic underperformance, so-called "cognitive interference." In his view, more than cognitive (that is, intellectual) issues were involved. He suspected that emotional ("affective") overactivity—an excess of fear, anger, or anxiety; he wasn't sure which short-circuited cognitive processing. Targeted learning fizzled out. He guessed that because of anxiety and fear, whether overt or disguised, such youngsters would once again find the classroom too threatening to bear and drop out for a second time. Moreover, he was worried: were these adolescents learning to hate learning?[iv]

He also wondered whether the affective turmoil in some cases was so concealed that some kids denied its existence. Thus they would be likely to lack insight into the motives for their behavior and would have difficulty understanding their behavior if their emotional conflicts caused them to tune out in the classroom or become truant or just give up and drop out. Fred speculated this might explain the high percentage of "don't know" answers to questionnaires surveying the motivation of

---

iv, Fred, of course, was speaking of the adolescent brain. However nowadays, some thirty-five years later, it is suspected that learning begins prepartum as the fetal nervous system is activated (learns) when maternal neurohormones and transmitters cross the placenta, most certainly postpartum. See volume 1, footnote ii, p. 138.

dropouts. Recalling our discussion of Winnicott[v] years earlier, he wondered whether other kids might express their conflicts via acting-out behavior or suppress them with drugs or alcohol. He summarized his concerns with the above aphorism, which I now adopt as the unifying concept for this volume.

Then his request: He had been encouraged to apply to the US Department of Education for a grant to bring public details of the WOC program, including his notion of "affective interference." Would I join with him and his team to develop a theoretical explanation of why and how affective interference undermined their work with some kids? I was both flattered and intrigued, so I signed up.

I will describe in detail my subsequent adventures as coauthor of what proved to be a failed grant application. Despite its collapse, my exposure to the vicissitudes of adolescent learning ignited an enduring curiosity in the subject. For example, I noted an issue that frustrated high-school educators and persists to date: high dropout rates. Was it a matter of inadequate funding? Also, what did the concept of "affective interference" involve? And was it true that school attendance for some kids simply taught them to hate learning?

---

v. In volume 1 I discuss conversations with Fred and his colleague, Richard Green, which took place years before when both were high school assistant principals and I was a staff psychiatrist at Anoka State Hospital, this at a time when we all were concerned with out-of-control behaviors demonstrated by their students and my patients. It was during these meetings with Fred and Richard, who later became Dr. Green and eventually Chancellor of New York City Public Schools, that I shared with them Donald Winnicott's interpretation of acting-out behavior as a signal for help. In return they introduced me to the notion of operant conditioning. Also, readers of volume 1 will recognize that its first case study—the composite "Dyllen"—incorporates the essence of Fred's "affective interference."

Introducing Volume 2

Inadequate Funding?

My first initiative as Fred's theoretician was to investigate whether graduation rates—the inverse of dropout rates—were a function of spending. Specifically, I wanted to determine whether there was a correlation between state-by-state graduation rates and certain measures of school resource allocation such as *teacher's salary, pupils per teacher,* and *spending per pupil.* Yearly spending figures are compiled and published by the National Center for Education Statistics, Common Core of Data. Devising a correlation of this requires constructing a table matching each state to its spending rank, then mathematically manipulating each ranked pair.

To honor my newly acquired responsibility as Fred's investigator-theoretician, I calculated by hand state spending for both 1972 and 1982. To my surprise the results clearly indicated that the correlations were insignificant at best and that some correlations even deteriorated despite increased spending during the ensuing decade. For example, the 1972 correlation of 0.26 between state-by-state graduation rates and *teachers' salary* had gone negative to -0.08 ten years later. Shocked by these figures, I rushed to reveal my discovery to Fred. His response was even more shocking. He just scoffed: "Everyone knows that." So here was one answer. It was clear that low graduation rates were not a function of inadequate funding. Spending was not the answer.

What Is "Affective Interference?"

Readers of volume 1 will recall that Fred's notion was instrumental in triggering my search for and investigation of its referents beyond the obvious. In volume 1 I describe in chapters 6 and 7 my subsequent professional adventures after Fred and I parted ways, a career during which for many years I did not directly address this issue and its relation to dropping out. Then in 2002 I accepted an offer to consult at the Elk River office of the Central Minnesota Mental Health Center, where one of my responsibilities was to provide outreach to area schools, and another was to provide consultation to the Focus Program, the district alternative school for middle and later grades.

My outreach experience with early elementary school teachers introduced me to the phenomenon of the student who is in the classroom but not really "there": a nascent dropout. This, plus working with Focus teachers Nancy and Shelia, served to put my years of dealing with adolescents in a different perspective. Their distrust, dissociative symptoms and difficulty learning from experience were not due to mental illness—a *"disease"*—but instead represented its consequences; that is, a *disability*. I realized that for years I had been witnessing and misdiagnosing as disease the enduring consequences of childhood trauma and neglect. I actually had been dealing with disability, which I subsequently dubbed "Attachment Disability," the understanding and management of which is the subject of volume 1. In short, Fred's "affective interference" proved to be both a manifestation of damaged attachment and a signal of potential dropping out.

Do Some Students Hate Learning?

This brings us to his other concern, which needs clarification. If we accept that certain youngsters bring to school an injured ability to attach, they will demonstrate difficulty learning new ways to deal with old problems. When they encounter the activation (challenge) of a novel situation—the nature of schooling, after all, is to present what is new—their tendency will be to fall back on former "solutions," such as avoidance behavior (skipping classes, truanting), substance use, or acting-out, or some combination thereof.[vi] It is not that such kids "hate" learning. Rather they find the formality of classroom instruction quite threatening. Another way to state the issue is that for these kids, *learning failure is only apparent.*

As professionals, parents, and sponsors, it is vital that we *learn*—notice the emphasis here on learning—in the course of our encounters with attachment and/or learning disabled youngsters and grownups to recognize and facilitate their adaptive behaviors while avoiding reinforcement of the maladaptive. This is why the major thrust of this volume—actually the logical progression of volume 1—is learning and its contingencies.

Recall in volume 1 my focus was twofold: (1) *identifying* Attention Disability and (2) *mitigating* its damage by avoiding making thing worse. However, even if we are fortunate enough to avoid the trauma of abuse or neglect, we will still experience the risk of abandonment or loss as loved figures die or move away or betray trust. And we all face death. We are never without anxiety susceptibility, hence never free of the possibility of experiencing disabling trauma. But there is a way to enhance our trauma resistance and inoculate or minimize evolution of Attachment Disability in response to life's inevitable traumas: developing adaptive flexibility.

Hence in volume 2 my focus is *preventing* Attachment Disability by developing a wide array of coping skills—a "bigger bag of tricks" is how I characterize it in the chapter on addiction. A more technical way to express this is that we need to promote *an enhanced behavioral repertoire* (EBR). I prefer this terminology because it expands the idea of a skill to imply the notion of reinforcement. In other words, the acquisition of a skill requires an environment to elicit and shape it via conditioning. A skill requires nurturing and care. Unlike Minerva bursting from Jupiter's brow, a skill does not emerge completely formed, but

---

vi. See the first case study of volume 1, "Dyllen," for a composite clinical presentation of the consequences of such maladaptive behaviors.

once formed it reduces the odds of maladaptive skills emerging in response to life's traumas. The idea is that by cultivating "good" habits, the "bad" are choked out before they can pop up.

So the question is, What can we do to smother maladaptive learning while promoting adaptive learning? I will address this in the following chapters

Chapter Overview

Part I—Review and Examples

Chapter 1: Brief review of volume 1. Reemphasize the fundamental Attachment Disability management technique: *avoid making things worse.* Again clarify that the issue is not learning failure but maladaptive learning. Summary of twenty-eight clinical cases.

Chapter 2: Learning theory review. Focus on learning by reinforcement to promote EBR. The cause of learning failure unknown. There is no universal reinforcer.

Chapter 3: Two examples of failure to learn adaptive skills.
Addiction: A clear-cut cause. Per Riesman, loss of rituals and rules that promote collective shame/guilt to guide behavior. No standards to define behavior, nothing to conform to or rebel against. Anxiety rules. Recent alarming increase in substance use, suicide, self-injurious behaviors (e.g., cutting) to manage anxiety.
Dropping out: A less clear-cut cause. Why is learning not sufficient to engage student interest? Hidden Attachment Disorder in part, but is that the whole story? Does the mandate to attend school extinguish curiosity for some? In any event, abolish the mandate. More funds not the answer. Standards must come

from leadership of parents and sponsors: not their words but their behavior. Cannot rely on the media for leadership.

Part II—Addiction

Chapter 4: Explosion of addictive behaviors, increase in suicide, overdose deaths, cutting.

Chapter 5: Anxiety now rules social behavior, per Riesman, rather than guilt or shame. The American teenager: something new under the sun?

Chapter 6: Addiction from perspective of learning theory; addiction as reduction of discomfort rather than getting high; that is, negative reinforcement. Suicide the ultimate reduction.

Chapter 7: Prevention of addiction begins the first day of school. Focus on kids learning anxiety management techniques other than substance use—adaptive skills to choke out maladaptive "solutions." Prevention of substance use in adolescents does not involve lectures. By the time users are using, the nonusers are not. Behavior patterns have already been established

Part III—Dropping out

Chapter 8: History of the concept, definition, figures, trends. Relation between incarceration and dropping out.

Chapter 9: My 1982 dropout research reveals no correlation between spending and graduation rates; obviously spending is not the answer. Sheridan's guffaw—"Everyone knows that!"—when, in the midst my naïveté, I reveal my conclusion. Still true thirty-five years later. Significance of his response: *exhaustion of the pedagogic imagination. Time to do something different.*

Chapter 10: Cause not clear. Survey of dropouts reveals high percentage of *don't know*. Truancy a tipoff of pending dropping out. No doubt attachment issues with some, but can't assume all. Dr. Sheridan's research leads to his innovation: learning contract, continuous education, no age segregation. Decreased likelihood of learning avoidance. Have to activate and nourish inborn curiosity.

Chapter 11: Schools not the default "solution" for youngsters with impulse control issues. By definition they are not responsive to verbal prompts and are therefore not responsive to standard teaching techniques that rely on verbal cues. Need drop-in centers per operant conditioning design we pioneered years previously at Anoka State Hospital.

Chapter 12: Advocate for reform. Volume 1 recommendation that the American Psychiatric Association scrap its *DSM (Diagnostic and Statistical Manual)* format of categorization, which is an expression of expert opinion rather than testable scientific statements. Here also advocate for reform: abandonment of mandated school attendance, a relic of a nineteenth-century America undergoing a transformation from rural to urban society. Any professional educator who still holds that children need to be forced to learn should never be allowed in a classroom or on a school board, or serve in the legislature until they have reread their Aristotle.

Chapter 13: Objections to eliminating the mandate. History of education in America, origins of the mandate.

Part IV—Are Antidepressants Effective?

Chapter 14: Continuing controversy re benefits of antidepressants. Review of my experiences, books by Dr. Peter Kramer, criteria for effectiveness. Conclusion: depends on what you are trying to manage. Not especially helpful with "Depression," *but of great potential benefit for anxiety,* therefore for today's teenagers as they grapple with the inevitable anxieties of our standardless society and its temptations to drop out or tune out via substance use.

About the Author

Dr. Curran is a graduate of Saint Mary's University of Minnesota and Columbia College of Physicians and Surgeons. He completed a medical surgical internship at Saint Luke's Hospital in New York City and a psychiatric residency at the New York State Psychiatric Institute, also in New York. He is certified by the American Board of Psychiatry and Neurology. His book is based on fifty years' experience providing consulting services at state and private mental hospitals, county and private mental health centers, nursing homes, and residential treatment centers for adolescent sexual offenders and adult alcoholics, as well as a few years of clinical research and forty-four years of private practice.